# EMT EXAM PREP

## Focused Prep for the NREMT Cognitive Exam

Sixth Edition

This publication is designed to provide accurate information in regard to the subject matter covered as of its publication date, with the understanding that knowledge and best practice constantly evolve. The publisher is not engaged in rendering medical, legal, accounting, or other professional service. If medical or legal advice or other expert assistance is required, the services of a competent professional should be sought. This publication is not intended for use in clinical practice or the delivery of medical care. To the fullest extent of the law, neither the Publisher nor the Editors assume any liability for any injury and/or damage to persons or property arising out of or related to any use of the material contained in this book.

© 2023 by Kaplan North America, LLC

Kaplan North America, LLC dba Kaplan Publishing
1515 West Cypress Creek Road
Fort Lauderdale, FL 33309

10 9 8 7 6 5 4 3 2 1

ISBN: 978-1-5062-8467-5

Kaplan Publishing print books are available at special quantity discounts to use for sales promotions, employee premiums, or educational purposes. For more information or to purchase books, please call the Simon & Schuster special sales department at 866-506-1949.

# TABLE OF CONTENTS

**GO ONLINE**

*kaptest.com/nremt*

## For Test Changes or Late-Breaking Developments

## kaptest.com/publishing

The material in this book is up-to-date at the time of publication. However, changes in the test may have been instituted after this book was published. Be sure to carefully read the materials you receive when you register for the test. If there are any important late-breaking developments—or any changes or corrections to the Kaplan test preparation materials in this book—we will post that information online at **kaptest.com/publishing**.

# ABOUT THE AUTHOR

**Jessica Discua, NRP**, began pursuing her interest in emergency services in 2005, when she first joined a volunteer fire department. She worked as an EMT for 10 years before moving forward to become an actively practicing paramedic. In her emergency services career, Ms. Discua has worked variously in Pennsylvania, Arizona, and Israel and as a paramedic on a cruise ship sailing around the world one country at a time. She hasn't looked back and hopes that her career will continue to be the adventure it has been thus far.

Since 2010, Ms. Discua has also served as an adjunct EMS instructor, an American Heart Association instructor for multiple disciplines, and a senior lead instructor for the EMT-Basic class at Gateway Community College in Phoenix, AZ.

Previous contributions by **Richard J. Lapierre**, MA,
EMT-Cardiac Director (Ret) of Brown University EMS

# HOW TO USE THIS BOOK

The book you have in front of you is not designed to reteach you the EMT curriculum, as you should have already successfully passed that portion of your path. It is instead designed to refresh and review key elements that are commonly asked on the cognitive portion of the National Registry of Emergency Medical Technicians (NREMT) exam.

By reading the chapters and taking the many practice questions and tests, at the end of the text you should feel confident in your ability to pass the exam.

As an emergency services professional, you may not always receive a thank you, but you may get to see people at possibly the worst or best moments of their lives. Our contact may be for a few minutes at a time, but what you choose to do in those moments will have a real impact on someone's overall care.

So, study hard and realize that you're not just studying to pass an exam. You are also going to be part of the medical care of another human being and have the potential to change people's lives.

## Step 1: Familiarize yourself with the exam.

The first chapter of this book, Inside the EMT-Basic Exam, covers the basics. From subjects covered, to how the test is administered and scored, this section is designed to hopefully lessen your anxiety as an EMT candidate.

## Step 2: Review the content chapters, paying special attention to any weak areas.

- Read the Learning Objectives at the start of each chapter. This gives a quick overview of the subjects explored in each chapter without having to shuffle through the entire book.
- Do the Test Yourself exercises throughout the book, and then check the answers at the back.
- Finally, do the Practice Sets at the end of each chapter. Read the explanations carefully to reinforce the material, especially those for any questions you got wrong. This review of the explanations and remediation is the most important part of answering practice questions, because focusing on the EMS content for the answers that you got incorrect is how you can identify your weak areas and fix them with targeted study.

## Step 3: Conclude with the EMT practice test, which covers the concepts tested on the exam.

After completing this exam, work through the explanations that follow it. Be sure to review the explanations for questions you got right as well as for those you got wrong. This will serve as a good review of the wide range of topics covered on the exam.

We recommend that you try to take the test all in one sitting with no breaks. Set a timer for 2 hours, and attempt to finish the exam in this amount of time. Doing a timed dry run will prepare you for what it is like on Test Day and get you in the right mind frame for when you are under a time limit.

## Step 4: Study a little bit every day before the exam.

This is especially important if you schedule the exam weeks or even months in advance. Once you have finished your course, it is critical to remain current on the topics you have learned.

With consistency and focused study, you should achieve your goal of becoming a practicing EMT. Good luck!

# THE BASICS

# INSIDE THE EMT COGNITIVE EXAM

---

**LEARNING OBJECTIVES**

- Identify the levels of EMS certification and the key differences in scope of practice
- Understand the steps to become certified as an EMT-Basic
- Understand the format of the NREMT Cognitive Exam
- Describe the principles of a CAT exam
- Implement CAT-specific exam strategies

---

Congratulations on your decision to become an emergency medical technician (EMT). While you haven't chosen an easy profession, it is an important and essential one—one that earns the respect of the communities you serve. Although no one really wants to need your services, you will be one of the most welcome sights in any emergency.

In the field of emergency medical services (EMS), there are various levels of certification:

- **EMT-Basic** (**most common**)
  - Entry-level patient care provider
  - Also called **EMT** or **BLS** (Basic Life Support)
  - Often used as a first step in career development for becoming a paramedic, firefighter, doctor, or nurse
  - Most limited scope of practice
- **EMT-Intermediate or Advanced** (EMT-I or EMT-A)
  - Currently, the NREMT offers advanced certification but not intermediate. (The intermediate level has been phased out, but those who already have EMT-I certification can convert their certification.)
  - More expansive in scope of practice: can begin IVs, perform EKGs, give some medications (often including certain narcotics for pain management), and use airway adjuncts such as a laryngeal mask (LMA), which sits above the epiglottis.
- **Paramedics**
  - Also called **ALS** (Advanced Life Support) or medics (their official lettering scheme is EMT-P or NRP for "Nationally Registered Paramedic").

– Highest level of certification in EMS, but there are specialties one may do such as flight or critical care level. These require additional schooling and certification.

– Broadest scope of practice that includes but is not limited to airway intubation, starting and maintaining IVs, administering over 30 different medications for various conditions, performing and interpreting EKGs, and many others.

The main difference between an EMT and a paramedic is that the paramedic has more advanced training and a broader scope of practice. For example:

- An EMT can perform CPR and utilize an AED for persons in cardiac arrest.

- An EMT can provide basic oxygen or assist with a prescribed inhaler for those with difficulty breathing.

- An EMT *cannot* provide treatment that involves invasive measures into the body, e.g., an IV. (Certain procedures are allowed in some states, e.g., providing an airway that goes beyond the back of the tongue.)

- A paramedic is an advanced provider of emergency medical care, whose work involves advanced resuscitation of patients beyond using an AED and compressions, including injecting IV medications and providing advanced airway assistance to patients.

While the different levels of EMS personnel have different certifications, these are commonly used only by health care personnel. This book reflects the common, more casual usage. For the remainder of this book, when the text uses the abbreviation "EMT," it is always shorthand for "EMT-Basic." It is true that a paramedic is also known as an EMT-P; however, in everyday language, an EMT-P is known as a *paramedic* or just a *medic*. It is understood that **when another EMS personnel states "EMT," that person is referencing someone who is certified at the Basic level.**

---

**NREMT Certification**: As of this printing, 45 states in the United States require EMT candidates to get initial certification through the National Registry of Emergency Medical Technicians (NREMT). In order to become a nationally registered EMT, you must have completed the following steps/courses:

- State-approved EMT course that meets or exceeds National Emergency Medical Services Education Standards for the Emergency Medical Technician

  – Course must have been completed within previous 2 years

  – Program director must verify course completion on the NREMT website

- National Registry cognitive (knowledge) and state-approved psychomotor (skills) exams (passed portions remain valid for 24 months provided all other eligibility requirements are met)

- CPR-BLS for "Healthcare Professional" or equivalent credential

---

## Becoming an EMT-Basic

Not everyone can become an EMT. In addition to the proper frame of mind and desire, there are also educational and physical standards. Whether you are a state-certified EMT or a nationally registered EMT, the certification process pathway has three required steps:

- Successfully complete a state-approved EMT course (150–300 hours)
- Pass a psychomotor exam (physical, hands-on knowledge)
- Pass a cognitive exam (computer-based knowledge)

Only after all of the components have been completed and passed can the student become a registered practitioner.

The purpose of this book is to prepare you for the **National Registry of Emergency Medical Technicians (NREMT)** exam.

### KEY TAKEAWAY

**State Certification:** A few states **do not require** NREMT certification as their initial pathway to becoming a practitioner. (As of this printing, those 5 states are Montana, Alaska, Illinois, New York, and North Carolina.) If you live in one of those states, you must follow the requirements by the state EMS office to gain your initial certification. However, it will closely follow the three steps listed above.

One downside to being only state certified is that it is less portable. If you wish to move to a different state that requires NREMT certification, you may be required to do additional testing. That is one of the main benefits of being an NREMT—it makes transferring certification much easier in the long run.

## Passing the Cognitive Exam

### Exam Structure

The NREMT cognitive exam is a computer-based, standardized test designed to measure your competence. The questions are written by a committee made up of EMS providers and other health and educational personnel; test scores are constantly monitored to assure accuracy and fairness.

**Registration**: To apply for the NREMT exam, go to **www.nremt.org**. You can register and pay online. After your training and state verification are complete, you can schedule your exam through the NREMT website.

Testing sites are available in most states through the testing company Pearson Vue. Since 2020, Pearson Vue has also started to offer online testing options, provided the candidate meets the technical requirements for the computer and webcam.

At press time, the EMT exam fee was $98 per exam attempt. This covers both registration and testing center cost, regardless of test location.

### Exam Format

- You will have 2 hours to complete the exam.
- There will be 70–120 questions, many of which are scenario based. These include:
  - Traditional, 4-option, multiple-choice questions in which only one option is correct
  - Technology enhanced items (TEIs), introduced in late 2020; these are multiple-choice questions in which more than one option may be correct
- There are 5 content domain areas (80% on patient care of adults; 20% on patient care of children):
  - **Airway, Respiration, and Ventilation**: 18–22% of exam
  - **Cardiology and Resuscitation**: 20–24% of exam
  - **Medical; Obstetrics and Gynecology**: 27–31% of exam
  - **Trauma**: 14–18% of exam
  - **EMS Operations**: 10–14% of exam

The format of the exam is a **computer adaptive test (CAT)**, a type of computer-based test that is assembled interactively based on the accuracy of to each test taker's response to the questions. Instead of having a predetermined mix of basic, medium, and hard questions, the CAT selects questions based on how well you have answered the previous questions. This ensures that the questions you are answering are not too hard or too easy for your skill level. You will see only one question at a time.

In other words, no two tests are alike.

- If you keep answering the questions correctly, the exam will get harder.
- If you answer some questions incorrectly, the exam will start to give you easier questions. If you get those easier questions right, it will pick up again giving you harder ones.
- You cannot return to a question once you've answered it, and you cannot skip around within a section; either action would throw off the CAT's sequence. Once you answer a question, it's part of your score, for better or worse.
- Once the CAT ascertains that you are competent in a particular area, it moves on to another area.

A CAT exam is structurally different from a paper-and-pencil exam. In a CAT, it is not the **number of questions** answered that determines whether you pass but, rather, the **difficulty of questions** (and your answers). One person may pass having answered 72 questions, while another person may fail having answered 72 questions.

## Scoring

- You will receive a **pass or fail** score, not a numerical score.
- Students who pass will receive a congratulatory message with a link to the official certification card. Passing the cognitive exam (in addition to the test of psychomotor skills) means you are a certified EMT, able to perform the procedures for which you have been trained in your state.
- Students who do not pass will receive a generalized report that indicates either "proficient," "below passing," or "near passing" for each of the 5 main areas of testing.
  - This breakdown is intended to help EMT exam candidates focus additional study on their specific weak areas (e.g., airway or medical emergencies) for a second attempt.
  - The test breakdown *will not* go over specific questions that the examinee answered incorrectly.

## Technology Enhanced Items (TEIs)

Since late 2020, the National Registry (NR) has been implementing new "technology enhanced items," or TEIs. These question types have been successfully used on many other professional certification exams and in academic settings. The NREMT may phase in additional TEI question types over time.

Here are some quick facts about technology enhanced items:

- TEIs are assigned to one of the 5 domains assessed by the NREMT and are administered like any other question on the exam.
- The number of TEIs varies from one test taker to another. You may see many TEIs or none!
- Exams are still limited to 2 hours.

The first TEI type to be implemented is **Multiple Response**. These questions reflect situations with simultaneous events and/or multiple priorities. For instance:

- A patient exhibits more than one main symptom
- A provider needs to account for two or more medical/trauma conditions when administering care

While Multiple Response questions still require test takers to identify correct answers, this question type also recognizes that there are "gray" areas in EMS calls.

Multiple Response questions ask you to choose *more than one correct answer* to a single question. For example, "Which of the following are used in airway management? Select the three answer options that are correct." The number of correct options in a Multiple Response question varies from item to item. However, these questions always take the form "Select the $(X)$ answer options that are correct," where $(X)$ represents the number of options to be chosen.

It is important to note that Multiple Response items are scored as either correct or incorrect, with *no partial credit*. Using the preceding example, if you selected 2 correct options and 1 incorrect option, the exam would count the entire response as incorrect.

This edition includes a sampling of Multiple Response questions to help you familiarize yourself with this question type.

## CAT-Specific Exam Strategies

Using these CAT-specific strategies can have a direct, positive impact on your score.

- Before you begin the live test, get comfortable with the exam interface. Use the computer tutorial to your advantage by spending as much time as you need, now. If you click on "Help" later, when the exam is underway, the time you use will count against your allotted time for that section.

- Be ready to answer questions correctly from the very beginning. There is no warm-up in a CAT, so every question counts. Be aware: the order of difficulty will not be predictable. The CAT *does not* begin with really easy questions that gradually get harder.

- Perform well early so that you are quickly given the hard questions. This is a key strategy for doing well on the CAT. Why? Because getting a hard question right will help your score a lot, but getting a hard question wrong will hurt your score only slightly. It pays to spend more time on those early questions and double-check each answer before you confirm it.

- Be as certain as possible that you have answered a question correctly before moving on. The CAT does not allow you to go back to questions you've already answered. It's up to you to double-check your work before you confirm it.

- If you cannot answer based on your knowledge, guess. The CAT does not allow you to skip questions. To improve the odds that your guess is the correct answer, first eliminate any wrong answer choices that you can spot. Then guess intelligently and strategically among the remaining choices, and move on.

- If a question stumps you, give up and move on to the next question. Sometimes it's necessary to give up on a tough, time-consuming question. It's difficult to do, but take a guess and let it go—and use your time on questions that you *can* answer. That's how you score points, not by agonizing over one question.

- Try to avoid getting several questions in a row wrong. If the previous question you answered was a blind guess, spend a little extra time on the next one.

- If you keep seeing really, really difficult questions, continue answering questions deliberately and with confidence. It doesn't mean the test is too hard for you. *It means you're doing very well on that section.* So don't get rattled. Keep up the good work!

## General Exam Strategies

The EMT-Basic exam is of fundamental importance in an EMT's career. To succeed, you've got to get enough right answers in each section of the test. Knowing the material is not enough. You have to manage your time and your mindset to apply your knowledge to as many questions as possible.

It's one thing to answer one question correctly. It's quite another to answer up to 120 of them in 120 minutes and get >70% right. To move successfully from doing individual practice at your leisure to handling dozens of questions under timed conditions, you need to practice in test-like conditions.

Good test-taking skills are crucial to exam success. Once you are comfortable with the content of the test, your next essential challenge is to gain test expertise.

## Use Process of Elimination for the Answers

Using a process of elimination is a way to answer questions both quickly and effectively. There are two ways to get all the answers right on the exam: you know all the right answers, or you know all the wrong answers. Since there are three times as many wrong answers, you should be able to eliminate some of them if not all. By doing so, you either get to the correct response or increase your chances of guessing the correct response. You start out with a 25% chance of selecting the right answer, and with each eliminated answer choice, your odds go up. Eliminate one, and you'll have a 33% chance of picking the right answer; eliminate two, and you'll have a 50% chance, etc.

Remember to look for wrong-answer traps when you're eliminating. Some answer choices are designed to distract you by distorting the correct answer.

## Remain Calm and Keep Track of Time

It's imperative to remain calm and composed while working through the test. You can't allow yourself to become so rattled by one hard question that it throws you off. When you face a tough question, remember:

- You won't be the only person having trouble with it.
- Having trouble with a tough question won't automatically ruin your score—but getting upset about it and letting it throw you off track will.
- When you understand that part of the test maker's goal is to *reward those who keep their composure*, you'll recognize the importance of not panicking when you run into challenging material.

Still, you can't let yourself run out of time. It's essential to pace yourself, keeping in mind the general guidelines for how long to spend on any individual question (<1 minute). Don't spend a wildly disproportionate amount of time on any one question.

## Be Aware of What's Needed on the Test

This test is like no other test you've taken before. If you took a test in high school or college and got a number of the questions wrong, you wouldn't receive a perfect grade. But on this test, you can get a number of questions wrong and still get a "perfect" passing score.

- The test is constructed so that only the very best test takers are able to answer every question. But even these people rarely get every question right.
- What does that mean for you? Since the test is challenging, you're likely to be unhappy with your answers to some questions. But don't let your negative feelings about one or two questions ruin your performance on the entire test! If you are preoccupied with your past answers, you'll be giving less attention to the new questions that are coming up next.
- Instead, pause for a moment to acknowledge that you feel dissatisfied or aggravated. Then choose to put aside that setback and give yourself a chance to prevail over the next question! Losing a few extra points won't do you in, but losing your cool will.

Remember, if you feel you've done poorly on a scenario, even one with more than one related question, don't sweat it. Remain calm and collected, and simply do your best.

## Build Stamina and Confidence

It's important to develop your test-taking stamina, because the exam is long and fairly challenging. It's also important to build up your confidence, because that leads to quick, sure answers and a sense of well-being—which translate into more points.

- Take the full-length practice test included in this book. You'll be able to review answer explanations and assess your performance. Be sure to go over your wrong answers! This is often the most important way to remedy your weak areas.
- If you lack confidence, you end up reading the sentences and answer choices two, three, and even four times, until you confuse yourself and get off track. This leads to timing difficulties, which only perpetuate the downward spiral, causing anxiety and a tendency to rush.

Focus all of your practice on the major goal of taking control of the test. When you've achieved that goal—armed with the principles, techniques, strategies, and approaches set forth in this book—you'll be ready to face the exam with supreme confidence.

## Have the Right Attitude

Don't waste energy making value judgments about the exam. It's not going to go away. Those who look forward to doing battle with an exam tend to score better than do those who resent or dread it.

It may be hard to believe, but take our word for it: attitude adjustment is a proven test-taking technique.

- Look at the exam as a challenge, but try not to obsess over it; you certainly don't want to psych yourself out of the game.

- Yes, the exam is obviously important. But contrary to what some exam candidates think, this one test will not single-handedly determine the outcome of your life.

- Try to have fun with the exam! Learning how to match your wits against the test makers can be a very satisfying experience, and the reading and thinking skills you'll acquire will benefit you in the EMS.

- Remember that you're more prepared than most people. You've trained with Kaplan. You have the tools you need plus the know-how to use those tools.

Try to think of the exam as "a celebration of learning." While this perspective may cause you some eye-rolling and groaning, it really helps to alleviate test anxiety.

## On Test Day

It should go without saying that on the day of the test, you should prepare by being totally rested and focused on the task at hand. Cramming at the last minute will not help you. Pulling an all-nighter a day or two in advance of Test Day will also not help you. (Plus, you run the risk of falling asleep during the exam.)

Here are steps and information that *will* help you on Test Day:

- Arrive at the test site at least 30 minutes before the announced start time. This will give you time to collect your thoughts. Arriving in a rush is distracting.

- Do not bring your notes with you. At this point, they will be more of a distraction than anything else. They also are not allowed in the test!

- Most testing sites will give you either paper and pen or an erasable writing board to use during the exam. While you may use these however you like during the exam, you may not take these with you when you leave.

- Some testing sites do not allow food or water. Eat and drink before the exam accordingly.

- If you start to feel distracted, overwhelmed, or tired: Pause. Close your eyes, and clear your mind. Take a few deep breaths. Eat some of your snack, and drink some water (if that is permitted at your testing center). Then continue. If these steps don't clear your mind sufficiently, follow the instructions given by the proctor to request a trip to the restroom. Usually no more than one person at a time is permitted to leave. If you can do so, go to the restroom and splash water onto your face. All of this will help you refocus on the task at hand.

- Keep an eye on the clock as you do not want to run out of time.

- If you cannot answer a question with certainty, analyze it and make your best guess. You will not be allowed to move on to the next question without answering the previous question.

# EMT REVIEW

# WELL-BEING OF THE EMT

---

**LEARNING OBJECTIVES**

- Understand the physical, emotional, and mental risks posed to the EMT
- Recognize the types of patient consent to treatment
- Understand how the law protects the medical provider
- Learn how to manage crime scenes as a medical provider

---

Prehospital emergency medicine is a tough, demanding practice. It requires not only physical strength and conditioning but mental and emotional stability as well.

To be able to go from a relaxed state of mind to one where you have just moments to make potentially critical decisions at any hour of the day involves the entire being. This chapter will discuss the many risks that EMTs face at any given time (on the job or off duty): physical, mental, and emotional.

## Risks of the Job

### Physical Risks

The most obvious danger to an EMT's well-being is physical danger. Physical danger can present in various ways: personal threats, environmental hazards (chemical spills, building collapses), and communicable diseases (hepatitis, COVID-19, etc.).

---

While heroics are common in the movies, the reality is that entry into an unsafe scene has the potential to cause you harm, which would complicate the response. It would also prevent you from being able to assist on the initial call.

---

The following are set as per national EMS operating guidelines:

- As an EMT, you are not allowed to enter any scene you believe to be dangerous or that presents a personal threat (e.g., a patient with a weapon). Such a scene must be secured by law enforcement prior to your entry. **Do not attempt to disarm anyone holding a weapon.** Call for police backup or defer to the police if they are already on scene.

- As an EMT, you must be aware of the dangers of blood-borne and airborne pathogens and know how to prevent contamination. You must also know how to handle articles exposed to bodily fluids that may be contaminated. Exposure to communicable diseases, such as hepatitis, tuberculosis, and HIV, is preventable with inoculation (vaccination) and the use of protective devices (masks, gloves).

- The proper use and disposal of hypodermic needles and syringes (often called "sharps") is paramount. One of the most common causes of prehospital exposure to pathogens among EMTs is the dirty needlestick. These are mostly preventable with proper use and disposal techniques.

## Mental and Emotional Risks

In addition to the physical danger, there is also the emotional trauma of being an EMT. Many EMS professionals can tell you that they have had at least one really tough call that has stuck with them to this day. For longevity in this career, the emotionally healthy EMT acknowledges this trauma, takes time to process it (with counseling if needed), and then moves forward.

On the job front, the formal response to an emotionally traumatic call may be a critical incident stress debriefing (CISD). These meetings are conducted within 24 to 72 hours of a critical incident by other public safety personnel, who may recommend one-on-one intervention for the affected EMS professional.

### KEY TAKEAWAY

While every EMT has wanted to resuscitate an apneic and pulseless patient, the fact is that death and dying are part of this profession. In her book *On Death and Dying*, Dr. Elisabeth Kubler-Ross clarifies 5 stages in dealing with death. These stages hold true for both the family members of the deceased and also the EMS providers on the scene:

- Denial and isolation
- Anger
- Bargaining
- Depression
- Acceptance

Many people entering the ranks of prehospital emergency medicine are young adults, whose experiences with death may be very limited. It is important for their mentors and officers to recognize the signs of PTSD and be prepared to intervene and assist as needed.

### Substance Abuse

Unfortunately, some EMS providers try to cope with the stress of the profession with substances such as alcohol or illicit drugs. Too often, someone may be struggling and no one knows until it's too late. This caution is not meant to scare you or anyone away from becoming an EMT but, rather, to raise awareness. As EMTs, we must actively look after our own well-being and our partner's.

If you or someone you know is struggling with substance abuse, please know that it is OK to reach out and ask for help. Many companies provide access to an employee assistance program (EAP), which can recommend and help coordinate assistance with many situations, including substance abuse. Consultation and treatment will remain confidential. EMS providers must be aware, however, that each company has the right to randomly drug test anyone they hire as a condition of employment. Companies expect EMS providers to be of clear mind and body in order to serve the public in their coverage area, so they have a strict no-drugs policy that can result in termination or legal action.

### Post-Traumatic Stress Disorder

Post-traumatic stress disorder (PTSD) is an anxiety disorder that can develop after experiencing a shocking or dangerous event, such as war or trauma. Symptoms usually arise within 3 months of the event but sometimes can take years to manifest. Various studies show that 20–55% of EMS providers will experience PTSD symptoms or are formally diagnosed with the disorder.

The signs and symptoms of PTSD include the following:

- Unexplained irritability
- Inability to concentrate or make decisions
- Difficulty sleeping, nightmares
- Anxiety
- Feelings of guilt
- Loss of appetite, sexual desire, interest in work
- Possible suicidal thoughts (in an effort to stop feeling any of the emotions noted)

Symptoms that persist for longer than a few days should be considered serious. Anyone experiencing these symptoms in themselves or witnessing them in a coworker should notify their superior immediately so that the situation may be dealt with either within the service or referred to a competent outside provider.

A good defense against serious PTSD is to share emotions in confidence with one's coworkers, especially those who were part of the difficult call and are familiar with the details, or with those who have been through something similar on other calls. Depending on the severity of the call, processing these emotions may take months or even years.

## Medical, Legal, and Ethical Issues

As an EMT, the particular state and service protocols under which you function will determine your scope of practice and standard of care. These protocols are the legal framework under which patient care is guided, so it is imperative that you know them well. Furthermore, deviating from these protocols could result in impaired treatment and/or legal action.

### Duty to Act

While the application of the rule varies from state to state, the duty to act is a legal requirement to take action that will prevent harm to another person or the general public. In the context of EMS providers, this means responding to calls in a rapid but safe manner, performing a thorough assessment, administering the necessary treatment, and transporting to a receiving facility when needed.

Legally, the EMT is bound by the following conditions:

- If an EMT is **on duty** as a prehospital medical provider, the EMT has a duty to act on any ill or injured patient dispatched to or encountered. It is not permissible to refuse an intervention, regardless of personal preference.
- If an EMT is **off duty** and encounters an ill or injured person, the EMT may feel an ethical duty to assist, but there is no mandate to do so. While wanting to assist is an admirable trait, use caution when deciding to proceed as liability coverage is usually very limited under these circumstances. This is not to discourage you from helping someone during leisure time, but be aware of the risks.

### Patient Consent

The issue of patient consent is one of the trickiest of all medical, legal, and ethical issues. It is a generally accepted legal principle that a competent individual age 18 or older has the right to permit or refuse any specific medical procedure.

A common example is when the EMT is confronted with a victim of a motor vehicle accident who refuses to allow the application of a cervical collar, which many states require of all trauma victims with a possibility of cervical trauma. Thus, the EMT is now faced with two conflicting ideas. The competent person's right of refusal will typically take precedence. However, it has been argued that a reasonable and prudent person would want the collar, and thus collars have been forced upon patients. The EMT has to be aware that such an action may well be considered assault and battery, should the patient choose to file a lawsuit. Patient consent falls into three different categories:

- **Expressed consent** is a verbal agreement to treatment by a competent patient.
- **Implied consent** means a patient who is unconscious, inebriated, or otherwise unable to express consent would reasonably agree to treatment that would be given to anyone in that situation.

- **In loco parentis** is a specialized term that is used for underage or pediatric patients whose parents/guardians are not present but would reasonably agree to treatment of their child in an emergency situation. It translates to "in the place of a parent."

---

### TEST YOURSELF 2.1

#### What type of consent is this?

A school nurse calls 911 for a child experiencing anaphylactic shock. The child has never had a prescription for an epinephrine pen. The parents were called right away, but they have not yet responded. The child is experiencing severe respiratory distress with hives present. Under what type of consent should the EMT act?

---

## Competency

When it comes to patient care, the word **competent** can also cause a dilemma in the emergency medical profession. It is a recognized legal fact that a person who is seriously intoxicated is not a competent person; however, there is no magic standard that defines the level of inebriation that creates incompetence. The EMT is thus thrust into the position of making this important determination on the scene and setting the level of medical care.

By utilizing various patient assessment tools such as the AVPU or alert and oriented scale or by speaking with medical command, the EMT can make the decision of whether or not a patient would be considered a competent person who could make reasonable decisions about the care received or refused.

---

A minor (under age 18) is held by most states to lack competence. So even if a 9-year-old bicycle accident victim refuses a cervical collar, the EMT can overrule that preference unless there is a parent on the scene who objects.

---

## Litigation and the Good Samaritan Law

It is important to know the defenses against being successfully sued in the performance of EMT duties.

Paramount among these is the **Good Samaritan law**. Generally speaking, this act provides a type of immunity against liability for someone who performs an emergency medical procedure for which they are trained and licensed/certified and are off duty, unless it is done in a manner that is grossly negligent. While on duty, the EMT has a duty to act and protocols to follow that provide a level of legal protection.

**Negligence** is defined by the *Oxford English Dictionary* as "failure to use reasonable care, resulting in damage or injury to another." In order to successfully sue an EMT, a plaintiff's lawyer must be able to prove that the EMT's actions caused harm to the patient.

For example, suppose an EMT is certified in CPR and use of an AED.

- The EMT was trained to use their hands placed on the lower half of the sternum, pushing down to a depth of 2–2.4 inches and at a rate of 100–120 compressions a minute per the most current AHA standards.
- If instead the EMT chooses to start care by providing compressions with their foot on the victim's chest or chooses not to use an AED that has been brought to them, the EMT could be considered grossly negligent.

Although these are extreme examples, they should give a clearer picture of actions that could be considered to cause due harm.

The usage of **medical direction** is another option to provide direction to the EMT. If the EMT is in doubt of whether or not to perform a particular procedure for which the EMT is licensed/certified, the first line of defense is the state protocols. After this is the use of medical control. Consulting with an emergency department physician for advice and orders for particular interventions is always the best course of action. Two forms of medical control are available to an EMT:

- The consultation is referred to as **online** medical control and essentially transfers patient care to the online physician with the EMT acting as their eyes and ears.
- If online medical control cannot be established, the written protocols become the **offline** medical control that are then followed and documented for the patient's care.

## Confidentiality

Numerous laws and court decisions have assured the confidentiality of medical information. What is told to the EMT by a patient is confidential and is to be told only to those to whom the EMT transfers patient care.

The passage of the Health Insurance Portability and Accountability Act (HIPAA) in 1996 secured the legal requirement by all health care professionals to handle protected health information confidentially. The EMT is bound by these requirements. It is never permissible to discuss a patient's history or care with anyone outside the medical community, unless compelled to do so by a legal order.

Some information that is asked of patients, known as protected health information (PHI), would disclose their identity to others not involved in their care. Therefore, the following information should be closely guarded from all except health care providers involved in the direct care or the appropriate billing services:

- First or last name
- Address or phone number
- Social security number or other identification number
- Date of birth
- Medical record number

This is not an exhaustive list; a variety of additional patient information is legally protected. However, these elements of PHI are the ones most commonly used for EMS purposes.

It can be hard to keep track of the various pieces of PHI. Nonetheless, it is important to remember when writing your patient care report or giving a radio report.

---

Extreme caution must be taken to protect the patient's identity.

---

In the field, keeping the HIPAA confidentiality requirements poses certain challenges. EMT assessments are routinely carried out in a public setting rather than a closed office. For example, someone is less likely to divulge a history of a sexually transmitted disease if there are coworkers standing nearby.

Legally speaking, certain information that a patient provides during the course of your assessment is considered protected. Remember the following:

- Assure the patient that everything is said in confidence and that only those in their direct care will have access to their answers. (Some services have this information in writing, so it can be handed to the patient.)
- While this information is often needed to fill out your patient care report (PCR) and allow the company to bill appropriately for services, the patient has the right to not answer these questions.

## Crime Scenes

When a medical scene is also a crime scene, care must be taken to disturb as little as possible. Documentation of patient care must also include any disturbances that were needed for the patient's treatment and transport.

Various state laws also address when medical personnel *must* notify law enforcement officials if they become aware of certain situations. If an EMT is aware that a child has been physically, emotionally, or sexually abused, failure to notify the proper agency may subject the EMT not only to civil but also to criminal penalties as well:

- If you suspect the abuse of a person or have identified physical indicators of such, you must document it in your patient care report and also let the receiving medical team know of your observations or suspicions.
- It is better to let the proper personnel know and have it turn out to be a false alarm instead of saying nothing and running the risk of further harm taking place later.
- Remember it is the EMT's duty to perform both medical care and patient advocacy.

Some states also provide for the notification of sudden death, overdoses of illicit drugs, gunshot wounds, spousal abuse, sexual abuse, elder abuse, and animal bites. Please follow your local or state protocols to make sure you are aware of when and whom to notify of such situations.

# Practice Set

1. A 25-year-old male who was involved in a car crash has a laceration on his forehead, which is approximately 2 inches long and oozing blood slowly. You stop the bleeding and bandage the wound. The patient's skin is warm, dry, and pink. His movement, sensation, and circulation are intact in all extremities, and you see no other visible wounds at this time. The patient is alert and oriented ×4. He tells you that the wound is minor, and he does not want to go to the hospital with you. Which of the following must happen before you can allow him to refuse further care or transport? Select the 2 answer options that are correct.

    A. The patient must read and understand the patient refusal form.

    B. You must contact and wait for law enforcement to sign as a witness.

    C. The patient cannot refuse, as he may have a head injury and probably has altered mental status.

    D. You must contact someone responsible who can come drive him from the scene, as he has a head injury.

    E. You must assess the patient's vital signs and record them on the refusal form.

2. You and your partner respond to a call involving the death of an infant. The following week, your partner tells you that he has been having nightmares involving the death of his own children and that he is not eating or sleeping well. Which of the following should be your next course of action?

    A. Slap your partner and tell him to snap out of it.

    B. Notify your immediate supervisor of your concerns.

    C. Do nothing, as your colleague's nightmares are his own problem.

    D. Drive him immediately to the nearest mental health facility.

3. You arrive at the scene of a "man down" call at a residential house with no other information. Once inside, your partner quickly assesses the patient, turns to you, and shakes his head. The patient is cyanotic, with full rigor and postmortem-dependent lividity clearly present in his torso. The man's spouse is anxious, peering into the room and asking, "Will he be all right?" You gently lead her into the living room and ask her to sit down. While looking directly at her, you quietly say that her husband has died and there is nothing that you can do. After a few moments without a reaction, the spouse wails loudly and throws herself into your arms, crying out, "He can't be dead; he was just talking to me!" What is this stage of the grief process called?

    A. Acceptance

    B. Anger

    C. Bargaining

    D. Denial

4. After discharging to the emergency department a patient who had been stabbed in the abdomen, you are removing your bloody gloves when you notice that they are torn and there is blood on your skin. When you wash the blood off, you further notice that you have a small, fresh laceration on your middle finger. What is your next course of action?

   A. Wash your hands a second time, as careful washing will resolve any contamination issues.

   B. Disinfect the wound with hydrogen peroxide, and bandage it with a sterile dressing.

   C. Sanitize the laceration with an alcohol-based hand sanitizer and vigorous hand rubbing, and repeat this process in an hour.

   D. Report a blood-borne-pathogen exposure to your immediate supervisor, and follow your service's protocol for exposure.

5. Which of the following situations violates a person's protected health information (PHI)?

   A. Documenting your patient's full name in your patient care report and submitting it to your service for billing

   B. Verifying through your lawyer that you treated a patient after being subpoenaed for a lawsuit concerning that particular person in question

   C. Attaching a copy of the patient's hospital information sheet to your patient care report for billing purposes

   D. Stating the patient's full name and your estimated arrival time while giving a prehospital radio report to the receiving hospital

6. You arrive on the scene of a "man down" call. Upon arrival, you observe a male in his mid-forties, lying faceup on the sidewalk. He is snoring, and you smell what you believe to be an alcoholic beverage on his breath. What legal doctrine allows you to begin treatment since he does not respond to your verbal questioning?

   A. Good Samaritan Act

   B. In loco parentis

   C. Implied consent

   D. Expressed consent

7. You are dispatched to an unknown-type medical call. You respond emergently and arrive at a residence. Police have secured the scene, and when you enter the apartment, you see a male in his fifties lying on a couch. He is semiconscious and smells of liquor. His response to your questioning is belligerent, and he repeatedly asks you to leave him alone and tells you that he is fine. He is unable to tell you what day it is or where he currently is. His breathing is rapid and shallow, and he appears pale and diaphoretic. You should now do which of the following?

   A. Have the patient sign a refusal form and go back in service.

   B. Advise the patient that he may be seriously ill, and continue to encourage him strongly to allow you to transport him to a medical facility.

   C. Physically remove the patient from the couch, have the police put him in handcuffs, and escort him out to your truck for transport.

   D. Advise the police that the patient must be transported due to his medical condition as he is incompetent to refuse transport due to suspected alcohol intoxication, and ask them to help you place him into the truck.

## Answer Key

| | | | | | | | |
|---|---|---|---|---|---|---|---|
| 1. | **A, E** | 3. | **D** | 5. | **D** | 7. | **D** |
| 2. | **B** | 4. | **D** | 6. | **C** | | |

## Answers and Explanations

### 1.  A, E

Not all car crashes involve police, and in most states, anyone over age 18 who is a neutral third party can sign as witness. Thus 100% of the time, you do not need a police officer to sign as witness (B). Unless they admit to being under the influence or you believe they are, car crash patients can and do sign refusal forms all over the US, so (C) is incorrect. While it is possible that the patient's head laceration indicates an underlying head injury (D), he presents as alert and oriented ×4. He is therefore considered competent and can refuse care. Only 2 answers remain that make sense to protect yourself and the patient, (A) and (E).

### 2.  B

Your partner is exhibiting symptoms of depression and anxiety brought on by post-traumatic stress. While nothing here suggests that the stress is critical at this time, you have a duty to act and seek proper care for him. Do this by notifying your supervisor of your concerns so that proper mental health care can be obtained. The "snap out of it" approach only works well in the movies. Doing nothing may allow the situation to resolve itself, but it may also allow your partner to slip into a clinical depression. Driving him to the mental health facility without having done a proper workup will likely be counterproductive and could damage your relationship.

### 3.  D

Denial is a common first reaction to difficult news, "If I don't believe it, it didn't really happen." News of tragic importance is often accompanied by a wide range of emotions as the mind attempts to absorb information it doesn't really want to hear. As such, the mind will process the emotions with whatever "controls" it can find to try to delay the final stage of grief (acceptance). Anger may also present as the first stage, and the EMT often may be the brunt of the attack, both verbal and physical, for instance, "They always save the patient on television; what did you do wrong?" Know that an angry response is a defense mechanism. Bargaining serves the same purpose, "If there is something I can trade for this bad news, I will."

### 4.  D

The combination of skin exposure to someone else's blood and an open wound means that blood-borne pathogens could have been introduced into your blood-stream. Possible pathogens include HIV and hepatitis, both of which can cause serious illnesses and are potentially fatal. Soap and water (A), hydrogen peroxide (B), and hand sanitizer (C) deal with external exposure and will not be effective if the pathogen has already been introduced into the bloodstream. Each service is required by law to have a exposure protocols in place, which include blood testing and medical consultation for treatments to minimize the risk of developing blood-borne illnesses; however, infection control protocols are effective only if they are implemented and the appropriate personnel are notified.

**5. D**

While prehospital radio reports may seem secure, they are in fact easily accessible by nonmedical personnel and can be heard by anyone who knows which frequency is being used. Revealing a patient's full name is not only *not required* to give a radio report, but it clearly identifies the patient to random individuals who have nothing to do with patient care. This is imperative for the EMT to remember at all times.

**6. C**

The correct answer is implied consent. The law allows the EMT (or any medical provider) to assume that the patient, if conscious, would consent to medical treatments. The Good Samaritan Act (A) covers the EMT while off duty, not when working in an official capacity at the time of incident. In loco parentis (B) is the type of consent used in pediatric cases where the parents or guardian are not on scene but would reasonably give permission to treat their child. Expressed consent (D) is the permission given by a conscious and competent patient for you to perform a medical procedure.

**7. D**

The key fact is that the patient does not know what day it is or where he is. These factors give you the criteria needed to overrule his rejection of a transport: the patient probably lacks the competence to refuse. Choice (A) is correct only if you are satisfied that the patient will be fine if he signs a refusal and you leave. It is always good to remember that somebody felt concerned enough to call EMS, and you should be extremely cautious in accepting a refusal from a patient who is presenting with serious symptoms. While encouraging the patient to permit transport due to his illness (B) is a correct step, the amount of time you should spend arguing with an intoxicated patient is limited. Physically removing an unwilling person (C) is not part of your job description and is properly done by law enforcement.

# CHAPTER 3

# ANATOMY AND PHYSIOLOGY

---

**LEARNING OBJECTIVES**

- Identify the prefixes, roots, and suffixes of commonly used medical terms
- Recognize the anatomical directions and planes of the body
- Identify the key structures and physiology of these body systems:
  - Musculoskeletal
  - Respiratory
  - Circulatory
  - Gastrointestinal
  - Genitourinary
  - Nervous
  - Endocrine
  - Integumentary

---

As a medical provider, the EMT must be familiar with the standard terminology of medical practice, including anatomical and physiological definitions. A good working knowledge of anatomy and physiology is necessary not only for the practice of prehospital medicine but also for communication with other medical professionals.

A large portion of the EMT exam focuses on the pathophysiology of the various body systems and how they contribute to various illnesses or accidents a patient may experience. The EMT must have a basic understanding of organs and structures in order to identify the correct treatments and recognize potential negative consequences if a wrong treatment is administered.

## Commonly Used Medical Terminology

Health professionals need a shared understanding of the meanings of terms in their field. Thus, the NREMT exam requires you to demonstrate a strong foundation in the use of medical terms. This section provides a brief list of some of the more commonly used medical terminology used in the EMS setting.

We'll begin by reviewing how to break down medical terminology into its component parts and then decode those parts. Many medical terms are composed of 3 parts: prefix, root, and suffix.

- The **prefix** is typically the descriptive part of the medical term, and it forms the beginning of the word.
  - It describes characteristics such as location, direction, number, quantity, amount, size, color.
- The **root** is the subject of the medical term, which may appear in a combining form that incorporates a vowel, typically "o."
  - It often pertains to a body part or system.
  - It forms the middle of the word when a prefix is present.
  - If the word has no prefix, the root forms the first part of the word.
- A **suffix** brings meaning to the medical term and forms the end of the word.
  - It indicates a disease, disorder, condition, procedure, process, specialty, test, or status.

**Table 3.1** Common Medical Prefixes

| PREFIX | MEANING | EXAMPLE |
|---|---|---|
| a-/an- | "not," "without" | **a**rrhythmia = without normal rhythm |
| bi- | "two," "double" | **bi**lateral = on both sides |
| brady- | "slow" | **brady**cardia = slow heart rate |
| hemi- | "half" | **hemi**paresis = muscle weakness or paralysis on one half of the body |
| hyper- | "more of," "excessive," "above" | **hyper**glycemia = excess glucose in the blood |
| hypo- | "less of," "low" | **hypo**thermia = low body temperature |
| tachy- | "fast" | **tachy**cardia = fast heart rate |

**Table 3.2** Common Medical Word Roots

| ROOT | MEANING | EXAMPLE |
|---|---|---|
| abdomin/o | "abdomen," "stomach" | **abdomin**al evisceration = abdominal organs outside of the cavity |
| arteri/o | "artery" | **arterio**sclerosis = thickening or hardening of the artery walls |
| bronch/o | "main air passages in the lungs" | **broncho**spasm = spasming of the bronchial tubes |

*(Continued)*

**Table 3.2** Common Medical Word Roots (*Continued*)

| ROOT | MEANING | EXAMPLE |
|---|---|---|
| cardi/o | "heart" | **cardio**genic shock = shock originating from the heart |
| cyan | "blue" | **cyan**osis = bluish tint of the skin |
| derm/o | "skin" | hypo**derm**ic = below the skin |
| em *or* hem | "related to blood" | ur**em**ia = blood in the urine |
| laryng/o | "larynx" | **laryngo**spasm = spasm of the larynx |
| my/o | "muscle" | **myo**cardium = muscle of the heart |
| nas/o | "nose" | **naso**pharyngeal airway = airway adjunct for the nose |
| neur/o | "nerves" | **neuro**genic shock = shock involving the nervous system |
| pnea | "breathing" | a**pnea** = cessation of (not) breathing |
| pulmon/o | "lungs" | **pulmon**ary edema = swelling of the lungs |
| therm | "heat" | hyper**therm**ia = elevated body temperature |
| vas/o | "vessel" | **vaso**dilation = widening of the vessel |
| ven/o | "vein" | intra**ven**ous = inside the vein |

**Table 3.3** Common Medical Suffixes

| SUFFIX | MEANING | EXAMPLE |
|---|---|---|
| -constriction | "narrowing" | vaso**constriction** = narrowing of the blood vessel |
| -dilation | "widening" | vaso**dilation** = widening of the blood vessel |
| -eurysm | "expanding," "widening" | an**eurysm** = expanding blood vessel |
| -ia | "condition of" | hypotherm**ia** = condition of low body temperature |
| -itis | "inflammation of" | bronch**itis** = inflammation of the bronchial tubes |

# Anatomical Terminology

In order to ensure that communication across health care is consistent, standard naming conventions are used to describe the locations and positions on the body. This is especially important for the EMT when assessing a patient, communicating with the receiving hospital staff, and writing a patient care report.

## Planes

Anatomical planes are imaginary lines that divide the body into sections. Knowledge of planes allows the EMT to communicate important information about the injury to other medical personnel. The exam will include a variety of questions about directions and planes.

Follow along with the labels in the graphic to make sure you understand each term presented. For instance, the question "the thumb is _____ to the wrist" will be presented with choices such as proximal, distal, lateral, or medial.

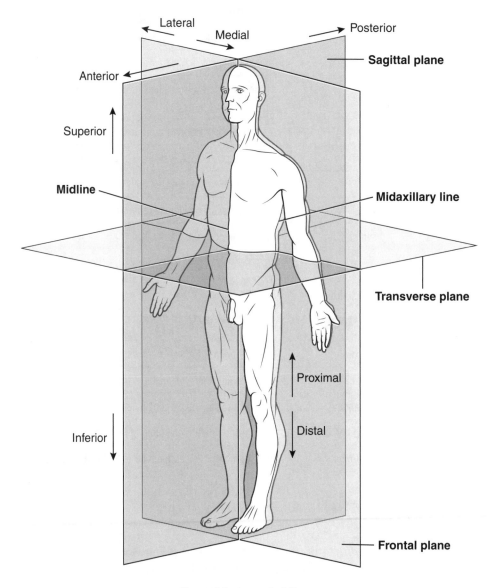

**Figure 3.1** Anatomical Planes

In practice, anatomical terms are patient oriented. For instance, "right side" refers to the *patient's* right side.

## Terms Explained

Anatomical and directional terms help to clarify where one body part is in relation to another.

**Table 3.4** Anatomical Terms

| TERMINOLOGY | DEFINITION | EXAMPLE |
|---|---|---|
| Anatomical position | Position where a person stands upright, with palms facing forward and thumbs facing away from the body | |
| Midline/sagittal plane<br><br>• Lateral objects go away from the midline<br>• Medial objects move toward the midline | Imaginary vertical line dividing the body into left and right side | • Lateral: the eye is lateral to the nose<br>• Medial: the nose is medial to the ears |
| Midaxillary line/frontal plane<br><br>• Anterior objects are on the front portion of the body<br>• Posterior objects are on the back portion of the body<br>• Ventral: toward the front of the torso<br>• Dorsal: toward the back of the torso | Imaginary vertical line dividing the body into front and back portions | • Anterior: the nose is on the anterior portion of the head<br>• Posterior: the gluteal muscles (buttocks) are located on the posterior<br>• Ventral: the naval (belly button) is ventral to the lumbar spinal vertebrae<br>• Dorsal: the shoulder blade is dorsal to the ribs |
| Transverse plane<br><br>• Superior: meaning above or up<br>• Inferior: meaning down or toward the bottom | Imaginary horizontal line dividing the body into top and bottom portions | • Superior: the head is superior to the feet<br>• Inferior: the foot is inferior to the patella (knee) |
| Limbs<br><br>• Proximal objects are closer to the torso<br>• Distal objects are farther (distant) from the torso | Extensions from the torso (trunk of the body) that include the arms (connected via the shoulder) and the legs (connected via the hips) | • Proximal: the elbow is proximal to the wrist<br>• Distal: the fingers are distal to the elbows |

Many other anatomical terms describe movement of the limbs. In the next section, we'll break down the movements that can occur in each plane of the body.

## Movements

Knowing how a limb moves within a certain plane of the body is immensely helpful for the EMT when trying to understand how an injury occurred or how to splint or bandage the affected part.

Using the following image and explanations, move your own body to grasp a deeper understanding of how each of these movements not only are made but also what injury patterns may occur if these movements are interrupted or injured somehow.

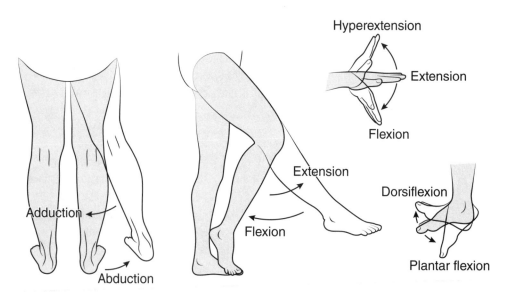

**Figure 3.2** Anatomical Movements

**Sagittal plane**—hyper ("more than") movements can occur in each way listed below:

- **Flexion**—decreasing the angle between two bones at a joint. An example is when you bend your knee toward your body.

- **Extension**—increasing the angle between two bones at a joint. An example is straightening the knee from a bent position.

- **Dorsiflexion** and **plantarflexion**—referring to movements the foot. An example of dorsiflexion is pointing your toes toward your head, while plantarflexion is pointing the sole of your foot toward the ground.

**Frontal Plane:**

- **Adduction**—moving a limb toward the midline. A helpful reminder is that you "add" to the body. An example is moving one leg toward your other leg.

- **Abduction**—moving a limb away from the midline. Think about how an abduction of something takes it away from somewhere or someone. An example is moving your leg away from your body as shown in the picture.

**Transverse Plane:**

- **Rotation**—the movement that turns around the vertical axis of a bone. You can have internal (inward) or external (outward) motion. An example is a hip fracture.

- **Pronation**—rotating a bone medially from another bone. An example is when you turn your foot toward the medial side of your body (inward, toward the center line) or "roll" an ankle and feel pain.

- **Supination**—rotating a bone laterally from another bone. Picture turning your wrist so that you can hold a bowl of soup in your hand. Soup = supination.

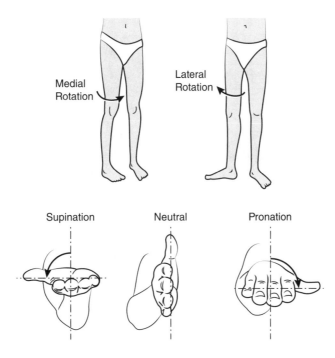

**Figure 3.3** Transverse Plane Movements

Now let's move to the review of individual body systems and physiology.

## Musculoskeletal System

### Skeletal System

The skeleton is a collection of bones that provides the framework of the human body. The bones also provide protection for the soft tissues and internal organs.

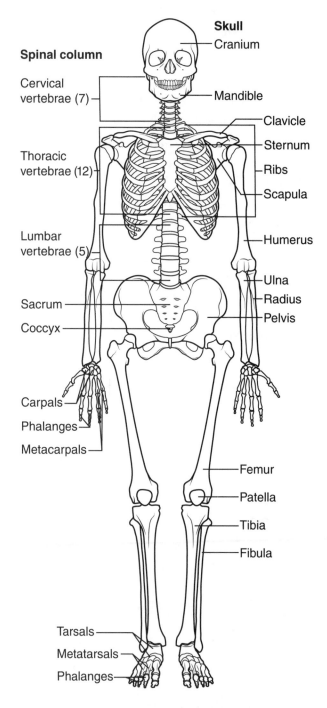

**Figure 3.4** Major Skeletal Bones

The skeletal system is divided into 6 sections: the skull (including the face), the spinal column, the thorax, the pelvis, the upper extremities, and the lower extremities.

The **skull**—also known as the **cranium**—is a cap of bone that serves to protect the brain. Different sections of the skull make up the cap itself:

- **Frontal bone**—located where the forehead is
- **Parietal bones**—located on both sides of the head and above the ears; these span toward the back of the head where they meet with the occipital bone
- **Occipital bone**—located on the posterior portion of the head; protects the cerebellum region of the brain
- **Temporal bones**—located superior to the ear, on both sides of the head
- **Sphenoid bone**—located posterior from the orbital socket
- **Sutures**—fibrous bands of tissue that connect the bones of the skull together
- **Fontanels** (found in pediatric patients)—located anterior and posterior; where the sutures have not yet fully closed; typically close by age 18 months
- **Facial bones**—include the orbit (eye socket), nasal bone, maxilla and mandible (jaw), and zygomatic bones (cheeks)

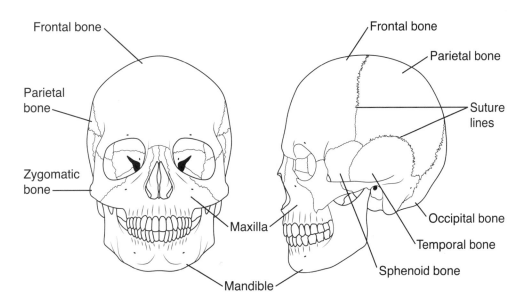

**Figure 3.5** Skull and Facial Bones

Next we have the **spinal column**, also known as the backbone. There are several sections of bones called the vertebrae:

- **Cervical** (neck)—has 7 vertebrae and is one of the most vulnerable portions of the spine due to its lack of protection from the rest of the body
- **Thoracic** (chest)—has 12 vertebrae; the thorax or thoracic cavity is located here as well
- **Lumbar** (low back)—has 5 vertebrae; a lot of the body's load pressure is placed here and is a common location for pain complaints

- **Sacral** (pelvis)—is a set of 5 fused vertebrae; located within the pelvic cavity
- **Coccyx** (tailbone)—is a set of 4 fused vertebrae; it is susceptible to trauma

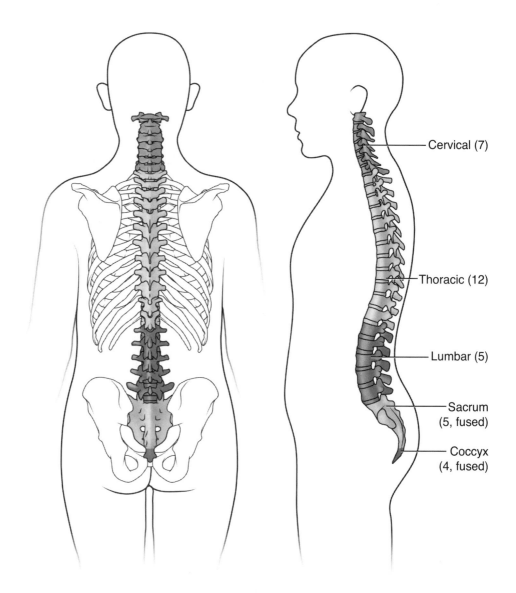

Cervical (7)

Thoracic (12)

Lumbar (5)

Sacrum (5, fused)

Coccyx (4, fused)

**Figure 3.6** Vertebral Sections of the Spinal Column

On the exam, you are almost sure to be asked about the number of vertebrae composing a particular section of the spinal column.

The **thorax or chest cavity** is comprised of 12 pairs of ribs, 10 of which are connected to the sternum or breastbone:

- The bottom two ribs are called "floating ribs" since they are connected in the back to the vertebrae but end before connecting anteriorly.
- The space between the ribs is called the **intercostal space.**
- The **sternum** is divided into three parts: the **manubrium**, or superior, portion of the sternum; the middle body; and the **xiphoid process**, which is the inferior tip of the sternum.

The **pelvis** is located in the inferior portion of the abdominal cavity and protects the internal reproductive organs, intestines, bladder, and rectum. Its major bones are as follows:

- **Iliac crests**—the wing sections of the pelvis
- **Pubis**—the anterior portion of the pelvic bone
- **Ischium**—the inferior portion of the pelvis

The **upper extremities** (arms and shoulder girdle) are comprised of the following bones bilaterally:

- **Clavicle**—collarbone
- **Scapula**—shoulder blade
- **Humerus**—superior bone of the arm
- **Radius**—lateral bone of the forearm; this is where your landmark is for a radial pulse
- **Ulna**—medial bone of the forearm; this is the thumb side of the lower arm
- **Carpals**—collective name of 8 tiny bones that make up the wrist
- **Metacarpals**—collective name for the 5 bones of the hand
- **Phalanges**—finger bones

**Lower extremities (legs and pelvic girdle)** consist of the following bones bilaterally:

- **Greater trochanter** (ball) and **acetabulum** (socket)—together form the hip joint
- **Femur**—thighbone
- **Patella**—kneecap
- **Tibia**—medial bone of the lower leg
- **Fibula**—lateral bone of the lower leg
- **Malleolus**—ankle bones on both medial and lateral sides
- **Tarsals** and **metatarsals**—12 bones that make up the foot
- **Calcaneus**—heel of the foot
- **Phalanges**—toe bones

Phalanges are in both the hand and the foot, so be specific about referencing their location.

## Muscular System

### Joints and Connections

A joint is a place in the body where two or more bones connect. There are 6 different types of joints: gliding, pivot, hinge, ellipsoidal, saddle, and ball and socket. Joints make a variety of motions possible. Two of the easiest joint types to visualize are **ball and socket** (like the hips and shoulders) and **hinge** (like the elbows and knees).

Two special fibrous connections called **tendons** and **ligaments** facilitate movement at the joint:

- Bones are connected to muscles by tendons.
- Bones are connected to other bones by ligaments.

Both of these connections provide motion ability, such as being able to bend your arm at the elbow or lift your leg and bend at the hip.

### Muscle Types

The body contains three types of muscle, which give the skeletal system the ability to move, give the body its shape, and supply protection for the internal organs of the body. Muscles are also differentiated by whether they are **voluntary** (requiring conscious control) or **involuntary** (cannot be voluntarily controlled or willed):

- **Skeletal** muscle (**voluntary**) connects to the skeletal bones and allows them to move in various ways. The actions of skeletal muscles are controlled by the brain and nervous system.
- **Smooth** muscle (**mostly involuntary**) is under the control of the autonomic nervous system. Smooth muscle functions as necessary for the body to exist. Examples of smooth muscle include the following:
  - The diaphragm, which controls lung inflation or deflation, works no matter the will of the individual but may temporarily be overridden by the person's conscious action, i.e., holding one's breath.
  - The digestive process muscles (e.g., esophagus and intestines) move the food particles along the path toward elimination and help the body absorb nutrients along the way.
- **Cardiac muscle** is involuntary but unique. It is classified by itself due to its ability for automaticity, or the ability to generate electrical impulses on its own. Cardiac muscle allows the heart to pump blood to the rest of the body and is found only within the heart itself.

# Respiratory and Circulatory Systems

## Respiratory System

The respiratory system provides the oxygen necessary for the body to metabolize fuel into the energy that is necessary for life. The word *pulmonary* refers to the lungs themselves, while the word *respiratory* refers to the structures that affect gas exchange (in this case, it includes the upper and lower airway structures).

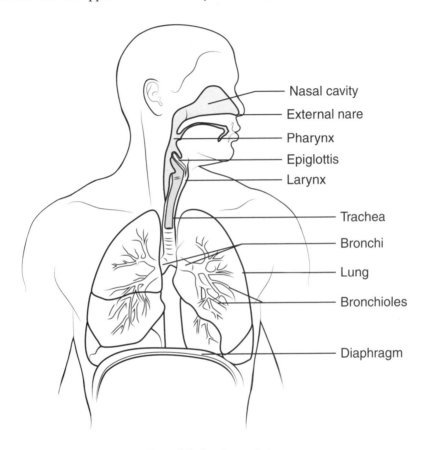

Nasal cavity
External nare
Pharynx
Epiglottis
Larynx
Trachea
Bronchi
Lung
Bronchioles
Diaphragm

**Figure 3.7** Respiratory System

The passage of air takes the path as follows:

- Air enters the nose through the **nares** and **nasopharynx**. Then it moves to the space behind the mouth called the **oropharynx**. *Pharynx* means space.

- At the inferior portion of the pharynx is the **epiglottis**, a leaflike valve that closes over the trachea during swallowing to prevent food and liquid from entering the trachea.

- The **trachea** (windpipe) is the tube that connects the pharynx to the **bronchi**, which are the two tubes that lead into the lungs. The bronchi are surrounded by bands of muscle that help constrict or dilate the tubes to allow air to flow in or out. Where the bronchi split into the left and right side is called the **carina**. Further branches off the bronchi are called **bronchioles**.

- Vocal cords are located in the **larynx** (voice box). When expiratory air passes through this area, sound is made.
- The **diaphragm** and **intercostal muscles** contract and relax in order to pull air into the lungs.
  - **Negative pressure** is created when the diaphragm moves downward and allows the lungs to expand, which pulls in oxygen-rich air.
  - **Positive pressure** is created when the diaphragm relaxes and allows the lungs to contract, which forces out carbon dioxide.
- Oxygen and carbon dioxide move through the alveoli (grapelike sacs at the end of the bronchioles) through the permeable walls of the capillaries. This is called **gas exchange**.

In order for gas exchange to happen properly, none of these pieces can be compromised in any way or else dysfunction begins to occur. Respiratory emergencies and how to assess them will be discussed later on in the airway chapter.

## Circulatory System

The circulatory (cardiovascular) system carries oxygen and nutrients to all the cells of the body. The main structure of this system is the heart, which functions as a 2-stage pump and provides the life-giving action of the blood supply.

The heart, which is approximately the size of a fist, has two sides that operate together at the same time, making a closed loop of continuous blood flow. The **right side** of the heart pumps blood to the lungs to be oxygenated, while the **left side** pumps blood to the rest of the body.

---

The adult human heart pumps 5–6 quarts of blood each minute, amounting to about 2,000 gallons per day.

- The heart contains 4 chambers that contract and relax at separate times, allowing blood to flow into the organ and become oxygenated before being recirculated to the rest of the body.
- Each chamber has its own pathway that sends blood to or receives blood from the body or lungs.

---

### Path of Blood Flow

Questions about blood flow are among the most commonly asked in class and on the NREMT exam. It is helpful to draw the pathway described below to help you memorize the route of blood:

1. Oxygen-poor blood enters the right atrium through both the superior vena cava and the inferior vena cava.

2. As the atrium contracts, blood flows downward through the open tricuspid valve and empties into the right ventricle.

3. The right ventricle then contracts and pushes the blood through the pulmonary valve, which leads to the pulmonary arteries.

4. The pulmonary arteries allow the blood to enter into either the left or right lung, where gas exchange takes place at the capillary level of the alveoli.

5. Oxygen-rich blood now returns through the pulmonary veins and enter into the left atrium.

6. The left atrium contracts and squeezes blood downward through the open mitral valve, which empties into the left ventricle.

7. The left ventricle then contracts and sends blood upward through the aortic valve into the aorta.

8. The aorta then delivers blood to the rest of the body.

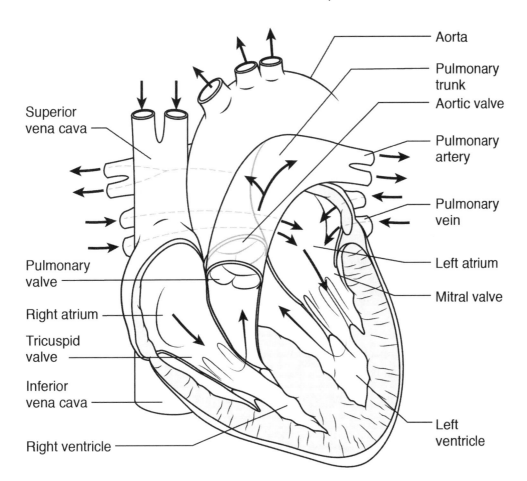

**Figure 3.8** Blood Flow Throughout the Heart

### Electrical Pathway of the Heart

Cardiac (myocardial) cells enable the heart to pump blood throughout the body correctly. Myocardial cells accomplish this by generating electrical impulses and directing the movement of these impulses throughout the tissue, which causes the mechanical function of the heart. These specialized properties are as follows:

- **Automaticity**—cell's ability to generate an electrical impulse spontaneously
- **Excitability**—cell's ability to respond to an electrical impulse
- **Conductivity**—cell's ability to transmit an electrical impulse to another cardiac cell
- **Contractility**—cardiac muscle cell's ability to contract after an electrical impulse is received
- **Rhythmicity**—cell's ability to send electrical impulses in a regularly and evenly paced manner
- **Refractoriness**—cell's *inability* to respond to another electrical impulse

To work properly, the heart's electrical impulses need to be generated and filtered through an electrical pathway to all sections of the heart. The pathway is as follows:

1. **Sinoatrial node (SA node)**—This "primary pacemaker of the heart" is located on the superior right side of the heart in the atrium and causes a contraction motion.
2. **Atrioventricular node (AV node)**—Signal is passed from the SA node to the AV node, which is located in the inferior portion of the right atrium, close to the right ventricle.
3. **Bundle of His**—This is located in the septal wall that separates the right and left ventricles. It splits the electrical pathway into two sides for each ventricle.
4. **Left and right bundle branches**—These are the two electrical pathways that stem from the bundle of His. They innervate either the right or left ventricle.
5. **Purkinje fibers** (small fibers)—These are located in the walls of the right and left ventricles. They cause the ventricles to contract and pump the blood into either the lungs or the rest of the body.

### Vessels of the Heart

The heart has a system of both arteries and veins in order to create a loop of continuous blood flow throughout the body.

**Arteries** are vessels that carry blood **away from the heart**. The major arteries are as follows:

- **Coronary arteries**—connect to the heart itself
- **Aorta**—main artery coming out of the heart, which then bends 180° into the trunk and divides at the navel into the two iliac arteries
- **Pulmonary artery**—carries blood from the right ventricle to the lungs
- **Carotid arteries**—supply blood to the brain
- **Femoral arteries**—supply blood to the lower extremities

- **Brachial arteries**—supply blood to the upper arms and are used to listen for blood pressure, the pressure being generated by the pumping action of the heart
- **Radial arteries**—provide the lower arms and hands with blood

**Veins** are vessels that carry blood **to the heart**. The major veins are as follows:

- **Pulmonary vein**—carries oxygenated blood from the lungs to the heart
- **Superior vena cava**—carries blood from the head and upper extremities back to the heart
- **Inferior vena cava**—carries blood from the trunk and lower extremities to the heart

### Sizing of Vessels

Vessels have different sizes throughout the body. From largest to smallest, sizing follows this pattern:

**Arteries → Arterioles → Capillaries**

**Veins → Venules → Capillaries**

The smallest blood vessels are the **capillaries**. Found throughout the body, capillaries allow oxygen to pass from the blood into the adjacent cells and permit carbon dioxide (the waste by-product of the metabolic process) to pass from the cells into the blood.

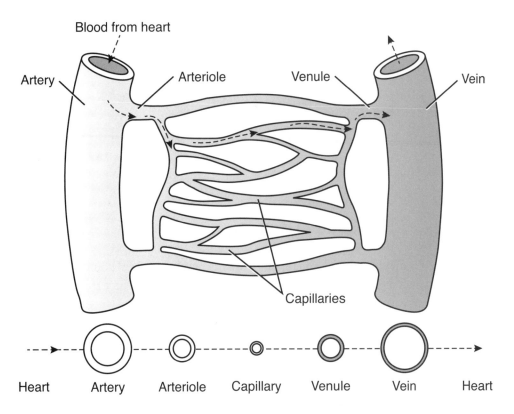

**Figure 3.9** Vessel Sizes

**Blood Components**

Blood is made up of different cell types, each of which has a unique function in the body:

- **Red blood cells (RBCs)** carry oxygen, nutrients, and waste by-products.
- **White blood cells (WBCs)**, which are only 1% of the blood, are part of the body's defenses against disease; they protect the body against illness and infection.
- **Platelets** allow blood to clot and thus stop leakage if a vessel has been damaged.
- **Plasma** (the clear fluid component of the blood that contains all the cells mentioned above) helps to deliver nutrients to various organs and to remove waste products from the body.

# Gastrointestinal and Genitourinary Systems

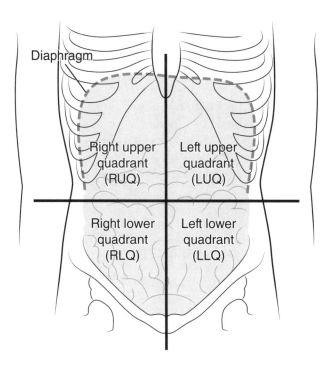

**Figure 3.10** Abdominal Quadrants

The abdomen is divided into four quadrants, with the navel as its focal point. The EMT must know which organs lie in each quadrant. In the event of blunt-force trauma to the abdomen, the location of rigidity and tenderness will indicate which organ is damaged:

- **Right upper quadrant (RUQ)**—liver, right kidney, colon, pancreas, gallbladder
- **Left upper quadrant (LUQ)**—liver, spleen, left kidney, stomach, colon, pancreas
- **Right lower quadrant (RLQ)**—colon, small intestines, ureter, appendix
- **Left lower quadrant (LLQ)**—colon, small intestines, ureter

The NREMT exam often includes questions about which organ lies in which quadrant, so do not skim over this section lightly. How to assess for various injuries in this area will be discussed in chapter 7 in Abdominal Injuries.

## Gastrointestinal System

The gastrointestinal (GI) system—the body's fuel-processing plant—is comprised of the hollow organs in the trunk and abdomen.

Digestion begins the moment food or liquid (sometimes referred to as a bolus) enters into the oral cavity. As the food or liquid moves along, the body pulls out nutrients or water as it sees fit, with waste products being expelled from the body in the form of fecal matter.

## Genitourinary System

The genitourinary (GU), or urogenital, system comprises the reproductive and urinary organs. Male and female GU organs are broadly similar, with certain exceptions.

### Urinary Organs

The urinary portion of both male and female systems includes:

- **Kidneys** (2)—responsible for filtering blood and producing urine
- **Ureters** (2)—stem off from the kidney; allow urine to pass through and flow into the bladder
- **Bladder**—has expansive properties; holds urine until it sends a signal through the nervous system to release
- **Urethra**—tube that carries urine from the bladder to the outside of the body; generally shorter in length in the female urinary system

---

Only males have a prostate gland, which surrounds the urethra. The gland's function is to secrete seminal fluid, which is needed for reproduction.

---

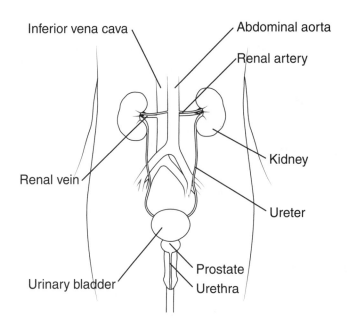

**Figure 3.11** Male Urinary System

### Reproductive Organs

Both male and female patients have reproductive organs that are very different from each other but have the same common purpose: to produce offspring in the form of an eventual fetus and subsequent child. Both genders have organs that are located inside and outside of the body.

### Male Reproductive Organs

- **Testicles** (2, also known as testes)—responsible for creating and storing sperm cells; also part of the endocrine system because they produce the hormone testosterone

- **Prostate gland**—secretes fluid that nourishes and protects sperm; during ejaculation, the prostate squeezes this fluid into the urethra, and it's expelled with sperm as semen

- **Seminal vesicles**—along with the prostate gland, responsible for secreting most of the fluid that makes up semen

- **Epididymis**—tube located in the scrotum that is attached to the testicles; responsible for the transport and storage of sperm cells that are produced

- **Vas deferens**—tube that transports mature sperm to the urethra; carries urine or sperm to the outside of the body in preparation for ejaculation

- **Scrotum**—loose, pouch-like sac of skin that hangs both behind and below the penis:

  - Holds the testes and acts as a "climate control system," bringing the testes closer to the body for warmth and away from the body for cooling properties

  - Houses many nerves and blood vessels

- **Penis**—functional unit of reproduction in males; cylindrical in shape, it is very vascular and made of spongy tissue that can become hard or soft depending on blood flow to the area; when the penis is erect, the flow of urine is blocked from the urethra, allowing only semen to be ejaculated at orgasm

Hormones produced during the male reproductive cycle are as follows:

- **Follicle-stimulating hormone (FSH)** stimulates the production of sperm.
- **Luteinizing hormone (LH)** stimulates the production of testosterone.
- **Testosterone** is responsible for the development of male characteristics (e.g., muscle mass, body hair, sex drive).

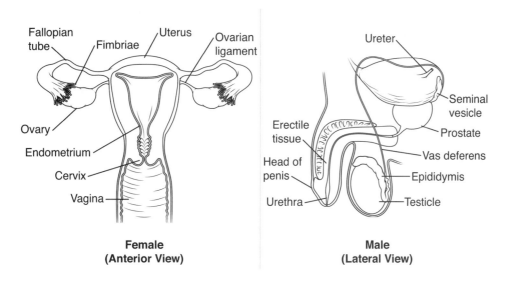

**Figure 3.12** Reproductive Organs

## Female Reproductive Organs

- **Labia majora and minora**—flaps of skin located on the outside of the vagina that protect the external organs:
    - Labia minora (interior facing)—surround the opening of the vaginal canal and urethra
    - Labia majora (exterior facing)—as puberty progresses, become covered with hair and contain sweat and oil-producing glands
- **Clitoris**—a small, sensitive protrusion where the labia minora meet; it houses many nerves and can become erect just like the penis
- **Vagina**—a hollow canal that joins the cervix (the lower part of uterus) to the outside of the body; also known as the birth canal

- **Uterus (womb)**—a hollow, pear-shaped organ consisting of muscle with an inner lining of vascular tissue (the endometrium) that grows thicker during the female reproductive cycle; this tissue then either:
  - Sheds monthly (in the case of non-fertilization) as a menstrual period
  - Remains in place in response to fertilization while the corpus (upper, main part of the uterus) expands to hold and help develop the fetus
- **Ovaries** (2)—small, oval-shaped glands located on either side of the uterus; responsible for producing eggs and hormones. When an egg is released, **fimbriae** (finger-like extensions) help push the egg from the ovary into the fallopian tube.
- **Fallopian tubes**—narrow tubes attached to the upper part of the uterus that carry the ova (egg cells) from the ovaries to the uterus. If the ovum is fertilized by sperm while still located in the fallopian tube, a dangerous condition called an ectopic pregnancy can occur.

Hormones produced during the female reproductive cycle are as follows:

- **Follicle-stimulating hormone** functions as in male reproductive systems, but in female systems it is responsible for egg growth in preparation for release from the ovary.
- **Luteinizing hormone** functions as in male reproductive systems, but in female systems it triggers ovulation and development of the corpus luteum in the ovary after a mature egg has been released.
- **Estrogen** is comparable to the role of testosterone in male reproductive systems, but in female systems it is responsible for the development of female characteristics (e.g., breast development, widening of the hips) and regulation of the menstrual cycle.
- **Progesterone** is secreted to prevent uterine contractions that may disturb the growing embryo. It also prepares the breasts for lactation for feeding infants.

## Nervous and Endocrine Systems

### Nervous System

The nervous system is the central communications system for how the human body operates. Think of it as the "master computer." It is responsible for both voluntary and involuntary actions:

- **Neurons** are the building blocks of the brain. The neuron is the basic working unit of the brain and is a specialized cell designed to transmit information to other nerve cells, muscle cells, or gland cells.
- **Dendrites** extend from the neuron cell body and receive messages from other neurons.
- **Synapses** are the contact points where one neuron communicates with another.
- A **nerve** is an enclosed, cable-like bundle of axons (the projections of neurons) in the peripheral nervous system (PNS).

Follow the layout of the flowchart below to understand the parts of the nervous system and how they relate to one another and interact.

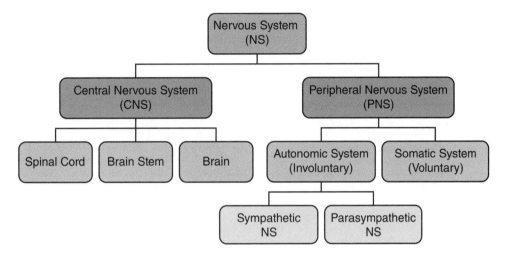

**Figure 3.13** Nervous System

## Central Nervous System

The first component is the **central nervous system (CNS)**. It consists of the following:

- **Brain**—this organ generates all the commands necessary for life, such as breathing and the pumping of the heart.
- **Spinal cord**—this long cord is connected to the brain and has hundreds of nerves that innervate various organs and tissues. It is responsible for passing all signals from the brain to its target tissues.
- **Brain stem**—this is the bottom part of the brain and connects to the spinal cord. It controls the flow of messages sent from the brain to the rest of the body. It is responsible for regulation of cardiac and respiratory functions, consciousness, and the sleep cycle.

## Peripheral Nervous System

The second component is the **peripheral nervous system (PNS)**, which is broken down into two systems, the autonomic and the somatic nervous systems.

The main function of the PNS is to connect the CNS to the limbs and organs, serving as an information highway between the brain, spinal cord, and the rest of the body. It includes 12 pairs of cranial nerves and 31 pairs of spinal nerves.

The **autonomic nervous system** is the part of the nervous system that controls and regulates the internal organs without any conscious recognition or effort; it controls involuntary functions and many reflexes. It has two parts:

- **Sympathetic nervous system**—responsible for the fight-or-flight response, which prepares the body to expend energy and deal with potential threats in the environment:
  - Will raise the heart rate, increase the breathing rate, and increase blood flow to muscles
  - Will activate sweat secretion
  - Will dilate the pupils
- **Parasympathetic system**—helps to maintain normal body functions and conserve physical resources:
  - Will lower the heart rate, slow down the breathing rate, and decrease blood flow to muscles
  - Will constrict the pupils

---

**Picture this example**: You are taking a walk in the woods and come across a bear who starts to walk toward you. Your sympathetic nervous system will kick in and start to prepare you to either fight the bear or run away fast. Once the bear is gone and you are safe, your parasympathetic nervous system is what allows you to calm down and come back to your normal resting state.

In other words, the parasympathetic nervous system "undoes" the work of the sympathetic division after a stressful event. The parasympathetic nervous system is responsible for the body's rest and digestion response when the body is relaxed, resting, or feeding.

---

The **somatic nervous system** is responsible for carrying sensory and motor information to and from the central nervous system. This is done by two main types of neurons:

- **Sensory neurons** (or afferent neurons)—these carry information from the nerves to the CNS.
- **Motor neurons** (or efferent neurons)—these carry information from the brain and spinal cord to muscle fibers throughout the body.

---

**Picture this example**: You touch a hot stove burner with your bare hand. Your sensory neurons register "that's hot!" and send that message to your brain, which then sends the order back through motor neurons to snatch your hand away from the burner in order to stop the burning process.

---

## Endocrine System

The endocrine system is made up of various glands that provide the body with the chemicals necessary for all bodily functions, such as insulin, adrenaline, and gender-specific hormones.

**Table 3.5** Endocrine Glands

| GLAND NAME | LOCATION | FUNCTION |
|---|---|---|
| Pituitary (master gland) | Between the hypothalamus and the pineal gland, inside the brain | Secretes hormones to control the other glands |
| Hypothalamus | Below the thalamus (a part of the brain that relays sensory information) and above the pituitary gland and brain stem | Secretes and metabolizes neurohormones that either stimulate or inhibit the pituitary gland |
| Pineal | Deep in the center of the brain, between the two halves of the brain | Secretes melatonin, which helps maintain circadian (sleep cycle) rhythm and regulate reproductive hormones |
| Thymus | Upper anterior part of the chest—directly behind the sternum and between the lungs | Stimulates development of T cells, a specific type of white blood cell that is a major component of the immune system |
| Thyroid | Anterior neck | Controls metabolism |
| Parathyroid | Posterior to thyroid | Produces parathyroid hormone (PTH) for the metabolism of calcium and phosphorus in the bones |
| Adrenal | Sitting on top of (superior) to each kidney | Produces the chemicals adrenaline and norepinephrine, which are used by the nervous system and muscles to control energy and respond to stimuli |
| Gonads (ovaries or testes) | Ovaries (located internally) are attached to the fallopian tubes; testes are located in the scrotum | Produce sex hormones |
| Pancreas (islets of Langerhans) | In both the upper left and upper right quadrants, posterior to the stomach | Produces insulin, which allows the body to metabolize sugar |

# Integumentary System

The integumentary system, which is more commonly known as skin, is the largest organ of the body. It is composed of three layers:

- **Epidermis**—outermost location and most exposed of the layers
- **Dermis**—deeper layer containing sweat and sebaceous (oil-producing) glands, hair follicles, capillaries, and nerve endings
- **Subcutaneous/hypodermis**—layer below the dermis that contains fatty tissue

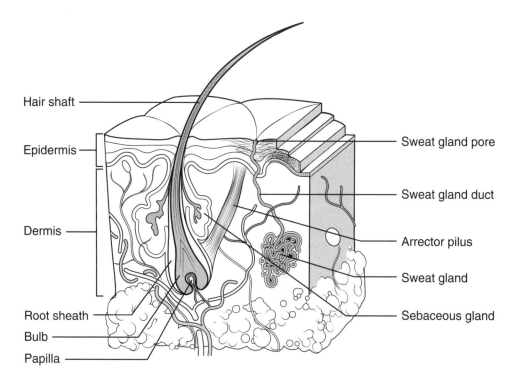

**Figure 3.14** Skin Layers

The functions of the skin are as follows:

- Serves as the outer layer of the body and holds everything in place
- Serves to protect the entire body from the environment and outside organisms
- Via its sensory functions, provides the central nervous system with most of the data required for the brain to function appropriately and helps the autonomic nervous system to regulate the body's temperature properly (crucial to cellular metabolism)

# Practice Set

1. The patella is located in which anatomical plane?

   A. Inferior/posterior

   B. Inferior/anterior

   C. Superior/posterior

   D. Superior/anterior

2. The direction away from the midline in anatomical position is

   A. distal.

   B. medial.

   C. lateral.

   D. proximal.

3. Another name for the mandible is the

   A. cheekbone.

   B. jawbone.

   C. nose.

   D. eye socket.

4. _____ connect bones to bones.

   A. Tendons

   B. Smooth muscle

   C. Skeletal muscle

   D. Ligaments

5. How many vertebrae are located in the thoracic section of the spine?

   A. 6

   B. 12

   C. 18

   D. 19

6. In respiratory inspiration, air passes through the pharynx into the

   A. nasopharynx.

   B. oropharynx.

   C. trachea.

   D. esophagus.

7. What is the name of a cardiac cell's ability to generate its own electrical impulse?

   A. Automaticity

   B. Elasticity

   C. Excitability

   D. Rhythmicity

8. Which type of muscle would be responsible for the digestion of food in the gastrointestinal system?

   A. Skeletal

   B. Smooth

   C. Cardiac

   D. Pulmonary

9. At which age do fontanels typically close in the skull?

   A. 6 months

   B. 12 months

   C. 18 months

   D. 24 months

10. Which of the following is NOT a part of the respiratory system?

    A. Aorta

    B. Nasopharynx

    C. Trachea

    D. Alveoli

11. Which of the following accurately describes the function of the peripheral nervous system?

    A. Transmits information from the central nervous system to the limbs and organs

    B. Processes information received from the sensory organs and orchestrates the appropriate action

    C. Regulates the excretion of epinephrine

    D. Responsible for the fight-or-flight response

12. Which organ is responsible for housing sensory nerves, regulating body temperature, and protecting the body's organs from the environment?

    A. Brain

    B. Kidney

    C. Liver

    D. Skin

13. The main artery coming from the left ventricle is called the

    A. aorta.

    B. pulmonary artery.

    C. inferior vena cava.

    D. superior vena cava.

14. Deoxygenated blood enters which heart chamber from the vena cava?

    A. Right atrium

    B. Left atrium

    C. Right ventricle

    D. Left ventricle

15. The focal electrical site that causes the ventricles to contract is called the

    A. sinoatrial node.

    B. atrioventricular node.

    C. Purkinje node.

    D. node of His.

16. What are the main functional units of the brain called?

    A. Neurons

    B. Nerves

    C. Synapses

    D. Dendrites

17. Which gland is most affected by diabetes?

    A. Adrenal

    B. Pituitary

    C. Pancreas

    D. Thyroid

18. Your ambulance responds to a motor vehicle accident. When you arrive, you find a male patient who was unrestrained and struck the dash. The upper left abdominal quadrant is tender and slightly rigid. You also note a large bruise in the upper left quadrant. The other abdominal quadrants are soft with no tenderness or rigidity. What injury should you suspect?

    A. Ruptured appendix

    B. Liver laceration

    C. Perforated bladder

    D. Spleen laceration

19. What plane divides the body into the left and right sides?

    A. Sagittal

    B. Frontal

    C. Transverse

    D. Midaxillary

20. The phalanges are _____ to the elbow.

    A. proximal

    B. superior

    C. lateral

    D. distal

21. Which hormone is responsible for stimulating sperm production in males and egg growth in females?

    A. Follicle-stimulating hormone

    B. Luteinizing hormone

    C. Epinephrine

    D. Growth hormone

22. Which layer of the skin is most susceptible to superficial damage such as an abrasion or burn?

    A. Hypodermis

    B. Subcutaneous

    C. Dermis

    D. Epidermis

23. You are dispatched to a call for a 77-year-old female with a broken hip. Upon arrival at her home, you find the patient lying supine on the floor of the bedroom. You notice that the patient's right leg is at a strange angle and appears to be turned inward. This injury would be a result of what type of movement?

    A. Pronation

    B. Rotation

    C. Supination

    D. Abduction

24. In an assessment, you ask the patient to point their toes toward the ground. This is a request to perform which movement and in which plane?

    A. Extension; sagittal

    B. Dorsiflexion; transverse

    C. Extension; frontal

    D. Plantar flexion; sagittal

25. You are called to the fifth floor of an apartment building for an unknown-type medical call. Upon arrival, you find a male patient in the tripod position and in obvious respiratory distress. After your partner administers oxygen to the patient at your request, you listen to the patient's lung sounds and hear wheezing bilaterally. Which of these lung structures is/are likely to be MOST affected?

    A. Alveoli

    B. Carina

    C. Capillaries

    D. Bronchi

26. In order from smallest to largest, what are the sizes of veins?

    A. Capillaries, veins, venules

    B. Venules, capillaries, veins

    C. Veins, capillaries, venules

    D. Capillaries, venules, veins

## Answer Key

| | | | | | | | | | |
|---|---|---|---|---|---|---|---|---|---|
| 1. | **B** | 7. | **A** | 13. | **A** | 19. | **A** | 25. | **D** |
| 2. | **C** | 8. | **B** | 14. | **A** | 20. | **D** | 26. | **D** |
| 3. | **B** | 9. | **C** | 15. | **B** | 21. | **A** | | |
| 4. | **D** | 10. | **A** | 16. | **A** | 22. | **D** | | |
| 5. | **B** | 11. | **A** | 17. | **C** | 23. | **B** | | |
| 6. | **C** | 12. | **D** | 18. | **D** | 24. | **D** | | |

## Answers and Explanations

**1.  B**

This question tests your knowledge of the anatomical planes and anatomical names. Once you have determined that the patella is the kneecap, you then can place it on the front (anterior) side of the leg, which is inferior to the horizontal midline of the body.

**2.  C**

*Distal* does mean "away from," but since the midline is the point in question, the correct answer is *lateral*. *Medial* means "toward the midline," and *proximal* means "next to." It is helpful to remember the pairs, such as lateral/medial, superior/inferior, etc., rather than try to memorize them individually.

**3.  B**

The cheekbone is the zygomatic bone. The nose is not a bone but consists of cartilage, and the eye socket is the orbit. A good way to learn anatomy is to purchase an anatomy coloring book.

**4.  D**

Ligaments connect bones to other bones in order to form joints. Tendons connect muscles to bones. The other two muscles exist in the body but have specific functions not related to connecting bones together.

**5.  B**

The correct answer is 12. This is a common question on the NREMT exam.

**6.  C**

The nasopharynx (A) and oropharynx (B) are parts of the pharynx located posterior to the nose and mouth, respectively. Oxygenated air then enters the trachea (C) through the vocal cords past the epiglottis. The epiglottis closes over the esophagus (D) to prevent air from entering the gastrointestinal system.

**7.  A**

The correct answer is automaticity. Elasticity (B) is not a term associated with cardiac cells. Excitability (C) is the ability to respond to an electrical impulse. Rhythmicity (D) may seem like a good answer, but it has to do with sending the pulses generated in an evenly spaced manner.

**8.  B**

The digestive process works without our having to manage it consciously. *Pulmonary* (D) is a word used to describe the respiratory system, not a type of muscle. We know that *cardiac* (C) means "heart," so we're left with either skeletal or smooth muscle. Skeletal muscle (A) is what moves our bones around, while smooth muscle (B) uses rhythmic contraction and relaxation to move fluids or broken-down food around the body.

**9.  C**

Remember that fontanels are specific to pediatric patients. They are where the sutures of the skull have not fully stitched themselves together yet to form the overall hard cranial cap. The correct answer is 18 months.

**10. A**

The correct answer is aorta, which is part of the heart.

**11. A**

The peripheral nervous system is responsible for transmitting information from the central nervous system to the muscles and various organs of the body. The other choices describe the functions of the autonomic nervous system.

**12. D**

The skin is the largest organ in the body and is responsible for housing sensory nerves, regulating body temperature, and protecting organs from the environment. The brain (A), kidney (B), and liver (C) do not perform these functions.

**13. A**

The superior vena cava and inferior vena cava are two of the largest veins in the body. So although they do help bring blood to the heart, they are not arteries and do not attach to the left ventricle. This leaves you with choice (A) or (B). The correct answer is the main artery supplying the body with oxygenated blood, the aorta.

**14. A**

The answer is the right atrium. Blood always enters into the atrium first on either side of the heart. Deoxygenated blood from the body enters the right side of the heart. Oxygenated blood from the lungs enters the left side. The ventricles are the bottom two chambers of the heart and are responsible for the strong contractions to push the blood to either the body (left side) or the lungs (right side).

**15. B**

*Sinoatrial* contains the word "atrial," which refers to the atrium, or upper part of the heart. So we can rule out choice (A). There is no such thing as the Purkinje node (C) or node of His (D). However, after the electrical command passes through the atrioventricular node, it then passes through the bundle of His into the Purkinje fibers. The only choice that contains the root "ventricle" is *atrioventricular node* (B), giving a high probability that this is the correct answer.

**16. A**

We can rule out nerves (B) because, although nerves are parts of the nervous system in general, they are not specifically located in the brain itself. Dendrites (D) are part of a neuron, but the entire neuron (A) itself is the functional unit of the brain. A synapse (C) is the connection point where two or more neurons "speak" to one another.

**17. C**

With diabetes, the body ceases to produce the hormone insulin. This affects the body's ability to metabolize sugar into energy and directly affects the islets of Langerhans, which are located within the pancreas. The adrenal gland produces epinephrine (adrenaline) and norepinephrine, which affect the nervous system; the pituitary gland secretes multiple hormones that control various glands and processes; and the thyroid helps regulate metabolism.

**18. D**

The spleen is located in the upper left quadrant, and there should be a high index of suspicion of damage to the spleen with any trauma to this abdominal quadrant. The liver is located mostly in the upper right quadrant. The bladder is located in the lower quadrants. The appendix is located in the lower right quadrant.

**19. A**

The correct answer is sagittal (A). The frontal plane (B) divides the body into anterior and posterior, and it also contains the reference point of the midaxillary line (D). The transverse plane (C) divides the body into superior and inferior portions. Refer to the table in the Anatomical Terminology section to refresh your memory if you got this question wrong.

**20. D**

The correct answer is distal (D). When speaking about limbs, we mainly use the terms proximal and distal to describe structures in relation to one another. *Proximal* means "closer to" the trunk of the body, while *distal* means "farther away from." Think of the word *distance* when trying to remember the difference between the two. Superior (B) refers to something above, while lateral (C) refers to something away from the midline.

**21. A**

Your first thought may have been growth hormone (D) since it contains the word *growth* in it; however, growth hormone is not specific to the reproductive system. Luteinizing hormone (B) is a reproductive hormone but is responsible for stimulating either testosterone production or ovulation. Epinephrine (C) is also a hormone but is not specific to the reproductive system. That leaves follicle-stimulating hormone (A), which is found in both male and female reproductive systems; it affects pubertal development and the function of ovaries and testes.

**22. D**

Hypodermis (A) and subcutaneous (B) are names for the same layer of skin, depending on which anatomical chart or textbook you use; it is the deepest layer of the skin. The dermis (C) is where most of the "parts" are, such as veins, arteries, nerves, sweat glands, etc. The key to this question is the word *superficial*, which means "occurring at or near the surface." This makes epidermis (D) the best choice as it is the top layer of skin.

**23. B**

Abduction (D) is a movement made in the frontal plane and involves moving a body part toward or away from the midline. Although this may seem like a good choice, you are looking for a rotational type of movement (B); remember that the hip uses a ball and socket joint in order to move. Both pronation (A) and supination (C) involve rotation, but those movements involve rotation around another bone.

**24. D**

The movement (pointing the toes) is happening with either the left or the right foot, which puts us in the sagittal plane. So, any answer that does not include the sagittal plane can be ruled out, leaving you options (A) and (D). Even if you are unsure which plane this movement is in, you may recall that both dorsiflexion and plantar flexion have to do with the foot in particular. This leaves you with choices (B) and (D). By putting these two strategies together, you arrive at the correct answer, plantar flexion and sagittal plane (D).

**25. D**

The correct answer is the bronchi (D), which are a pair of tubes with bands of muscle that either constrict or dilate to allow airflow in or out of the lungs. In this case, this patient's bronchi are being constricted, creating a smaller space for air to pass and producing a wheezing sound. This patient needs a bronchodilator medication to relieve the bronchial constriction. Although the rest of the answers are also located in the respiratory system, they are not the MOST affected, as the question asks.

**26. D**

(D) is the correct answer. Please refer back to the Circulatory System and Sizing of Vessels portion of this chapter to review a visual aid if you got this question wrong.

[ CHAPTER 4 ]

# PATIENT ASSESSMENT AND DOCUMENTATION

---

**LEARNING OBJECTIVES**

- Understand what to consider in the scene size-up
- List the components of an initial patient assessment
- Implement the SAMPLE mnemonic
- List the steps used to obtain baseline vital signs
- Perform a focused history and physical exam for a medical call
- Implement the OPQRST mnemonic
- Perform a focused physical exam for a trauma call
- List the components of a detailed physical exam
- List the priority steps of ongoing patient assessment
- List the components of a prehospital care report

---

It is just after midnight when your radio beeps and dispatch announces, "Rescue 1, respond to 123 Main Street, unknown-type medical call, no other information available." You pull on your examination gloves and respond with lights and sirens to the call.

An unknown-type medical call is a truly random event. You can encounter something as simple as a splinter in a finger or as dangerous as an ongoing gun battle. Dispatchers are trained to try and get as much information as they can from a caller, but the information they are given may be fragmented or incomplete, especially if the call is coming from a third party.

## Patient Assessment

Patient assessment is the most important part of your toolbox as an EMT. Observing symptoms or signs visually is of course part of this, but by itself it's not enough. You must also know how to ask specific questions to determine the true issue afflicting the patient. It's like being a medical detective. Furthermore, assessment is not a one-time event but, rather, an ongoing process that's running from the moment you are dispatched to the moment you clear yourself from a call. Let's review the different parts.

## Scene Size-Up

The information gained from assessing the scene may be critical to patient care or even a police investigation. Here are some guidelines.

### Assess for Hazards

As an EMT, you must judge to the best of your ability whether a scene is safe, and you always want to err on the side of caution. When you see a person down, likely your first impulse is to run right over and render care. However, even before you get out of the truck, you must scan the area for any hazards that would endanger your safety or the safety of your crew, including:

- People who present a danger, such as a person with a weapon
- Hazardous materials, such as toxic or dangerous chemicals
- Environmental hazards, such as unstable ground, ice, or snow

If you determine a scene is unsafe, it must be made safe before you and your crew enter.

### Observe the Scene

Once the scene has been made safe, you should remain watchful and observant of all that is around you. Your observations will help you determine the nature of this call—medical versus trauma—which directly influences how you assess and treat your patient:

- When you approach a scene, you must act as a medical detective. Look for the clues that enable you to respond appropriately to the situation. If conscious and alert, the patient is usually the best source of information. If this is not the case, bystanders become your next best source. Don't ignore the people standing around. Engage them to help you ascertain what the problem is.
- Immediately figure out how many patients there are. The number of patients and the severity of injury or illness will help determine how many additional units will be needed at this scene.
- If this is a **medical call**, first establish that the patient has an airway, is breathing, and has a pulse demonstrating blood circulation (the ABCs). Then determine the nature of the illness.
- If this is a **trauma call**, again first check the ABCs. Then determine the mechanism of injury. In other words, answer the question, "How did this patient become injured?"

---

### KEY TAKEAWAY

Don't get tunnel vision when encountering a seriously injured patient. An open femur fracture is sure to get your attention. However, if you treat it with a traction splint and forget to check for an open airway, you may deliver a dead patient (with a properly applied traction splint) to the ED.

Injuries such as these are referred to as **"distracting injuries."** They may look bad, but they will cause you to miss other, more important, life-threatening injuries.

---

## Initial Patient Assessment

### Remember Your ABCs

As you approach, ideally from the feet, observe the patient to determine priority, age, gender, and overall appearance:

- Introduce yourself as an EMT and ask the patient's name.
- If the patient is conscious and responsive, that will tell you right away that they have airway, breathing, and circulation (ABC).
- If the patient is unconscious, first check the airway. Open it if necessary, ventilate if apneic, and assess for a pulse.

---

Always treat life-threatening situations as you encounter them. If the patient has no pulse, commence CPR immediately.

---

### Level of Consciousness

If the patient has no immediate life-threatening conditions, you must then determine the patient's level of consciousness. The acronym **AVPU** is a shorthand for assessed level of consciousness:

- Fully **A**lert (responds appropriately to a normal voice)
- Responsive to **V**erbal stimuli (responds if spoken to in a loud voice)
- Responsive to **P**ainful stimuli (responds to a vigorous rub of the sternum or something similar)
- **U**nconscious (does not respond to any of the above)

### Bleeding Control

With ABCs taken care of and level of consciousness established, the EMT must next check for gross hemorrhage, or major bleeding. If it is present, steps must be taken to control the bleeding. (See the section Focused Physical Exam: Trauma for a discussion of specific techniques.)

### Pulse Check

The most common pulse point checked is either the radial or the carotid in adults and the brachial in pediatric patients. However, you should be familiar with the all major anatomical points for palpating a pulse. These include:

- Radial (wrist)
- Brachia (upper arm)
- Posterior tibial, dorsalis pedal (feet)
- Carotid (neck)
- Femoral (upper leg)

Knowing your pulse-taking options is valuable. If one of the more common points is not available for some reason (e.g., trauma, inability to find a palpable pulse), you will still be able to assess this aspect of your patient's status.

### Temperature

As you are assessing, feel the patient's forehead and, if appropriate, exposed areas of skin on arms and legs for temperature. The back of your hand is ideal for this assessment.

The skin should be warm and dry. If it is hot to the touch, the patient may be running a fever or have been exposed to high temperatures. If cold, the patient may be hypothermic from cold exposure or have circulation impairment. Is the skin dry or moist? Dampness may be due to **diaphoresis**, or sweating, which is a symptom of many medical problems.

### Transport Priority Decision

The initial assessment is performed primarily to indicate whether the patient should be transported immediately or if there is time to perform a more thorough assessment and any applicable treatment protocols on scene. A patient who presents as being in serious condition should be transported immediately, with any further assessment and/or intervention done en route to the emergency department (ED).

In addition, the following are considered "load and go" patients based on the primary assessment:

- Unresponsive with no gag reflex
- Responsive but unable to follow commands
- Dyspnea (difficulty breathing)
- Hypoperfusion syndrome (shock)
- Childbirth with complications
- Chest pains with pallor and dyspnea
- Uncontrolled hemorrhaging
- Severe pain

Any of the conditions listed would require a priority transport. Immobilize the patient and transport to the nearest emergency department. Depending on the situation, you may also consider requesting an ALS intercept to initiate advanced protocols with less loss of time to the patient. (Since the primary consideration is *time lost*, if you can get to the emergency department faster than it would take for ALS to arrive, then of course do that.)

If the situation is not a priority transport, proceed to the appropriate focused assessment and physical examination. This is sometimes called a "stay and play" situation, where the word *play* refers to treatments or focused assessments that may be done on scene without immediate danger of the patient degrading.

**Be alert for an evolving need to transport.** At any time, the patient's condition may change or the focused assessment may discover a condition that necessitates advanced measures. If that happens, transport without delay.

Initially, the EMT should determine the chief complaint. There are various ways to ask for this information, but watch your tone and body language. Your goal is not only to get all the vital information needed but also to make the patient feel comfortable about your intervention:

- **DO NOT ask**, "Why are we here?" while standing over the patient and having your hands on your hips.
- **DO ask**, "How can I help you? Can you explain what happened?" while sitting/squatting at the patient's eye level and showing kindness in your voice.

### KEY TAKEAWAY

Keep that in mind that questions you ask should not be simply a "checklist" of facts. You need to understand the *story* of what happened. Piece together the different details you learn to get a larger picture so that you can determine the proper course of treatment.

Once the immediate problem is stated, you need to gather more information about the situation and the patient's needs. If the patient is unconscious or otherwise unable to respond, bystanders and/or family members are the best resource for this assessment. A helpful tool is the **SAMPLE** history. This set of 6 questions is a concise way to get a lot of information about the patient and understand the reason why 911 was called for assistance.

Let's assume your patient is a female who says she has abdominal pain. The following are appropriate questions to ask using the SAMPLE mnemonic:

- Signs and symptoms
  - **Is it like anything you've had before?**
  - **Can you point to exactly where it hurts? Does anything make the pain better or worse?**
  - Focus your questions on the multiple causes for female abdominal pain, e.g., a gastrointestinal, vascular, or gynecologic condition. If the patient says that she developed a sharp pain in her right lower quadrant an hour ago and she is holding her hand on the right lower abdomen just superior to the right leg, you would consider appendicitis. Do not assume anything, however, and ask the remainder of the questions.

- Allergies
  - **Do you have any allergies?**
  - This is pretty straightforward. Most people are willing to share this information.

- Medications
  - **Are you on any medications?**
  - This starts to get confidential. Some patients will provide a negative answer and then, in the privacy of the emergency department, tell the nurse the truth. This is especially true for medications for sexually transmitted diseases, HIV, hepatitis, or erectile dysfunction.
  - Ask about any over-the-counter (OTC) medications such as pills, powders, or tinctures as well as homeopathic medications and home remedies. Although patients may not think of these as "medications" because they are not prescribed by a medical doctor, they may be causing the problem.

- Pertinent history
  - **Are you being treated for any medical conditions?**
  - If the patient with abdominal pain now says that she has a history of ulcerative colitis, you might reconsider your assumption about appendicitis. Again, patients may avoid telling you the truth about certain conditions. Be alert for signs of lying, such as the inability to maintain eye contact or a sudden change in demeanor.
  - If you think that the patient is telling a serious lie, be sure to share your suspicions with the triage nurse at the emergency department. The goal is not to catch someone in a lie but, rather, to ensure that a true clinical picture emerges for the physician who will treat your patient.
  - Keep your patient focused on her major and most recent medical history. This is especially important when the patient has conditions that could lead to an extensive history (e.g., older adult, patient with psychological issues).

- Last oral intake
  - **When and what did you last eat?**
  - If the patient says that she ate "two large orders of super-hot chicken wings a few hours ago," you might now consider indigestion as the cause of her gastric pain.

- Events leading to this episode
  - **What happened just prior to the pain starting?**
  - This answer may give you a clue to the current condition. Using a different example, suppose you are treating a person experiencing chest pain who responds, "I was lifting weights." This response helps you understand why the patient is experiencing this particular type of pain. Dispatches for chest pain always cause the EMT to think of cardiac-related conditions. However, given this context and in the absence of any other cardiac symptoms, the problem may be a pulled muscle caused by exercising.

## Baseline Vital Signs

A common question on the NREMT cognitive exam begins with a scenario including vital signs and asks either which vital sign would be most indicative of a certain condition or which is the most concerning given the patient's presentation. The following are 7 points you should keep in mind when assessing the patient's baseline vital signs:

1. Level of consciousness
2. Pulse rate
3. Respiratory rate
4. Blood pressure
5. Skin condition
6. Capillary refill
7. Pupils

**Level of consciousness (LOC).** The following table shows key points you are assessing and provides sample questions you can ask to ascertain just how "with it" your patient is. (Do not confuse this with *loss of consciousness*. If you use the acronym "LOC," make sure you clearly document which situation you are describing.)

**Table 4.1** Level of Consciousness Key Points to Note

| COMPONENT | QUESTIONS TO ASK OR KEY POINTS TO NOTE |
|---|---|
| Conscious or unconscious? | • If conscious: determine HOW conscious<br>• If unconscious: assess ABCs, maintain airway, determine whether resuscitation is needed |
| Orientation to person | Ask questions such as:<br><br>• "What is your name?"<br>• "Can you tell me who you are?"<br>• "What would you like me to call you?" |
| Orientation to place | Ask questions such as:<br><br>• "Do you know where you are?"<br>• "Can you tell me where we're at?"<br>• "Where are we at right now?" |
| Orientation to time | Ask questions such as:<br><br>• "Do you know what time it is right now?"<br>• "What day is it?"<br>• "What year (or month) are we in right now?"<br>• "How long ago did this happen?" |
| Orientation to event | Ask questions such as:<br><br>• "Can you tell me what happened?"<br>• "What made you call 911 today?"<br>• "Do you know what happened to bring you to this situation?" |

If the answers to the questions are satisfactory, the patient is said to be **alert and oriented times 4**. Conversely, if the answers to the questions are unsatisfactory (for example, if the patient is unable to state what happened), you would record that the patient is **alert and oriented times 2, with confusion as to present event**.

**Pulse rate** in an adult patient is usually measured by finding the pulse at the point where the radial artery crosses the wrist bone:

- You may count the number of beats for 15 seconds and multiply by 4.
- You may also count for 30 seconds and multiply by 2.
- If the pulse is irregular, count the pulse for a full minute and make a notation that it is irregular.

**Respiratory rate** is calculated by watching the rise and fall of the patient's chest wall for 15 seconds and then multiplying by 4:

- If the rate is irregular, take the measurement for a full minute.
- A useful technique for counting respirations is to fold the patient's arm at the elbow, placing it against their chest, as though you are taking a radial pulse. You can then feel the chest rise and fall and count respirations without having to stare at the person, who may become self-conscious and breathe at a different pace or pattern.
- Breathing that is shallow, deep, or labored or noises in the patient's breathing (e.g., wheezing, snoring sounds, or high-pitched whistling) indicate a potentially serious medical problem.

**Blood pressure** is measured by placing a blood pressure cuff (sphygmomanometer) on the patient's upper arm and listening with a stethoscope over the brachial artery inside the elbow. Inflate the cuff to 200 mm Hg, and then slowly release the pressure while you listen for Korotkoff sounds (the "thumping" noises):

- The point at which the pulse sound begins to be heard is the *systolic blood pressure*, or the pressure in the arteries as the ventricles in the heart contract and push blood into the system.
- As the pressure in the cuff continues to drop, the sound grows louder and then begins to diminish.
- When the sound cannot be heard any longer, *diastolic pressure*, or the pressure in the arteries while the ventricles are at rest, is taken.

**Skin condition** documentation should note skin color, temperature, and condition. **Skin color** is often the most useful diagnostic tool available to the EMT, because it conveys a variety of information about the patient's status. The table lists some potential causes for differences in coloration. It is not exhaustive, and a thorough assessment may uncover reasons other than those listed.

**Table 4.2** Skin Colorations and Potential Conditions

| SKIN COLOR | POTENTIAL CONDITIONS | ADDITIONAL CONSIDERATIONS |
|---|---|---|
| Pale (light or white) | <ul><li>Shock</li><li>Blood loss (hypovolemia)</li><li>Anemia</li><li>Hypothermia</li></ul> | Ask what the patient's normal skin color is. Some people are naturally pale and may have nothing wrong with them medically. |
| Cyanotic (blue/gray/ purple) | <ul><li>Hypothermia</li><li>Shock</li><li>Hypovolemia</li><li>Respiratory distress/failure</li><li>Asphyxia</li><li>Hypoxia</li></ul> | Cyanotic technically means bluish. Depending on a person's natural skin color, however, it may present as gray or even purple. |
| Flushed (red/deeper shade of pink) | <ul><li>Burns</li><li>Hyperthermia</li><li>Skin conditions (e.g., rosacea, eczema, psoriasis)</li><li>Certain medications (e.g., nitroglycerin, beta-blockers, diltiazem, adenosine)</li><li>Extreme emotions (e.g., embarrassment, anger, shyness)</li></ul> | Is this the patient's normal coloration?<br><br>If unsure whether the flushing is caused by a medication, check a search engine (e.g., Google) for common side effects. |
| Jaundiced (yellow) | <ul><li>Liver inflammation or failure</li><li>Blocked bile duct</li><li>Hepatitis A/B/C</li><li>Long-term alcohol abuse</li><li>Reabsorption of a large hematoma</li></ul> | Jaundice is common in newborns because the baby's body is newly filtering out excess bilirubin on its own; in the womb, the mother's body did this. Typically, it resolves after a week or so.<br><br>Persistent jaundice is cause for concern. |

In addition to making your own observations, it can also be helpful to ask patients themselves (or someone who knows them) if their color appears different from usual.

In patients with little or no pigmentation, changes in skin color may be more easily observed due to the lack of melanin in the skin. In patients with deeply pigmented skin, changes in skin color may be apparent only in certain areas, such as:

- Fingernail beds
- Lips
- The mucous membranes in the mouth
- The underside of the arm/hand
- The conjunctiva of the eye

Finally, determine skin's temperature and condition:

- Is the skin dry, or is the patient sweating (diaphoretic)?
- Is the patient's skin cool, normal temperature, or warm to the touch?

**Capillary refill** is a measure of how the patient is perfusing, i.e., how well oxygen is being transferred from the red blood cells to the tissues:

- It is measured by depressing the nail bed and noting how many seconds elapse before the color returns.
- Normal return of color should be 2 seconds or less; longer than that is considered delayed.

**Pupils** often give clues about the condition of the patient's nervous system. Shine a pocket flashlight into each eye and note the following:

- Do the pupils contract and then dilate as you move the light out of the pupil?
- Are the pupils of equal size and shape?
- Can the patient follow the moving light from side to side with the eyes?

Documenting the pupils can be done in various ways:

- **PERL**: Pupils Equal and Reactive to Light
- **PERRL**: Pupils Equal, Round, and Reactive to Light
- **PERLA**: Pupils Equal, Round, Reactive to Light, and Accommodating

## Focused History and Physical Exam: Medical

Regardless of whether you have decided to prioritize transport or not, the next step is to conduct a focused history and physical exam of the patient.

### Vital Signs

If you have not already done so, take a baseline set of vitals now. A blood glucose level (BGL) reading may also be taken at this time if permitted by local protocol, especially in cases of altered consciousness.

### Patient Complaints

Next assess the patient's complaints as well as signs and symptoms. Naturally, these questions cannot be answered in an unresponsive patient unless a witness/family member can assist.

The acronym **OPQRST** is helpful for remembering what to ask about the condition that has brought EMS to this patient:

- **O**nset—when did the pain start?
- **P**rovocation—did the patient do anything to aggravate the problem?
- **Q**uality—can the patient describe the pain?
- **R**adiation—does the pain move in any direction?

- **S**everity—how bad is the pain on a scale of 1–10 (with 10 being worst)?
- **T**ime—how long has the pain persisted, and is this the first time it is happening?

Suppose you are responding to a patient with chest pain. Scene safety, universal precautions, and ABCs are all done. The primary assessment does not indicate a need to expedite transport, and your patient is conscious and alert. *Now is the time to ask the OPQRST questions*, which will facilitate a discussion about what the patient is experiencing.

---

**TEST YOURSELF 4.1**

Use the OPQRST questions to label the patient's response for each letter in the following scenario:

"The pain started right after I finished exercising an hour ago. I was lifting weights, and all of a sudden, I felt a sharp pain right here [points to left chest superior to left nipple]. If I raise my left arm, it gets a lot worse, and it feels like a tearing sensation. The pain doesn't move. I would rate it about 6 on a scale of 1 to 10. I've never had anything like it before."

**What type of condition do you think this patient is suffering from, given his answers for chest pain?**

---

At this point, you should have a general clinical picture of the patient's condition and be ready to conduct a thorough physical exam:

- It is not necessary to palpate the entire body of a patient; however, it is necessary to physically examine the area of complaint.
- Palpating with the fingertips is often revealing of the ultimate diagnosis. Does the area of complaint appear normal in relation to the surrounding body areas? When you feel it with your fingers, does it feel the same as the surrounding tissue, or is it abnormally rigid?
- When you palpate, does the patient complain that the area you are touching is tender or painful? Pain that is increasing or decreasing is a sign of something wrong.

At the conclusion of the focused medical assessment, position any patient who is unconscious in a manner to protect the airway, and transport the patient to the hospital emergency department. Remember that assessment is constant and repeated often. During the transport, be alert for changes in the patient's status and be prepared to respond accordingly.

## Focused Physical Exam: Trauma

The detailed physical exam (or the head-to-toe exam) enables the EMT to get a clearer picture of what is going on with the patient. In the past, the purpose of the exam was to identify and treat life-threatening conditions and stabilize the patient. Now, however, a more complete exam is used to reveal conditions that will be of help to the receiving physician so that a definitive diagnosis can be made and treatment can be started.

Each EMT will develop a personalized system for performing a complete physical assessment. The goal should always be a methodical and thorough checking of the entire external body.

### Head-to-Toe Exam

The mnemonic **DCAP-BTLS** is used as each section of the body is closely examined both visually and by touch:

- **D**eformities, **C**ontusions, **A**brasions, **P**unctures/Penetrations
- **B**urns, **T**enderness, **L**acerations, **S**welling

A thorough exam includes the following, checking for DCAP-BTLS at each section.

**Table 4.3** Detailed Physical Exam

| BODY SECTION | PALPATE/CHECK FOR | POSSIBLE INJURY OR CONDITION |
|---|---|---|
| Head | • Cranial plate instability<br>• Fluids coming out of ears, nose, or mouth<br>• Bruising behind one or both ears (Battle sign) | • Skull fracture<br>• Internal cranial injury |
| Face | • Traumatic injury and bleeding<br>• Pupil response, color, and foreign bodies | • Internal head structural injury<br>• Internal head bleed<br>• Concussion<br>• Increased cranial pressure<br>• Poisoning<br>• Overdose |
| Nose and mouth | • Fluids<br>• Loose or broken teeth<br>• Foreign odors | • Fluid buildup: saliva or blood<br>• Lacerations from broken teeth<br>• Airway obstruction from loose teeth or difficulty getting a good mask seal if needed<br>• Odors (could indicate alcohol intoxication or ketones in diabetic emergencies) |
| Neck | • Jugular vein distension<br>• Tracheal shift<br>• Subcutaneous emphysema (bubbling sensation under the skin) | • Tension pneumothorax<br>• Underlying air leakage from the respiratory system secondary to chest trauma or illness |
| Chest | • Rib tenderness, crepitus<br>• Paradoxical motion (an area of the chest moves in the opposite direction of normal motion) | • Rib fracture<br>• Flail segment ($\geq$2 ribs are broken in $\geq$2 places) |

*(Continued)*

**Table 4.3** Detailed Physical Exam (*Continued*)

| BODY SECTION | PALPATE/CHECK FOR | POSSIBLE INJURY OR CONDITION |
|---|---|---|
| Abdomen | • Bounding or visible pulsation around the navel<br>• If patient complains of pain, start palpating away from the pain first<br>• Palpate all 4 quadrants, feeling for rigid or soft feeling | • Rigidity (could indicate intra-abdominal bleed)<br>• Bounding or visual pulsation (could indicate an abdominal aortic aneurysm, which could be fatal if ruptured) |
| Pelvis/genitalia | • Pelvic stability—gently compress and press down on either hip<br>• Genital bleeding<br>• Priapism (persistent erection; males) | • Hip fracture, including "open book" fracture (would cause a lot of blood to collect in pelvic cavity)<br>• Internal or external bleeding of genitalia must be padded and controlled by pressure<br>• Priapism could indicate spinal injury in males |
| Arms/legs (extremities) | • Pulse and capillary refill in each extremity<br>• Motor function—"Squeeze my hand" or "Wiggle your toes"<br>• Sensation—"Can you feel this?" or "Which finger or toe am I touching?" | • Circulatory compromise if delayed capillary refill<br>• Dislocated bones/joints<br>• Impaired motor or sensory function (could indicate spinal injury ) |
| Back/posterior | • Injury to the spine or back<br>• Must be done while log rolling patient onto the backboard (not while patient is secured on the backboard) | • Spinal injury<br>• DCAP-BTLS injuries |

The final step in the detailed assessment is to retake vital signs and especially note any wide divergence from the initial vital signs taken during the focused assessment.

## Scores

There are two methods used in EMS to score an assessment. Either one can help you to monitor changing conditions in the patient and to determine transport priority and destination. Since the patient's status can change at any time, you must be diligent in your reassessment to catch any developing issues.

The **Glasgow Coma Scale** (GCS) assesses a patient's level of consciousness in both medical and traumatic injury. Calculate GCS by assigning the following index numbers as appropriate. The range is 3–15 total points. A patient who is unconscious and unresponsive would receive a score of 3, while a patient who shows no deficiencies would receive a score of 15.

**Table 4.4** Calculating the Glasgow Coma Scale

| TYPE OF RESPONSE TESTED | POINTS ASSIGNED |
|---|---|
| Eye response | • Spontaneous (4)<br>• To verbal stimuli (3)<br>• To painful stimuli (2)<br>• No response; eyes will not open (1) |
| Verbal response | • Oriented conversation (5)<br>• Confused conversation (4)<br>• Inappropriate conversation (3)<br>• Incomprehensible conversation (2)<br>• No response (1) |
| Motor response | • Obeys commands (6)<br>• Localizes pain (5)<br>• Withdraws from pain (4)<br>• Flexes extremities/decorticate position (3)<br>• Extends extremities/decerebrate position (2)<br>• No response (1) |

The **Revised Trauma Score (RTS)** is a numerical index based on the severity of injury and patient condition in a traumatic injury. The RTS calculation takes into account the systolic blood pressure, respiratory rate, and GCS score. The range is 1–12 total points.

**Table 4.5** Calculating the Revised Trauma Score (RTS)

| MEASUREMENT TAKEN | POINTS ASSIGNED |
|---|---|
| Respiratory rate | • 10-29 breaths per minute (4)<br>• >29 breaths per minute (3)<br>• 6-9 breaths per minute (2)<br>• 1-5 breaths per minute (1) |
| Systolic blood pressure | • >89 mm Hg (4)<br>• 77-89 mm Hg (3)<br>• 50-75 mm Hg (2)<br>• 1-75 mm Hg (1)<br>• No pulse or no blood pressure (0) |
| GCS score | • 13-15 (4)<br>• 9-12 (3)<br>• 6-8 (2)<br>• 4-5 (1)<br>• <4 (0) |

**TEST YOURSELF 4.2**

**Calculate the Revised Trauma Score for the following patient:**

- Conscious; alert and oriented ×4
- Fell from a stepladder; no loss of consciousness
- Has abdominal pain; guarding with right hand
- Respiratory rate 20/min
- Blood pressure 80/60 mm Hg

## Ongoing Reassessment

A patient who is stable one minute can easily become unstable in the next. Apnea, for instance, can occur without any struggle or outward sign—and should that happen, the EMT must be ready to deal with this new medical problem. The EMT is responsible for the patient for as long as the patient remains in the care of that EMT, even after initial and focused assessments are complete. This is the portion of the call during which the patient's condition can change and not be noticed, often with tragic results. You must reassess.

As a general rule:

- Repeat vital signs every 5 minutes for unstable patients and every 10–15 minutes for stable patients. (Enter these checks chronologically in the patient documentation care report.)
- Repeat the focused assessment anytime you detect a change in patient condition.
- Repeat the focused assessment if a downgrading trend is noticed, whether vital signs or mental status.

Treat new conditions encountered as they occur, and immediately relay the new information to the receiving facility.

## Documentation

More than just a legal requirement to fulfill, good documentation is also a prerequisite for good patient care. "Documentation" goes by various names depending on what service you work for, where you live and practice, and even what state you are in. Whatever terms are used, they all refer to the same thing: the set of information that is collected on a patient, records events that occurred during the call, and is submitted to your service (in either paper or digital format) for billing purposes.

## Prehospital Care Report

The documentation of an EMS encounter is called a **prehospital care report (PCR)** but is commonly referred to as a **run report** or just a "chart." Many agencies have moved away from paper charting and now utilize electronic versions, also called EPCRs or ePCRs.

It is your responsibility to be familiar with the format of charting that your agency uses and be able to fill out a report on every patient you treat. Remember the general rule of documentation: if it's not written down, it didn't happen.

---

The bane of any job is paperwork, and EMS charts are no exception. Since you, as an EMT, are in a medical profession and the United States is the most litigious country in the world, good documentation is a skill that is almost as necessary as good patient care:

- Your medical report may be subpoenaed for a criminal or civil action, and an attorney may subpoena you as well to testify about the events in question.
- Civil actions often take up to 7 years to reach a jury trial, which would require you to recount facts 7 years after they occurred.
- The documentation is your official record of what happened. You may *remember* inserting an oropharyngeal airway (OPA), but the written report of the event carries legal weight. If it says only, "No breathing, started CPR," the attorney will suggest to the jury that the OPA was never inserted.

---

## Good Documentation Is Good Patient Care

As an EMT, you are often the first medical provider to interact with a patient. Thus your observations may be critical in the patient's course of treatment. The physician who ultimately becomes responsible for a patient's care will have been far removed from the initial point of care. The PCR may be the only way the physician can picture the situation that brought the patient to her care. Consider the following scenario:

You arrive on the scene of a "man down" call. The patient is a 40-year-old male who is actively seizing, with his hands clenched and rotated inward. As you reach the patient's side, the seizure subsides, and his hands relax to a normal position; he is now unconscious. There is no indication of trauma, so you perform an initial assessment that is unremarkable. The bystanders are not aware of any medical history. You transport to the nearest emergency department. While en route, the patient begins to regain consciousness but is confused and disoriented. His vitals remain stable, and he becomes more lucid as you discharge him to the emergency department.

By the time the physician sees this patient, he may have completely returned to normal, with no memory of the events that brought him to the hospital. The physician would thus lack information about the patient's seizure and the important detail of decorticate posturing (with hands clenched and rotated inward), a possible indication of brain injury. The EMT's PCR is crucial to the patient's treatment in this case.

## Run Report or "Charting"

The run report will contain the following information:

- Current date
- Patient's name, address, phone number
- Gender
- Date of birth and possibly social security/insurance number (not required by all services)
- Medical history
- Current medications and known allergies
- Narrative of events and treatment
  - Gives the story of the encounter and paints a picture that will allow the reader to visualize what you saw and experienced
  - Provides the context for why you took the actions you did in treating and transporting the patient
  - Includes any findings made during the patient assessments, including baseline vital signs
  - States clearly and definitively the chief complaint
  - Includes specific patient comments on scene, such as, "I had too much to drink," which should be put in quotation marks
  - May include some abbreviations as governed by local medical usage
- Patient's and provider's signatures

---

The run report is a confidential medical document. **Completed run reports must be secured** and not be left out where they can be read by anyone nearby. If a run report is used for training or educational purposes, you must remove any information that could identify the patient.

---

Since the PCR is a legal document, it should state only the actual facts of a call as the EMT records them. False statements on the run report—including omissions of protocol steps—should never be made and could have several serious consequences:

- Could place you in danger of losing your license or certification to practice
- Could open the service (and potentially you) to increased legal liability, including possible criminal charges
- Could cause the patient to be given inappropriate follow-up care at the receiving facility, with possible adverse effects

If any error is made on the paper PCR, it must be corrected, noted, and signed. A correction is usually marked by placing a horizontal line through the incorrect information, neatly adding the correct information, and noting the date and time of the correction with the initials of the report writer.

If utilizing an ePCR format, information may be deleted and rewritten just as you would on a computer, as long as the run report is still in progress. If the run report has been closed for editing and submitted and the EMT then realizes that a mistake has been made or information has been left out, an addendum may be written with the correct information and attached to the chart. Alternatively, a supervisor may have to "reopen" the chart for the errors to be fixed.

Patient refusal issues are increasingly problematic to EMS, so the documentation of refusals must be especially thorough. Proceed as follows:

- An adult patient of sound mind can refuse medical treatment or transport. If you believe that a specific treatment or hospital transport is appropriate, you must explain the rationale to the patient; if the patient continues to refuse, you must document both your explanation and the patient's refusal.
- Your documentation should include a note that the patient was informed of the potential consequence of not following the EMT's recommendations.
- Once the documentation is complete, have the patient sign the refusal, witnessed by an impartial third party (ideally a police officer if one is on scene).
- If the patient refuses to sign the release, ask an impartial third party to witness that you explained the procedures and consequences.

In addition to the PCR, you must also be familiar with the written documents in use by your service. These include injury reports for EMS personnel in the line of duty, auto accident reports for incidents involving the EMS vehicle, infectious disease exposure reports, and police witness statements (if you have witnessed a criminal act or are the victim of a crime). Any of these reports should be attached to the PCR for the incident during which they occurred as well as placed in the appropriate personnel and service files.

Many states and services require submission of the run report (whether paper or electronic) within 24 hours of the completed call. Some services require submission of the chart before the EMT can be made available to take the next 911 call. Keep this in mind for time management purposes. Delayed chart completion can leave the EMT out of service when a serious call comes in. If the EMT is not able to respond, patient care is delayed.

**TEST YOURSELF 4.3**

**Can this patient refuse care?**

You are dispatched to an unknown medical call and told that the caller (bystander) has stated the patient is "confused." Upon arrival, you find a 32-year-old male who is stumbling around the living room of the dwelling and slurring his words; however, he is cooperative when asked to take a seat. BP is 128/72 mm Hg, respiratory rate is 14/min, and pulse rate is 92. Blood sugar level is 68 mg/dL. He states that he does not want to go to the hospital. He is able to answer your questions but at a slower rate than normal. His friend states he has diabetes.

After oral glucose administration, the patient's blood sugar rises to 76. He still slurs his words, but he is becoming more clear. He still does not want to go to the hospital. Does the patient have the right to refuse care at this point?

# Practice Set

1.  Which of the following are part of the primary survey? Select the 2 answer options that are correct.

    A.  Asking about prescribed medications

    B.  History of present illness

    C.  Determine alertness level (LOC)

    D.  Determine scene safety

    E.  Detailed physical exam

    F.  Assess airway and breathing

2.  You respond to a fight in progress. The police advise the scene is secure, and you are wearing suitable protective equipment. Your patient is a male, thirtyish, seated on the steps of a residence, bent over, and clutching his chest. He is making noisy respiratory sounds and groaning in pain. You can smell the odor of alcohol. You check his carotid pulse and find that it is strong, with a rate of 80. There are no signs of gross hemorrhage. Your next step is to perform which of the following assessments?

    A.  Focused medical assessment

    B.  Focused trauma assessment

    C.  Initial assessment

    D.  Medical insurance assessment

3.  You are dispatched to a motorcycle accident on the freeway. You respond emergently and arrive on scene. You observe 3 police cars on scene, a destroyed motorcycle lying on its side, and a man lying supine next to the motorcycle with a large piece of the front fork of the motorcycle sticking out of his abdomen. The scene is safe, and you are wearing suitable protection. You approach the patient. Which of the following is the next thing you do?

    A.  Check his airway.

    B.  Stabilize the large piece of metal with cravats and bandages.

    C.  Request a physician to the scene to perform a surgical removal.

    D.  Transfer the patient to a backboard and transport immediately.

4.  You arrive on scene to find a patient lying supine on the ground, eyes closed. As you approach the patient, you can hear her breathing and observe her chest rising and falling. The scene is secure, and you are wearing appropriate protective equipment. The patient's eyes are closed, and you shake her shoulder and ask her name. There is no response. You shout, "Are you all right?" and the patient opens her eyes and groans. You ask her what happened, and she does not appear to understand at all. You rub her sternum, and she yells, "Ow!" Which of the following best describes this patient's level of consciousness?

    A.  Conscious and alert

    B.  Responsive to pain

    C.  Responsive to verbal

    D.  Unresponsive

5. You are writing your BLS patient chart for a call that you just completed of a 16-year-old male with a hypoglycemic diabetic emergency. Which of the following components should NOT be included in the chart? Select the 2 answer options that should not be included.

   A. Patient's full name

   B. The paramedic's interpretation of the EKG, told directly to you after arriving on scene

   C. Patient's date of birth

   D. 2 sets of vital signs taken at 15 minute intervals

   E. Your impression that the patient was high on marijuana despite his denial of any illicit drugs

   F. Patient's parent's or guardian's name and phone number, as they are next of kin

6. Which of the following patients would be given a priority transport?

   A. 20-year-old female in second-stage labor of a first birth

   B. 18-year-old male with a suspected radius fracture from a fall during a soccer game

   C. 12-year-old female with difficulty breathing and a history of asthma

   D. 2-year-old male who fell out of his crib and is crying loudly

7. Which of the following patients would be given a priority transport?

   A. Male patient conscious and alert with a blood pressure of 210/110 mm Hg

   B. Female patient in labor with respiratory rate of 20/minute

   C. Male patient with a pulse rate of 110/minute

   D. Female patient with a pulse rate of 20/minute

8. Immediately following a rapid physical exam on an unresponsive medical patient, which of the following should you do next?

   A. Find out when the patient last saw a doctor.

   B. Check the scene for any medications.

   C. Perform a focused physical exam.

   D. Obtain baseline vital signs.

9. Which of the following conditions noted during the focused trauma assessment would indicate immediate transport?

   A. Unconscious

   B. Low blood sugar

   C. Tracheal shift to the right

   D. Pedestrian struck by a car

10. You are dispatched for a bicyclist struck by a car. On your arrival, your patient is lying supine on the ground, motionless. You approach your patient from the feet, take manual stabilization of the head, and check the airway. The patient is breathing, and you can palpate a carotid pulse, which appears rapid. You ask in a loud voice, "Are you OK?" and get no response. Your partner rubs the patient's sternum with her thumb, and your patient opens his eyes, groans, and moves his hand to his chest to push your partner's hand away. There is a large bruise with swelling on the right side of his head and no other apparent injuries. The patient's vital signs are BP 160/100 mm Hg, pulse 60/min, and respirations 15/min. What would be his Revised Trauma Score?

    A. 8

    B. 9

    C. 10

    D. 11

11. You arrive on the scene of a motor vehicle accident. Your patient is a 25-year-old female who was ejected from her vehicle when it struck a telephone pole. The car is totally demolished. Your initial assessment is that your patient is unconscious and unresponsive. Due to the mechanism of action and patient ejection, you determine that this is a "load and go," immobilize your patient, and begin transport. As you do your focused trauma assessment, you notice that the patient's left upper quadrant is now rigid, whereas in the initial assessment it appeared normal. What should be your next action?

    A. Nothing; continue with the assessment and see what else comes up injury wise.

    B. Place a non-rebreather mask at 6 liters per minute onto the patient's face.

    C. Request your driver to expedite as you suspect your patient has an intra-abdominal bleed.

    D. Perform a modified jaw thrust to open the airway.

12. You are dispatched to a report of an intoxicated female. The scene is secure, and you are wearing suitable precautions. You arrive on scene and find a female in her forties lying supine, unconscious, and responsive (groans) to painful stimuli. You detect an odor of alcohol, and her friend confirms that she has been drinking vodka shots heavily all evening. There is no indication of trauma, and your initial assessment is unremarkable. You place the patient into the truck, administer 10 liters per minute oxygen via non-rebreather mask, and begin priority transport to the nearest emergency department 15 minutes away. You notify the hospital of the patient's condition and vital signs. After disconnecting from the hospital, you begin to reassess your patient and now notice that she is not breathing. Which of these is your next step?

    A. Advise the driver to expedite transport to the hospital.

    B. Insert an oropharyngeal airway and ventilate at 10–12 times per minute.

    C. Continue the assessment to try and discover any other conditions.

    D. Retake pulse, respiratory rate, and blood pressure.

13. The patient tells you that his symptoms started 20 minutes ago. What letter is this represented by in the mnemonic OPQRST?

    A. Onset

    B. Present event

    C. Situation

    D. Time

14. What do the letters B and P stand for in the mnemonic DCAP-BTLS?

    A. Burn, puncture

    B. Bruise, pain

    C. Bruise, penetration

    D. Burn, pain

15. You are dispatched to a call for a 34-year-old fall victim. Upon arrival at the scene, you note a strong odor of alcohol on the patient's breath and see multiple beer bottles on the table near where he is sitting. His girlfriend, who called 911, states that he had been drinking when he tripped on the rug and fell onto the table, striking his head. She says that he did not lose consciousness, and you do not see any major bleeding from the patient's head. The patient is slurring his words as he tells you he does not want to be transported to the hospital, "I'm fine. She shouldn't have called." What is your next step?

    A. Get your partner to take a baseline set of vitals. If all of the patient's vital signs are in the normal range, have the patient sign a refusal; then leave the scene.

    B. Call for police backup. You may have to take the patient to your ambulance forcibly.

    C. Explain that the patient cannot refuse at this time due to his level of inebriation and the blow to his head, and it is in his best interest to be evaluated at the hospital.

    D. Confirm that the girlfriend will remain there caring for the patient, have the girlfriend sign the refusal form, and leave the scene.

16. When the patient is a competent adult who is conscious, alert, and oriented times 4, who should sign the refusal form?

    A. The patient only

    B. The patient and an impartial third party who is present

    C. The patient and the patient's spouse, who is the family member that is present

    D. The patient and the patient's 17-year-old, who is the family member that is present

17. Falsification of a run report can result in which of the following?

    A. Nothing, as long as it was never submitted in the first place

    B. Arrest of the EMT and jail time up to 7 years

    C. Incorrect care of the patient at the hospital

    D. Possible legal action, loss of right to practice as an EMT, and possible damage to the patient with follow-up care

18. You arrive on the scene of a one-car motor vehicle accident. The car left the lane of travel and struck the soft shoulder, where it appears to have rolled over at least once. The driver is a female, approximate age 40, who is conscious, alert, and oriented times 4. Your partner applies head stabilization from the backseat while you conduct the assessment. The patient states that she's fine and just wants a ride to the hospital. The windshield is cracked and the patient, who is not wearing a seat belt, has a bruise on her forehead. You explain that you want to apply a cervical collar to protect her spine and then use a Kendrick Extrication Device (KED) to remove her from the vehicle. The patient becomes agitated. "All I wants is a ride to the hospital. I don't want you to do anything else!" she announces, and she begins to get out of the car. Which of the following actions is MOST appropriate to take next?

    A. Let the patient walk herself to the truck, and transport her to the hospital.

    B. Caution the patient that unless she permits you to take these precautions now, the police will place her in protective custody, and then you will be able to do whatever you want.

    C. Explain the risks of spinal injury unless you take these precautions now. If the patient still refuses, document your explanation and her refusal in the narrative, and have her sign it in the presence of the police.

    D. Disregard the patient's protests, and apply the cervical collar and KED.

19. You respond emergently to a call to the police station for a male with chest pains. You arrive on scene with appropriate BSI precautions and find a male in his forties seated in a chair clutching his chest, in obvious distress. He is pale, diaphoretic, and having difficulty breathing. There is no indication of trauma. The patient is not in police custody but is the victim of a crime. He states that he's fine and refuses all treatment and transport options. Which of the following actions is MOST appropriate to take next?

    A. Explain the consequences of his refusal, enlist a police officer to serve as witness, and have the patient sign the refusal form.

    B. Disregard his objections, administer oxygen via non-rebreather, and transport priority to the nearest hospital emergency department.

    C. Patiently explain the seriousness of his condition, and continue to encourage the patient to allow you to treat him and transport him to the hospital.

    D. When his eyes are closed, administer 0.4 mg nitroglycerin sublingual (1 tablet) to the patient as your service's protocols permit EMTs to give this treatment.

20. Your patient is an unresponsive adult female patient lying on her bed. There is an empty pill bottle lying next to the bed, and when you look up the medication, you discover it is a powerful sedative. The prescription on the bottle is for the patient's husband, who is not present to answer questions about the medication. What should you do next and why?

    A. Document the empty pill bottle. It may provide important clues to the patient's current condition.

    B. Document the empty pill bottle. It is obvious that the patient took the pills.

    C. Do not document the pill bottle. You cannot prove that the patient took the pills.

    D. Do not document the empty pill bottle. It doesn't belong to the patient.

THIS PAGE INTENTIONALLY LEFT BLANK

## Answer Key

| | | | | | | | | | |
|---|---|---|---|---|---|---|---|---|---|
| 1. | **C, F** | 5. | **B, E** | 9. | **C** | 13. | **A** | 17. | **D** |
| 2. | **C** | 6. | **C** | 10. | **D** | 14. | **A** | 18. | **C** |
| 3. | **A** | 7. | **D** | 11. | **C** | 15. | **C** | 19. | **C** |
| 4. | **C** | 8. | **D** | 12. | **B** | 16. | **B** | 20. | **A** |

## Answers and Explanations

### 1. C, F

Determining alertness level (C) and assessing airway and breathing (F) are parts of the primary survey. Both deal with threats to life and determine whether the patient is able to participate in the interview phase of a call. While scene safety (D) is always important, it is part of the scene size-up, not the primary survey. Medications (A), history of present illness (B), and the physical exam (E) are all in the secondary phase of assessment.

### 2. C

The temptation is to answer (B), as this is probably a trauma, but taking shortcuts compromises the EMT's ability to make the correct determinations. An initial assessment covers the ABCs first, regardless of how the potential injury or illness happened. The noisy respirations are a cause for concern and need to be addressed before a more focused assessment and head-to-toe exam are done.

### 3. A

Even though this is a "load and go" situation due to the magnitude of the patient's injuries, a patient without an airway will arrive at the ER dead. If the patient has a patent airway, is breathing, and has a pulse, then stabilize the metal (B) and prepare for immediate transport. Requesting a physician to the scene (C) would take too much time and would further endanger the patient. The metal can be removed best in an operating room.

### 4. C

When assessing for level of responsiveness, we take the best and highest level of response the patient has. Here, the patient did not respond to normal stimuli, so she is not conscious and alert (A). The next level is verbal (C), and this is where the patient responded by opening her eyes and groaning when you shouted her name. While she also responded to pain (B), the higher level (verbal) applies, because she did initially respond to your shouting. She responded to both verbal and pain stimuli, so she is not considered unresponsive (D).

### 5. B, E

Good documentation is good patient care. We must include factual statements in our charts, such as the patient's full name and date of birth. In this case, we would also include the parent's or guardian's information, as the patient is under the age of 18 and cannot legally give consent in most cases. The prehospital or in-hospital health care providers must attempt contact until they reach the parent or guardian. Opinions must be left out of the chart unless they are relevant to the call itself and you can provide follow-up information to justify your opinion; thus you would leave your suspicion of marijuana use (E) out of the chart unless, for example, you found marijuana near the patient. EKG interpretation is done by a higher level of care, so you would not include the paramedic's EKG interpretation (B), which the paramedic will include in their own patient chart. Out of the choices given here, this answer is one of the 2 best choices needed.

**6.  C**

While all the choices are possibilities if secondary assessment finds something significant or conditions change, the patient with difficulty breathing needs to be expedited. The ABCs must always be addressed first.

**7.  D**

A patient with a pulse of 20/min will present with symptoms of low perfusion, including pale skin and diminished level of consciousness. The other vital signs may be out of normal range but in the absence of a life-threatening condition would be considered a nonpriority transport.

**8.  D**

We need a baseline set of vitals (D) to begin the trending process and see if the patient is getting better or worse with any treatment that we give. Although the date of the patient's last doctor visit (A) could be useful for your patient chart and report, it is not the best answer for this scenario. Checking for medications (B) is a good option if baseline vitals can't be taken and is still a good idea with an unconscious patient, but there is a more correct answer listed. If you have ruled out anything in a rapid physical exam and if the patient were conscious, a focused physical exam (C) would be appropriate. In this scenario, however, the patient is unconscious and you need to know if resuscitation is needed.

**9.  C**

Tracheal shift to either side is indicative of a tension pneumothorax, which is a collapsed lung that is pushing against other organs and may lead to other organ failure or damage. It can be relieved only by placement of a chest tube, which is beyond the EMT scope of practice. Unconsciousness (A) is a condition that should have been found in the initial assessment and by itself does not indicate immediate transport. Neither does low blood sugar (B), which can be treated by the EMT in the field in some services or by calling for an ALS assist. A pedestrian struck by a car (D) has a high incidence of suspicion due to the nature of the injury but, again, by itself does not indicate an immediate transport.

**10.  D**

The first thing you must calculate is the Glasgow Coma Scale (GCS) score. The patient's eyes open to pain (2 points), his words are incomprehensible (2 points), and he localizes pain (5 points). So total GCS is 9, making the Revised Trauma Score (RTS) index a 3. In calculating the RTS, this patient gets 4 points for respiratory rate between 10 and 29, 4 points for systolic blood pressure >89 mm Hg, and 3 for the GCS. This gives the patient a Revised Trauma Score of 11. Use care in calculating mathematical questions like this one since one of your choices is 9, which is the GCS. It's always a good idea to run calculations twice to be sure.

**11.  C**

While you suspected a serious injury before, the development of a rigid left upper quadrant is fairly indicative of a ruptured spleen, which will result in the patient's bleeding intra-abdominally. The only treatment for this condition is removal of the spleen in an operating room. Doing nothing (A) is inappropriate; you must recognize this as an injury that will benefit the most by getting the patient to a hospital sooner rather than later. Your goal is getting this patient to an operating room as soon as possible. Oxygen at 6 liters per minute is not the appropriate liters per minute rate to be used with a non-rebreather mask (B). Jaw thrust (D) should have already been done on the scene, not at this time.

**12.  B**

A patient needs oxygen to live, and if she is not breathing, she will die. You must first secure the airway and then ventilate the patient (B). Once this is done, you can advise the driver to expedite (A). Continuing the assessment (C) and retaking vital signs (D) can be undertaken only if you have another EMT in the back of the truck. If you are alone, your concern must be for the patient's airway and respirations.

**13. A**

The correct answer is onset (A). Onset is when the symptoms started, whereas time (D) is how long the symptoms have been occurring or whether the patient has experienced this type of symptom before. Situation (C) appears as part of the SAMPLE questions in the events leading up to situation, and present event (B) is not part of either mnemonic.

**14. A**

The correct answer is (A). While P stands for either puncture or penetration, none of the other choices gives the correct answer in its entirety.

**15. C**

The correct answer is (C). Under the circumstances, due to the patient's level of intoxication (evidenced by the strong odor of alcohol on his breath, slurred words, and the scene survey of multiple empty beer bottles next to him) and the head strike, this patient is considered not competent to make a decision about his transport. Having the patient sign a refusal at this point (A) would put you in a precarious position if this chart ever went to court. An EMT in this situation may need to request police assistance (B). Before resorting to this, however, you should try to state your position calmly and persuade the patient yourself, unless you feel unsafe at any time or doing so is outside your protocols. Leaving this patient in his home, even in the care of the girlfriend (D), could lead to further complications such as a head bleed or even death.

**16. B**

The correct answer is (B) because it is the most legally protective. The third party is impartial, whereas a family member may not be impartial. Note, however, that some systems may allow the patient's spouse (C) to witness as a last resort if there is no other suitable option. The 17-year-old child of the patient (D) is unable to sign due to being underage.

**17. D**

The EMT should never falsify the run report for any reason at any time. If an honest mistake is made in charting, whether it is electronic or written, the proper correction method must be used. Failing to submit the run report (A) is a bad mind frame to get into in the long run. The EMT is not always arrested and jailed (B). Incorrect hospital care (C) is one of the possible consequences, but (D) provides the most thorough answer of all the choices given.

**18. C**

Explaining and documenting the risks of refusal (C) is the appropriate course of action here. If this patient walks herself to the truck (A) before you have explained and documented the treatment options, you may become liable for injuries. Unless the police have probable cause for doing so, they will not place a person in protective custody (B). Proceeding with the cervical collar and KEC despite the patient's protests (D) may be considered assault and battery.

**19. C**

The potential seriousness of the situation really requires you to stand by as long as possible. (A) is legally correct, but if the patient's condition changes as soon as you drive out of the parking lot, a jury might consider it abandonment. (B) is assault and battery, and possibly kidnapping. (D) is also assault since you do not have the patient's permission to give treatment, even if it is allowed by your protocols.

**20. A**

Clues in the scene, especially if there are no bystanders, can be vital in how or why our patient is in her current condition. In this case, the pill bottle found next to your patient is a clear clue as to why she may be unconscious, so you should document it (A). Although the prescription doesn't belong to the patient (D) and you can't prove that she took the pills (C), you should document the empty pill bottle. Though answer (B) is similar, if you pay careful attention to the wording, you will realize that it includes an opinion, "It is obvious that the patient took the pills." Even if you strongly suspect the patient took the pills, you did not witness this.

# RESPIRATORY EMERGENCIES AND AIRWAY MANAGEMENT

**LEARNING OBJECTIVES**
- Understand how respiratory emergencies happen
- Identify the signs and symptoms of a respiratory emergency
- Identify breath sounds and interpret what they mean
- Describe the steps to take to open the airway
- Identify different airway adjuncts and when they would be used
- Describe diseases that contribute to respiratory emergencies
- Understand artificial ventilation techniques and equipment
- Understand the function and use of oxygen delivery systems

In order to live and breathe, every patient needs an airway—that is, a pathway for oxygen to travel from the outside environment to the alveoli of the lungs, where it can enter the bloodstream to be used in the metabolic process. If any part of this pathway is interrupted, whether by a disease process or trauma to its structures, a person has great difficulty breathing, if they can breathe at all. The EMT must be able to recognize when a respiratory emergency is happening and take decisive, quick steps to remedy the situation—or else they will soon have a deceased patient on their hands.

## How Respiratory Emergencies Happen

In a healthy person, normal airflow is a continuous cycle of oxygenated air that is brought in through the oropharynx and nasopharynx and introduced into the lungs by the acts of respiration and ventilation.

Remember that **respiration** is the act of gas exchange of oxygen and carbon dioxide that happens at the capillary level. This is different from the act of **ventilation**, which is simply the movement of air in and out of something, such as the human body, either under its own power or through artificial means such as a bag-valve-mask device.

When there is an interruption of the airflow or gas exchange at any level of the respiratory system, the body will become distressed. The brain's respiratory centers, located in the brainstem, will recognize a problem and trigger the body to either speed up or slow down the person's breathing pattern in response. But circumstances can overwhelm the body's ability to compensate for respiratory distress. When the burden becomes too great for the person to handle on their own, emergency services are called. In fact, respiratory distress is one of the most common EMS calls you will receive.

The EMT must not only be able to recognize the different levels of respiratory distress but also have a strong understanding of *why* the emergency is happening to enable swift steps toward reversing it.

The different levels of respiratory emergencies are distress, failure, and arrest.

## Respiratory Distress

In respiratory distress, the person is experiencing **tachypnea** (fast breathing), is experiencing **bradypnea** (slow breathing), or has an obstruction of some sort. In this level of respiratory emergency, your quick actions can prevent the problem from progressing to something worse. You may see the following signs of respiratory distress:

- Patient is in a tripod position or propped up with pillows to facilitate breathing (because breathing is more difficult while lying supine)
- Has difficulty speaking in full sentences
- Lowered pulse oximeter ($SpO_2$) reading
- Skin color changes
- Delayed capillary refill time (takes >2 seconds to return to normal)
- Is becoming or already is very anxious as a result of **hypoxia** (low levels of blood oxygen)

## Respiratory Failure

In respiratory failure, either too little oxygen passes from the lungs into the bloodstream or the lungs can't properly remove carbon dioxide. In either case, there is too much carbon dioxide in the blood, which can harm the body's organs:

- Patients in acute respiratory failure need ventilatory support or else they will quickly progress into respiratory arrest.
- Patients with chronic respiratory failure are often being treated with home oxygen and/or taking medications prescribed to manage this condition. These patients have a baseline lower level of oxygen saturation.
- People experiencing either acute or chronic respiratory failure may display "pursed-lip breathing," inhaling through the nose and exhaling through puckered lips (as if they are trying to kiss someone). Pursed-lip breathing helps create pressure that keeps the airways open, and a person may do it consciously or subconsciously.

## Respiratory Arrest

In respiratory arrest, the body has ceased to breathe properly on its own. People in respiratory arrest absolutely need artificial ventilatory support done by the EMT. In this final stage of respiratory emergency, the heart will soon stop beating if respiratory function is not restored immediately:

- Color changes in the skin will range from gray to blue to white.
- Be prepared to perform CPR if necessary.

With these warning signs of the various levels of respiratory emergencies in mind, let's review how to do a proper assessment.

## Respiratory Assessment

To assess respiratory function properly, observe and note the following signs and symptoms:

- Observe the rise and fall of the chest as the patient breathes.
- Look for accessory muscle usage, particularly in the neck and intercostal spaces.
- Check body positioning, i.e., is the patient tripoding or propped up?
- Check for adequate volume, i.e., is the patient breathing deeply or taking shallow breaths?
- Listen for any speech, i.e., is the patient speaking in full sentences without difficulty or are breaths required between words?
- Measure the oxygen saturation ($SpO_2$) level using a pulse oximeter.
- Auscultate (listen by stethoscope) the lungs.

When a patient presents with respiratory difficulty, *always check the airway first* to see if there is an obstruction.

To use time efficiently, you may place the pulse oximeter onto the patient's finger and let it begin to calculate while you attempt to listen to lung sounds. Remember that if a patient is able to speak to you in full sentences without distress, they most likely have an open airway.

Three steps on this list require further clarification: checking for breath sounds, measuring oxygen saturation, and checking for an open airway.

## Checking for Breath Sounds

Textbooks differ on the best locations to listen for breath sounds. Since there are 5 lung lobes, or sections—3 on the right and 2 on the left—a comprehensive assessment should include them all. The best way to do so is to locate the following 6 anatomical landmarks and place a stethoscope on each of them:

- Left chest, proximal to the clavicle at the midclavicular line—listen for the breath sound, which should be the sound of air flowing in and out without obstruction
- Right chest, proximal to the clavicle at the midclavicular line—always listen to one side and then the other (bilateral auscultation) to compare the sounds in opposite fields
- Left lateral chest on the midaxillary line
- Right lateral chest on the midaxillary line
- Left back below the scapula, opposite the midclavicular line
- Right back below the scapula, opposite the midclavicular line

Abnormal (or adventitious) breath sounds can help the EMT understand not only why the patient is breathing a certain way but also how to proceed with treatment. You must be able to identify the breath sounds in the following table. If you are struggling to tell them apart, review the sounds in a multimedia library online until you can.

**Table 5.1** Abnormal Lung Sounds

| LUNG SOUND | DESCRIPTION OF SOUND | PATHOPHYSIOLOGICAL DETAILS |
|---|---|---|
| Crackles or rales | Rattling, crackling, clinking, or popping | • Described as "fine" or "coarse" to indicate degree of loudness<br>• Caused by fluid in the small airway passages or collapsed alveoli<br>• Can be heard on both inspiration and expiration<br>• Occur when the smaller airways open suddenly during inspiration |
| Wheezes | Squeaky, musical, or moan-like | • Potential causes include air moving through airways narrowed by constriction, swelling of the airway, partial airway obstruction, or excess secretions<br>• Can be heard on expiration in early stages, but on inspiration and expiration as the airways become more compromised<br>• Frequently heard in the bases of the lungs; be sure to identify the correct auscultation site |
| Rhonchi | Low-pitched, clunky, rattling, or snore-like | • Caused by obstruction or buildup of mucus in large airways<br>• Often cleared when the patient coughs |
| Stridor | High-pitched and whistle-like, like a seal barking | • Caused by obstruction or blockage of the upper airway, e.g., foreign object or inflammation of upper airway anatomical structures such as epiglottis<br>• Can be heard on inspiration<br>• Commonly associated with pediatric patients (e.g., in croup) but possible in patients of any age |
| Pleural friction rubs | Low-pitched grating or creaking, like the squeak of a leather couch when sat upon | • Caused by inflamed pleural lung surfaces rubbing together during respiration<br>• Can be heard on both inspiration and expiration<br>• Often very painful due to inflamed tissue, producing shallow breathing and consequently inadequate tidal volume or lowered pulse oximetry in the patient |

Once you understand how to conduct a respiratory assessment, you need to know the signs and symptoms of adequate (and inadequate) breathing. The 4 criteria for this are rate, rhythm, quality, and tidal volume:

- **Rate** is counted as the number of breaths per minute. What constitutes a "normal" adult respiratory rate is subject to debate. Some textbooks say 8–24, others 12–20. We recommend splitting the difference for your rule of thumb: regard rates >22 as tachypnea and <9 as bradypnea.

- **Rhythm** is determined by noting the times of inspiration, exhalation, and pause between. They should be equal in each cycle.
- **Quality** is determined by use of the accessory muscles. If the patient is utilizing the accessory muscles of the intercostal spaces and neck in order to breathe, or is having some type of difficulty, this must be noted.
- **Tidal volume** (or depth of ventilation) must be sufficient for the person to speak normally, and the chest should rise and fall with each breath cycle.

If everything appears to be within a normal range (does not raise any red flags), you can then move to assessing the next part of the body. However, if the airway is not **patent** (open), the patient is in distress, or they require ventilatory assistance, the EMT must continuing exploring WHY and fix problems here before moving on with the assessment.

## Measuring Oxygen Saturation

To measure oxygen saturation, the EMT uses a pulse oximeter, which is a noninvasive tool that measures the amount of oxygen being carried in the body. This device helps determine the patient's need for oxygen and how best to deliver it:

- Oximeter types include handheld monitor, separate corded unit on a cardiac monitor, and fingertip-only unit with a built-in screen.
- The device sends 2 wavelengths of light through the finger to measure both the pulse rate and the amount of oxygen in the body system.
- Once the oximeter finishes its assessment, the screen displays the percentage of oxygen.

Generally, oxygen saturation for a healthy patient should be 94–100%. Anything <94% oxygen saturation should be explored and potentially corrected, but keep in mind that certain patients live with a baseline of lowered saturation rates. Be sure to do a full assessment and ask good questions.

---

Be careful to monitor the patient and not just the pulse oximeter. Check whether the patient is wearing nail polish, the patient's hands are cold, the batteries are charged, the reader is properly placed on the finger, or (if you do not have a dual reader) the person had carbon monoxide exposure. Any of these situations can skew a true oximeter reading.

If the patient is not presenting with any respiratory distress, take the whole picture into account. Treat the patient, not the equipment.

---

## Checking for an Open Airway

With an occluded (or blocked) airway, the EMT's first order of business is to open it to enable the patient to breathe. Assuming you have deemed a scenario safe and are wearing the proper protective equipment, do the following:

1. Approach the patient (usually from the feet if the patient is lying down), and scan the area for anything that may indicate a change in scene status or that may have caused the emergency to which you are responding.

2. If there is no response, kneel at the patient's head and hold the cervical spine in place. Bend down over the patient's nose and mouth to see if you can hear breathing sounds or feel exhalations on your cheek. Watch the patient's chest to see if there is any breathing motion.

3. If these signs are negative, your next move must be to open the patient's airway.

Opening the patient's airway is a lifesaving maneuver. It involves you being able to diagnose an occluded airway and then using both gloved hands to open and clear the oropharynx to let air into the trachea.

### Trauma Considerations

If you suspect a traumatic event, the most important concerns are to stabilize the neck and provide an open airway for breathing. Using the jaw-thrust maneuver is the most appropriate way to minimize cervical movement while achieving an open airway.

**Figure 5.1** Jaw-Thrust Maneuver

Be aware that you may need another EMT to complete the rest of the body assessment while you continue to secure the airway. Be sure spinal precautions have been properly taken and a properly sized cervical collar (C-collar) has been secured to the patient.

The purpose of the jaw-thrust maneuver is to minimize cervical spine movement by stabilizing the neck and to provide an open airway for breathing. Any other problems noted at this time should be addressed later. Proceed as follows:

- Hold the patient's head, placing your ring and little fingers underneath and your thumbs alongside the head.

- Place the first and middle fingers of both your hands beneath the jawbone (mandible) and push upward. This action will lift not only the mandible but also the tongue—which is attached to the structures of the mouth—by pulling the tongue away from the posterior larynx.

- Look into the mouth for anything physically blocking it (if there is, have your partner remove it), and begin artificial respirations if spontaneous respirations do not begin.

### Nontrauma Considerations

If you have ruled out or do not suspect a trauma scenario, the actions are essentially the same except that the airway can be opened by using the head-tilt, chin-lift method.

**Figure 5.2** Head-Tilt, Chin-Lift Maneuver

To perform the head-tilt, chin-lift maneuver, do the following:

- Lift the chin using the first and middle fingers of one hand, and with the other hand push the forehead back. This will move the tongue away from the posterior larynx.

- Maintain this position by placing a rolled towel/blanket underneath the patient's shoulders, which will allow you to have your hands free.

- If the airway is blocked by solids, clear it by removing the object (assuming it can be seen) with forceps. If the person is unresponsive or was known to be choking prior to becoming unresponsive, you may also elect to do chest compressions to try and relieve the unseen object, as per the most recent AHA guidelines.

- If the airway is blocked by fluids (such as vomit), suctioning may be indicated.

### Suctioning the Airway

If the EMT determines that there is a solid or fluid obstructing the airway, suction may be indicated. If so, it should be used in the patient early to avoid **aspiration**, or the movement of fluids or solids into the trachea or lungs.

Suction units come in both handheld nonelectric and electric/battery-powered models. Most EMS units carry both. It is up to you to know where your equipment is and how it works prior to going on your first call of the shift.

---

Lack of a working suction unit in the field could have devastating consequences for your patient. **Check your equipment** at the beginning of every shift.

---

There are 2 types of suction catheter: hard tip (or Yankauer) and soft, flexible tip:

- **Hard-tipped suction catheter** (Yankauer) is designed to allow effective suction without damaging surrounding tissue:
  - Firm plastic with large opening at the end, surrounded by bulbous head
  - Appropriate for most scenarios, except for cases of clenched teeth or where the EMT cannot fit the suction tip into the orifice to be suctioned (e.g., tracheostomy or nostrils)

- **Soft-tipped suction catheter** is more flexible; it comes in various sizes that can be inserted via the mouth, nose, or tracheostomy port:

  - Latex-free material, flexible, with a small diameter
  - Appropriate for more challenging scenarios (e.g., clenched teeth)

No matter the type of catheter you use, the steps for **suctioning the mouth** remain the same:

1. Make sure proper PPE is on (this includes gloves and protective glasses in case of splatter of bodily fluids). Aprons should also be made available.

2. Open the airway using the proper technique (trauma vs. nontrauma), and visualize the airway to see if suctioning is needed.

3. Select the proper suction catheter, and attach it to the suction tubing that is on a working suction unit.

4. Turn on the unit if indicated. (Hand-powered models do not have a power button and rely on manual squeezing of the bulb.)

5. Place the suction catheter tip into the patient's mouth no farther than the base of the tongue.

6. Place your finger over the designated vent hole on the suction catheter to create the vacuum seal.

7. Suction for no more than 10–15 seconds, backing the catheter OUT of the mouth and using a back-and-forth motion to reach all corners of the mouth.

8. Remove the catheter from the mouth, and clear the tip by suctioning up a small amount of water to flush the catheter.

9. Repeat the steps above as necessary to clear the oropharynx.

---

**Never suction for more than 10–15 seconds** at a time since suctioning removes oxygen from the oropharynx.

---

**Suctioning a tracheostomy tube** is similar; however, a soft-tipped catheter tip is more appropriately sized for the opening of the tube:

- Insert the suction catheter into the tracheostomy until you feel resistance, and then draw it back about 1/2 inch.

- Suction no more than 10–15 seconds at a time, as suctioning removes not only airway obstructions but also oxygen from the patient's system.

**Suctioning the nasopharynx** calls for use of a soft-tipped suction tip, which you must lubricate prior to insertion. The steps and cautions are like those in the previous methods but with these exceptions:

- If the patient is conscious, try to keep the patient at a 45° angle to facilitate the process of insertion.

- Once the tip is lubricated, advance the catheter tip until it induces a gag reflex in the patient or you meet resistance.

## Airway Adjuncts

There will be cases when you will need to insert an airway adjunct in order to maintain a patent airway and ensure proper oxygenation. Airway adjuncts come in both adult and pediatric sizes.

Note that this device is to be used only after the patient has a patent airway.

### Oropharyngeal Airway

An oropharyngeal airway (OPA) is a device hooked underneath the tongue that holds the tongue away from the posterior larynx. Various shapes and sizes are available:

- Measured for length by measuring from the tip of the ear to the corner of the mouth

- Inserted backward (rotated 90° or 180°) to the normal anatomical position and twisted into position

- Alternatively, inserted in anatomical position as a tongue depressor holds down the tongue while OPA is moved into position behind the tongue; if patient gags during insertion, withdraw immediately and use another method

**Figure 5.3** Measurement of an Oropharyngeal Airway (OPA)

### Nasopharyngeal Airway

A nasopharyngeal airway (NPA) holds the nasopharynx open and lifts the tongue with the use of a soft tube inserted into the nasopharynx through the nose:

- Can be used on patients with a gag reflex or whose teeth are clenched because of seizure or other medical condition

- Measured for length from the tip of the patient's nose to the tip of the ear

- Lubricated with sterile, water-soluble lubricant and inserted into the larger nostril with the bevel toward the septum using a back-and-forth twisting motion; once the flange of the NPA reaches the nostril, stop inserting and evaluate your patient

- Contraindicated in patients with facial trauma or possible skull fracture in whom there may be an opening that would allow the NPA to enter the cranial compartment

**Figure 5.4** Measurement of a Nasopharyngeal Airway (NPA)

---

**TEST YOURSELF 5.1**

**What airway tools would you use with this patient?**

Your patient is a 19-year-old female who was driving home after a party and smashed her car into a tree. She had been drinking heavily. Her friend, who was a passenger in the car, self-extricated and is now being assessed by your partner. Your patient says, "I think my nose is broken" and then coughs up some bright-red blood. She faints at the sight of the blood and collapses to the ground, hitting legs first. You immediately check for a pulse and find it present. You notice a large amount of blood leaking from the mouth and note her breathing rate to be at 10.

Which airway opening maneuver should you use and why? What type of suction tip would you use? What airway adjunct would you use?

---

# Respiratory Emergencies

The severity of respiratory emergencies can range from simple dyspnea to apnea (cessation of respiratory function). This section will discuss the more common respiratory diseases.

---

This is a good time to review the anatomy and physiology of the respiratory system, which is necessary to recognize and treat the various conditions that come under this heading.

---

## Dyspnea

One of the most common EMS dispatches is for difficulty breathing (dyspnea). The causes and manifestations of this broad-based condition include conditions such as asthma, bronchitis, and emphysema.

The signs and symptoms of dyspnea may include any of the following:

- Shortness of breath (SOB), restlessness, increased pulse rate, changes in respiratory rate (>20 or <12 breaths/min in adults)
- Changes in skin color (bluish gray, pale, or flushed)
- Noisy respirations (wheezing, gurgling, snoring, or stridor)
- Inability to speak
- Breathing that uses accessory muscles or the abdomen, or breathing that has an irregular rhythm
- Altered mental status
- Patient in tripod position (hunched forward with arms rotated outward) and barrel chest

### Emergency Care of Dyspnea

If the patient is conscious and able to answer, asking questions is appropriate at this time:

- Begin with the **OPQRST questions**: Onset, Provocation, Quality, Radiation, Severity, Time of onset
- Follow with the **SAMPLE questions**: Signs and symptoms, Allergies, Medications, Past history, Last oral intake, and Events leading to this condition

In addition, ask if the patient has an inhaler or other self-administered therapy. If so, ask whether the patient has used one of these interventions since the onset of the current symptoms and whether there was any resulting change in condition. If the patient is unconscious or unable to speak, a family member or other bystander may have to be the source for this information.

If the patient is unconscious, you must take swift steps to secure the airway and be ready to deliver artificial ventilations if necessary.

If the patient experiencing dyspnea is conscious, assess and treat as follows:

1. Take a set of baseline set of vitals, including pulse oximetry ($SpO_2$).
2. Based on patient presentation and $SpO_2$ readings, apply oxygen via the appropriate device in accordance with local protocols.
3. Auscultate the chest, noting normal or abnormal breath sounds.
4. If indicated and approved by local protocol, administer a breathing treatment or assist with a bronchodilator inhaler.
5. Consider calling for ALS assistance; call ALS if you believe the patient may need advanced care beyond your scope of practice.

6. Reassess the patient, and repeat vitals every 5–15 minutes as indicated by the patient's severity of distress.

7. Begin preparations for transport if indicated; keep in mind that a focused assessment may be done en route to the hospital.

---

If the patient has used an inhaler prior to the arrival of EMS, the number of times and amounts administered must be relayed to the medical control as the patient may have reached or exceeded the maximum dose for that particular medication.

---

Since most states allow EMTs to administer bronchodilators, you must be familiar with these medications and the methods by which they are administered. Most states will allow, with medical control, the assistance of the EMT in administering the patient's own prescribed inhaler.

Always make sure you follow the **5 Rights** before administering any medication:

1. Is this the right **patient**?

2. Is this the right **medication**?

3. Is this the right **dosage**?

4. Is this the right **route** of administration?

5. Is this the right **time** to administer the medication?

### Bronchodilator Inhalers

Medications such as albuterol (including brand names Ventolin and Proventil) are beta-agonist bronchodilators, which quickly and effectively dilate the bronchioles. This dilation reduces airway resistance and allows air to pass more easily and quickly into the alveoli of the lungs.

Bronchodilators are used only for patients experiencing dyspnea at the EMT level of care. The patient must already be prescribed an inhaler by their physician, as EMTs do not carry one in their drug box. Thus, if no inhaler is present with the patient, the EMT's only choice of medication is oxygen or continuous positive airway pressure (CPAP) if indicated. ALS may deliver medication through a nebulizer treatment. However, the EMT must weigh the option of traveling to a close hospital or waiting for ALS to arrive on scene if they were not previously called.

If medical control gives the order for administration of a handheld metered-dose inhaler (MDI), first verify the 5 Rights, and then administer as follows:

1. Shake the inhaler vigorously several times, and confirm that the inhaler is at room temperature.

2. Remove any oxygen adjuncts from the patient, such as a non-rebreather (NRB) mask on the face.

3. Ask the patient to exhale deeply.

4. Ask the patient to place the lips around the mouthpiece of the device and close them, creating a seal.

5. Depress the container as the patient inhales deeply.

6. Ask the patient to hold their breath for as long as possible to allow time for the medication to be absorbed into the tissues of the lungs.

7. Allow the patient to exhale when ready, and replace the oxygen adjunct if needed.

8. Reassess the patient.

A patient with a prescribed inhaler has usually received detailed instructions on its use and may not need all of these details.

Be aware of the possible side effects of these medications, including tachycardia, tremors, and increased anxiety. Be prepared to manage these if and when they occur.

Indications for administration of a prescribed inhaler **must include all of the following criteria**:

- Patient must be exhibiting signs and symptoms of a respiratory emergency
- Patient's physician must have prescribed the inhaler
- EMT must have authorization from medical control to administer the medication (unless EMT works in an area that allows administration without medical control permission)

If these conditions are not met, the use of the inhaler is contraindicated.

### Conditions That May Lead to Dyspnea

The EMT must be familiar with the various diseases and conditions that may lead to dyspnea. Common conditions include:

- Asthma
- Chronic obstructive pulmonary disease (COPD), which includes emphysema and chronic bronchitis
- Diabetic ketoacidosis
- Hyperventilation syndrome (can sometimes be psychological)
- Overdose (illicit drugs or otherwise)
- Pneumonia
- Pneumothorax (spontaneous, hemo [blood], or tension based)
- Pulmonary embolism
- Pulmonary edema (often secondary to congestive heart failure [CHF])
- COVID-19

Regardless of why the dyspnea is occurring, oxygen saturation must be monitored and corrected as necessary. If respiratory distress begins to progress into failure, more aggressive measures must be taken, such as insertion of an OPA/NPA or use of a bag-valve mask (BVM) or CPAP.

If BLS medications are indicated for the presenting conditions and no contraindications are present, deliver the medications and note whether or not improvement is gained. Be prepared for respiratory or cardiac arrest if they occur.

## Asthma and COPD

Both asthma and COPD can cause similar symptoms when aggravated: airway constriction, excess mucous production, and shortness of breath. However, they are two distinct disease processes:

- **Asthma** is a lifelong inflammatory condition. It is often diagnosed in early childhood but may not present until later in adulthood. There is no cure, but its symptoms can be controlled.  Each person is different, and what may trigger one asthmatic may not affect another.
    - For some, asthma is a minor nuisance, and a few puffs of rescue inhaler are all it takes to resolve symptoms.
    - For others, asthma can be a major problem that interferes with daily activities and could lead to a life-threatening asthma attack (typically when 911 is activated).
- **Chronic obstructive pulmonary disease (COPD)** is a chronic inflammatory lung disease that causes obstructed airflow from the lungs. It is most commonly seen in patients who have both emphysema and chronic bronchitis.

The asthma disease process can be broken down as follows:

- The main problem is that inflammation causes the bronchial airways to narrow, swell, and produce extra mucus.
- Symptoms include coughing, wheezing, and shortness of breath.
- Common triggers  are pollen, dust, mold, exercise, and even cold weather and humidity.

Treatment of severe asthma attacks requires supplemental high-flow oxygen or possibly use of CPAP if no other contraindications exist. ALS treatment includes nebulized breathing medications and possible intubation. The EMT must be able to recognize signs of degrading respiratory efforts, but other factors such as the time waited before a patient called 911 or what medications they have used prior to EMS arrival also matter. The EMT must decide on a course of treatment that not only manages current symptoms but also accounts for possible decompensation if BLS efforts are not successful. This often means an ALS intercept or rapid transport to a hospital for stabilization.

The COPD disease process can be broken down as follows:

- The main problem is that chronic inflammation causes narrowing of the bronchial airways and excess mucus production.
- Symptoms include difficulty breathing, cough, mucus production, and wheezing.
- Common triggers are tobacco smoke, fumes from chemicals, dust, preexisting asthma or respiratory infection, exercise, and hot/cold weather.

Treatment is the same as for asthma. Some people with a long-term diagnosis of COPD are very familiar with the use of CPAP during an exacerbation (worsening) of their symptoms and may request that you use that treatment. They may even already know their mask size, which can save you valuable time.

People with COPD often have 2 additional, simultaneous disease processes:

- **Emphysema** is a lung disease that destroys the thin walls and elastic fibers of the alveoli. This causes the small airways to collapse during exhalation, which then impair airflow out of the lungs.
- **Chronic bronchitis** is long-term inflammation of the bronchial tubes. The lungs respond to the irritation by producing more mucus, which increasingly blocks the already narrowed tubes. The patient develops a chronic cough in an attempt to clear the airways.

The common symptoms of these separate disease processes can combine to increase the difficulty of a respiratory distress patient. That is why patients are often on multiple medications at the same time—to help manage the dyspnea.

---

Most people with asthma do not develop COPD, and likewise, many people with COPD do not have asthma. However, a few people do have both conditions (called **asthma-COPD overlap syndrome [ACOS]**) and require multiple medications.

---

## Pulmonary Edema and Embolism

Another word associated with the respiratory system is *pulmonary*. Specifically, the term refers to the lungs themselves, while the word *respiratory* refers to the entire system, including the upper and lower airways.

**Pulmonary edema** is excess fluid in the lungs. It builds up when the capillaries in the lungs become more permeable, or "leaky," and collects in the numerous air sacs in the lungs, making it difficult for the patient to breathe. Pulmonary edema can be an acute condition or build up gradually over time. If left untreated, it can cause death as patients drown in their own lung fluids.

Typically, heart problems such as CHF are the cause of pulmonary edema. However, fluid can accumulate for other reasons, including pneumonia, exposure to toxins or certain medications, trauma to the chest wall, drowning or near-drowning incidents, and visiting or exercising at high elevations.

Signs and symptoms, which vary depending on whether the condition is acute or chronic, are as follows:

- **Acute**
  - Extreme shortness of breath (SOB) that worsens with movement or lying down
  - Wheezing or gasping for air

- Cold, clammy skin
- Anxiety or restlessness
- Frothy sputum that may be pink and tinged with blood
- Rapid, irregular pulse
- Rales/crackles lung sounds—these are discontinuous, short, bubbling sounds that correspond to the splashing of the fluid in the alveoli during breathing
- **Chronic**
  - More than normal shortness of breath when active
  - Difficulty breathing with exertion or when lying down
  - Possible waking up suddenly with shortness of breath
  - Wheezing, rales, or crackles
  - Swelling of lower extremities
  - Fatigue

Treatment is supplemental oxygen delivered by either nasal cannula or non-rebreather mask and monitored with pulse oximetry. Consider ALS and CPAP treatment. Transport the patient to the closest, most appropriate hospital; if the condition is caused by high altitude, a hyperbaric chamber–capable hospital would be a great choice, if available.

**Pulmonary embolism (PE)** is a blockage in one of the pulmonary arteries in the lungs. Most instances are caused by blood clots that travel to the lungs from deep veins in the legs; such a blood clot is called a deep vein thrombosis (DVT). Rarely, the clot arises from veins in other parts of the body. Other potential causes of PE are air bubbles, fatty marrow clots resulting from a broken bone, or tumor particles that have broken off and traveled.

Typically, multiple clots are involved in a PE episode. The parts of lung served by each blocked artery are deprived of blood, causing the tissue to die in a phenomenon known as pulmonary infarction. Just like in cardiac infarction, the death of tissue makes it more difficult for the lungs to provide oxygen to the rest of the body.

When conducting your assessment of pulmonary embolism, do the following:

- Ask if the patient has undertaken travel within the last week, particularly the last 48 hours, that involved long periods of sitting.
- Ask if the patient has recently had prolonged bed rest (surgery, pregnancy, nursing home patient), which increases the risk of pulmonary embolism.
- Check whether the patient is wearing compression stockings; this could help to differentiate between a heart attack, simple dyspnea, or something more complex such as pulmonary embolism.
- Obtain a thorough medication history; certain birth control medications make women more prone to pulmonary embolism.

Signs and symptoms to watch out for are as follows:

- Shortness of breath of sudden onset that worsens with movement
- Chest pain, often sharp, when breathing in deeply
- Cough, which may produce a  bloody sputum
- Rapid, irregular heartbeat
- Light-headedness or dizziness
- Clammy, diaphoretic, or cyanotic skin
- Fever
- Leg pain or swelling, particularly in the calf

Treatment is much the same as any other dyspnea episode: administer supplemental oxygen using either a nasal cannula or non-rebreather mask, monitor pulse oximetry, and transport to the most appropriate hospital. Consider ALS if there is serious deterioration of the patient and if ALS would be closer than a hospital. Be prepared to provide artificial ventilations if necessary.

## COVID-19

In 2020, the novel coronavirus SARS-CoV-2 was introduced to the world and caused a global pandemic of COVID-19. The medical community, including EMS, was quickly overwhelmed at the sheer number of people contracting the virus.

Over time, scientists were able to determine the genetic sequence of the virus and identified different strains such as Alpha, Delta, and more recently Omicron. In late 2020 into early 2021, vaccines were developed, tested, and deployed to the public and health care professionals. In 2021, vaccination boosters also became available to protect recipients from the most serious health consequences of the disease.

### COVID-19 Infection Control

At the time of this writing, three-quarters of the U.S. population has been fully or partially vaccinated against COVID-19, with 1 shot or more. A substantial number of Americans remain unvaccinated for a variety of reasons. In addition, some fully vaccinated people have nonetheless been infected with COVID-19. Consequently, EMS providers who are called to help a person with respiratory distress and "COVID-like symptoms" are at risk of becoming infected themselves.

COVID-19 infection is spread predominantly by respiratory droplets. This is why there is so much focus on having both the patient and the provider wear protective respiratory barriers.

Providers should be wearing proper PPE as required by their organization; this typically includes respiratory protection of a surgical mask or N95 mask and possibly goggles or a face shield as well. Some companies are also requiring their employees to wear gowns and/or higher levels of PPE (e.g., hazmat suit). As knowledge about COVID-19 has increased throughout this pandemic, many companies have been modifying their PPE requirements in a fluid manner.

Besides PPE, providers should keep in mind the respiratory impact of all their equipment. For example, using a bag-valve mask (BVM) or CPAP may expel additional respiratory droplets from the patient or spray them into the air more forcefully than does simply breathing.

## Symptoms of COVID-19

Symptoms of COVID-19 infection typically appear 2–14 days after initial exposure to the virus. The table lists common symptoms to look for in patients. **Note that a patient does not need to have all of the symptoms listed to be positive for COVID-19.** It has also been shown that some people are infected despite having no symptoms at all.

**Table 5.2** Signs and Symptoms of COVID-19

| TYPICAL SYMPTOMS | EMERGENCY SYMPTOMS |
|---|---|
| • Chills or fever (typically $>100.4°F$) <br> • Persistent cough <br> • Shortness of breath or difficulty breathing <br> • Fatigue <br> • Muscle or body aches <br> • Sore throat <br> • Congestion or runny nose <br> • Nausea/vomiting/diarrhea <br> • Headache <br> • Loss of smell or taste | • Persistent respiratory distress <br> • Persistent pain or pressure in the chest <br> • Confusion or altered mental status <br> • Inability to wake up or stay awake <br> • Pale/gray/cyanotic skin, which may be more noticeable in the lips or nail beds |

## Treatment of COVID-19

The COVID-19 pandemic has caused widespread disruption and engendered strong personal feelings and political stances. Regardless your own beliefs on vaccination or COVID-19 science, remember that a patient infected with COVID-19 is your priority and is due the same respect and dignity as any other respiratory distress patient. Patients experiencing the effects of COVID-19 infection may have strong beliefs regarding this virus; it is not the EMT's job to engage in a debate on the merits of those beliefs. Treat the symptoms, and deliver the patient to definitive care at the hospital.

BLS treatment includes the following:

- Monitor $SpO_2$ and reassess frequently to make sure the patient's airway and breathing remain adequate.
- Give supplemental oxygen as necessary.
- Gather a focused medical history on possible COVID-19 exposure events, when symptoms started, vaccination status, and symptoms experienced.

If the patient is in severe respiratory distress or failure and ALS is not already present, call for them as soon as possible. The patient may require advanced airway management.

### Decontamination for COVID-19

Providers must properly disinfect their unit after transport of a positive or suspected COVID-19 patient. Procedures may include:

- Airing out the patient compartment for a minimum of 15–20 minutes by leaving the doors open, allowing for natural airflow
- Cleaning all surfaces touched and/or used in unit with industrial-strength disinfectant wipes or sprays
- Using UV lamps designed to kill bacteria and viruses

Regardless of the equipment used, be sure to follow your company's procedures and be familiar with all products being used.

## Apnea

Apnea is the cessation of breathing. No matter the cause, prompt action must be taken by the EMT, or the heart and the rest of the body will cease to function shortly thereafter:

- If a patient is found not breathing, check for a pulse immediately in the carotid artery. If there is no pulse after 5–10 seconds, begin CPR starting with chest compressions.
- If working alone, you can use a face mask with a one-way valve to provide breaths after every 30 compressions.
- Ideally, you should use a bag-valve mask (BVM) to deliver ventilations with the proper tidal volume (seen with a rise and fall of the chest wall).
  - Once chest rise has occurred, stop squeezing the bag; this helps to prevent overinflating the lungs or allowing excess air into the stomach.
  - If there is no chest rise, reposition the head, press down on the mask, and attempt to ventilate again. After 2 breaths (or 10 seconds) without a chest rise, resume compressions.
- If you find that squeezing the BVM bag is becoming increasingly difficult but you are still getting chest rise, report this to your partner. An internal issue such as a tension pneumothorax or an airway obstruction may be causing the resistance. If ALS has not already been contacted, this is the decision point to do so or begin to emergent transport.
- If you suspect an obstruction is the cause of the apnea, open the mouth and look for the object. However, do NOT perform a blind finger sweep of the mouth if you do not see it, per AHA standards. When chest compressions are being performed, the pressure within the chest cavity may build up enough to force the object out of the airway. The person administering the ventilations should view the airway periodically. If the object does not appear, leave further visualization and removal of the object to ALS or the hospital, which has tools for these tasks.
- When the apnea has a medical cause such as drug overdose or anaphylaxis, medication such as naloxone or epinephrine could prompt the patient to begin breathing on their own. If you suspect this and the patient still has a pulse, you may need to administer one of these medications.

No matter the cause of the apnea, it is up to the EMT to correct it as soon as possible, before the patient is beyond revival.

# Airway Management

## Artificial Ventilation

In the event of poor or absent respirations, artificial ventilation of the patient may be required. This is accomplished by forcing air into the lungs, utilizing a technique known as positive pressure ventilation (PPV).

There are multiple ways to perform PPV: mouth-to-mask, bag-valve mask, oxygen-demand valve, and CPAP.

### Mouth-to-Mask

Mouth-to-mask (or pocket mask) ventilation is used when no other EMS equipment is available to sustain a patient's oxygen saturation level until more effective ventilation can be achieved. It is commonly used in EMS.

The mouth-to-mask is available as an individual package or as a set with a bag-valve mask. If packaged individually, it should come with a one-way valve to help protect the rescuer.

To provide effective breaths mouth-to-mask, it is imperative that the mask be tightly sealed to the patient's face:

- Use an E-C clamp where the thumb and index finger hold the mask down over the nose and mouth of the patient, forming a C.
- The other 3 fingers of your hand should grasp the patient's mandible, forming an E.

Then tilt the head back using the other hand (or use the jaw-thrust maneuver if trauma is suspected):

- If the person has a pulse and requires only rescue breaths, give 1 breath every 5–6 seconds.
- If the person is pulseless and not breathing adequately on their own, do CPR in conjunction with breaths.
  - Use a 30:2 rhythm, i.e., 30 compressions and 2 breaths.
  - Deliver each breath over 1 second, with each breath producing visible chest rise.

---

With the increase in communicable diseases that can be spread by intimate contact, mouth-to-mouth resuscitation is now used less and less. Practically speaking, the only time it is used today is when the EMT is reasonably certain that there is no risk of contamination.

---

### Bag-Valve Mask

Bag-valve-mask (BVM) ventilation provides a higher concentration of oxygen than exhaled air and lessens the contact with biological hazards for both the patient and the EMT. A tight seal is also imperative between the mask and the face:

- Use a one-handed C technique, as described for the pocket mask.
- Connect the bag to the opening at the top of the mask if this has not already been done.
- Use the other hand to squeeze the bag and push air into the patient.
  - Be careful to squeeze the bag only until you see chest rise, and then stop.
  - That will reduce the chances of barotrauma, overinflation of the lungs, or air entry into the stomach.
- The most efficient way to use a BVM is to use the 2-person technique—one person maintains a mask seal, while the second person ventilates with the bag.

**Figure 5.5** Parts of a Bag-Valve Mask (BVM)

The BVM also comes with an oxygen inlet port, which allows the patient to be ventilated with 100% oxygen. An experienced EMT can feel in the resistance of the bag the efficiency of the ventilation effort as well as note the patient's chest rise and the exhalation of air after inspiration.

If the bag becomes increasingly harder to squeeze, reassess the airway, as a number of things could be wrong:

- Check the mask seal to make sure it is still intact with the face.
- Check the airway to make sure it is not obstructed by fluids or objects. Suction if necessary.
- Check whether the airway is positioned properly, and readjust if needed.
- Consider the possibility of a tension pneumothorax or other complications.

- If the patient is intubated by an ALS provider, have that person check the position of the tube placement. Communicate that you are feeling resistance and it is becoming harder to squeeze the BVM.

### Oxygen-Demand Valve

The oxygen-powered ventilation device provides the same type of ventilation but with less physical exertion, as it is does not require one to squeeze a bag to inflate the lungs. This method uses a demand valve that is controlled by respiration rate, allowing increased oxygen flow in response to increased demand. However, the mask must be sealed on the face as with both the pocket mask and the BVM.

Many EMS services have discontinued the oxygen-powered device. Many EMTs feel that the BVM gives better control of artificial ventilation and that with an oxygen hookup, the amount of oxygen delivered with either device is 100%.

### Continuous Positive Airway Pressure

Airway collapse can result from many conditions. One of the tools now available to many EMTs (state dependent) is the use of CPAP.

Via a specialized face mask, CPAP forces a small amount of air pressure through the bronchioles and into the alveoli, causing them to reopen. The pressure created by CPAP is held constant throughout the breathing cycle. During inspiration, the patient may feel a small amount of pressure (versus a regular breath); during exhalation, the patient may feel the same thing.

---

For patients using a CPAP for the first time, it can be a very strange feeling—one that may require convincing to accept. Moreover, the patient may not be thinking clearly (often due to hypoxia). Even though you know that CPAP will help alleviate the breathing, it might feel suffocating to the patient. This is when a good patient rapport and patience can go a long way in gaining compliance.

---

In conditions that cause excess fluid in the lungs, such as heart failure, drowning, and pulmonary edema, the gas exchange between carbon dioxide and oxygen occurs within the lung's alveoli. Each alveolus has a liquid called **surfactant**, which reduces water surface tension within the pleural space and keeps the alveolus open. If the fluid balance is disturbed, this will cause the alveolus to collapse, a condition called **atelectasis**. That, in turn, will compromise the gas exchange process, and the patient will start to experience respiratory distress.

CPAP may also be indicated for several other conditions where the gas exchange process is disrupted:

- Bronchoconstriction, e.g., asthma and COPD in moderate to severe distress
- Toxic gases, e.g., chemicals or smoke inhalation that cause bronchoconstriction and swelling

- Flail chest—insufficient chest rise as a result of broken ribs and pain (CPAP can support proper tidal volumes)
- Lung infections, e.g., pneumonia and any other infection that occurs within the lungs

A main concern with CPAP is that it can lower blood pressure. (As pressure increases inside the lungs, the pressure on the heart chambers and great vessels also increases, thus causing cardiac output to drop.) Contraindications for CPAP use are as follows:

- Reduced level of consciousness or being unconscious
- Inability to protect their own airway
- Cardiac or respiratory arrest
- Facial trauma that would prevent a good mask seal (broken bones, burns, etc.)
- Copious secretions in the mouth
- Severe nausea with vomiting

## Oxygen Delivery Systems

### Oxygen

Oxygen is the most widely used drug by EMS and is indicated in almost all protocols for difficulty breathing, as well as many other conditions such as chest pain. Consequently, it is carried aboard all EMS vehicles and is used routinely by EMTs:

- The **onboard system** is stored in an "M" cylinder, which contains 3,000 liters of oxygen.
- The **portable system** (carried to a patient) is stored in a smaller "D" or "E" cylinder, which carries 350 and 625 liters of oxygen, respectively.
  - Cylinders are filled to a maximum pressure of 2,000 pounds per square inch and must be handled with great care.
  - If heated, a full cylinder may rupture and cause an explosion that can easily kill a bystander.
  - Keep at least one hand on the cylinder at all times, as it may also become a projectile if dropped at a certain angle.

To be used for EMS purposes, the pressure must be reduced by a pressure regulator, which is attached to the valve of the tank. This regulator can then be adjusted to provide the proper flow to the patient in liters per minute (LPM).

### Masks

Oxygen is delivered to the patient through a mask that fits over the nose and mouth or through a prong that fits into the nostrils. Masks come in different styles, as per the percentage of oxygen required:

- A **full non-rebreather mask (NRB)** at a flow rate of 10–15 liters/minute delivers almost 100% oxygen.
- A **simple face mask** at a flow rate of 6–10 liters/minute delivers 40–60% oxygen.

- A **nasal cannula (NC)** at a flow rate of 2–6 liters/minute delivers 20–40% oxygen.
- A **Venturi mask** is an adjustable type of mask with a flow rate from 2–15 liters/minute and delivers 24–60% oxygen depending on which of the color-coded valves is chosen.

The choice of device is predicated on the patient's degree of **hypoxia** (low oxygen). A pulse oximeter is very useful for this task. A patient who presents with cyanosis requires more oxygen than one who presents with normal skin color and an inability to catch their breath:

- A patient who complains of difficulty breathing yet has normal color and pulse oximeter reading in the high 90s may be given an NC.
- A pale patient with saturation below 90% probably needs a higher concentration device, such as an NRB.

---

Treat the patient, not the equipment. Look at the overall patient presentation to determine the proper treatment sequence:

- A potential carbon monoxide victim may produce a false reading of 100% $SpO_2$ if you do not have a dual-reader for both oxygen and carbon monoxide.
- Be careful in cases of stroke and myocardial infarction. Studies have shown that 100% oxygen rates may be harming patients; instead, the ideal pulse oximeter reading is 92-98% with a flow rate 2-4 liters/min.

---

### TEST YOURSELF 5.2

**What type of oxygen would you provide to this patient?**

You respond to your local nursing home facility for a patient who has fallen. Upon arrival, you find an 87-year-old male lying on the floor next to his bed and a staff member who hands you paperwork. The staff member states that she doesn't know what happened as she "just came on shift and when doing her rounds, found him on the floor like this and was afraid to move him." The patient is normally on 2 liters per minute (LPM) of oxygen with a nasal cannula (which is not on his face at this time). Vital signs are BP 118/58 mm Hg, pulse 82, respiratory rate 14, and pulse oximetry 93%. He is not in any obvious respiratory distress.

Do you give this patient oxygen? If yes, what delivery device would you use and how many liters per minute would you provide?

# Practice Set

1. Your patient is a 24-year-old male with respiratory distress. He states he has a history of asthma. His respiratory rate is 26, $SpO_2$ is 94% on room air, blood pressure is 128/90 mm Hg, and pulse is 102. You have placed him on supplemental oxygen and gained medical command to administer his prescribed albuterol inhaler for 2 puffs. Which of the following 3 characteristics describe asthma? Select the 3 answer options that are correct.

   A. Bronchospasms

   B. Stridor lung sounds

   C. Destruction of alveolar walls

   D. Edema of the airways

   E. Thickening of bronchial walls

   F. Increased sensitivity of lower airways to irritants

2. You are dispatched to a residence for a child not breathing. The scene is safe, and you are wearing gloves. Upon entering the living room, you see a 4-year-old child lying on his back and his mother nearby screaming, "My baby, my baby!" You approach the child, take stabilization of the head, and look, listen, and feel for air exchange; none is noted. You perform a modified jaw-thrust maneuver and again look, listen, and feel; air exchange is still negative. You instruct your partner to attempt to ventilate, and she advises you that there appears to be an obstruction. You reposition the airway, and she tries again with no success. What is your next instruction?

   A. Call 911.

   B. Examine the airway.

   C. Perform a blind finger sweep to feel for an object.

   D. Roll the patient over and perform 5 back blows.

3. What occurs during the exhalation portion of the breathing process? Select the 3 answer options that are correct.

   A. Air exits the thoracic cavity.

   B. The intercostal muscles contract.

   C. Pressure inside the chest increases.

   D. Diastolic blood pressure rises.

   E. The diaphragm relaxes.

4. The correct landmarks for sizing a nasopharyngeal airway are

   A. tip of ear to tip of nose.

   B. tip of ear to corner of mouth.

   C. corner of mouth to tip of nose.

   D. corner of mouth to temple.

5. Which of the following is a contraindication for use of a nasopharyngeal airway?

   A. Apnea

   B. Seizure

   C. Facial trauma

   D. $SpO_2$ <90%

6. Which of the following is true concerning the procedure for inserting a nasopharyngeal airway (NPA)?

   A. It can be placed only in the right nostril since that one is straighter.

   B. Measuring the length is less important than when placing an OPA.

   C. The bevel should be turned toward the septum, or base, of nostril.

   D. If a water-soluble lubricant isn't available, a silicone spray may be used.

7.  Your 57-year-old female patient is sitting leaning forward and exhaling with her lips pursed together. When asked, she says she has a history of emphysema and uses an albuterol inhaler. You auscultate and hear wheezes and rhonchi in all fields. Vital signs are pulse of 110, respiratory rate of 27, blood pressure of 134/92 mm Hg, and SpO2 of 95% on home oxygen 3 liters per minute (LPM) by nasal cannula. Which of the following are actions you should take next? Select the 3 answer options that are correct.

    A.  Administer oxygen by non-rebreather mask.

    B.  Increase the nasal cannula rate to 6 LPM.

    C.  Assist the patient with her prescribed inhaler.

    D.  Immediately take a second set of vitals.

    E.  Begin to ventilate with a BVM at 10–12 breaths per minute.

    F.  Make her a priority patient and begin transport.

8.  You respond to a residence for a call for difficulty breathing. In the bedroom is a 40-year-old female sitting up in bed in severe respiratory distress. She is pale, and you note that her neck muscles are protruded. She is breathing at a rate of 30. The patient tries to say, "Can't breathe," but is barely able to speak. Her pulse oximetry is 72% on room air. Her husband explains that she has a history of emphysema, for which she takes medication. She is not on supplemental oxygen. She has no other pertinent history and no allergies. Auscultation of her chest, sides, and back reveals the presence of rhonchi in all fields. Which of the following is the most appropriate first treatment?

    A.  Administer 2 puffs of her albuterol inhaler.

    B.  Administer liquid albuterol through a nebulizer mask.

    C.  Administer oxygen via nasal cannula at 6 LPM.

    D.  Administer oxygen via non-rebreather mask at 15 LPM.

9.  You are transporting the patient in question 8 to the emergency department. Her pulse oximetry has risen to 92% with supplemental oxygen, and her respiratory rate is now down to 20 breaths per minute. Suddenly, the patient becomes unconscious, and you notice she has stopped breathing. You open her airway, but she still does not breathe spontaneously. She also has no gag reflex, and you do not see any secretions. What devices, in the correct order, would you utilize next?

    A.  CPAP, OPA, NPA, suction

    B.  Suction, NPA, BVM

    C.  OPA, BVM

    D.  BVM, NPA, OPA

10. You respond to a residence for a call for difficulty breathing. You enter the bedroom of a 60-year-old female, seated with her shoulders hunched forward in respiratory distress. Her pulse oximetry is 78%, her respiratory rate is 30, and she is pale and diaphoretic. Auscultation of the lungs reveals a crackling sound in the posterior bases. This type of breath sound is referred to as which of the following?

    A.  Rales

    B.  Rhonchi

    C.  Stridor

    D.  Wheezing

11. While attempting to ventilate a patient who has stopped breathing en route to the hospital, you insert an OPA, place a BVM over the patient's mouth and nose, and squeeze the bag. You note that there is not much resistance and that the patient's chest does not rise. Which of the following is the most likely cause of this failure?

    A. Inadequate oxygen supply

    B. Equipment failure

    C. Failure to preoxygenate the patient

    D. Failure to seal the mask against the patient's face

12. Which of the following patients should NOT have their airway opened using a head-tilt, chin-lift maneuver?

    A. A 47-year-old woman with diabetes who became unresponsive in the driver's seat before leaving her driveway

    B. A homeless person of unknown age found lying unresponsive in an alley with no bystanders present

    C. A 16-year-old male who is still unresponsive after experiencing a grand mal seizure in his bed

    D. A 38-year-old female who choked on a piece of food in a restaurant and was lowered safely to the floor by a waiter

13. While conducting your truck check at the beginning of your shift, you notice that the onboard oxygen system tank has no pressure left. What size tank should you replace it with?

    A. D

    B. E

    C. M

    D. X

THIS PAGE INTENTIONALLY LEFT BLANK

## Answer Key

| | | | | | | | | | |
|---|---|---|---|---|---|---|---|---|---|
| 1. | **A, D, F** | 4. | **A** | 7. | **A, C, F** | 10. | **A** | 13. | **C** |
| 2. | **B** | 5. | **C** | 8. | **D** | 11. | **D** | | |
| 3. | **A, C, E** | 6. | **C** | 9. | **C** | 12. | **B** | | |

## Answers and Explanations

### 1. A, D, F

Asthma is a condition that causes normally functioning airways to become more sensitive to irritants (F), which in turn cause bronchospasms (A) leading to bronchoconstriction. The increased sensitivity and resulting bronchospasms produce edema (swelling), which worsens the spasm (D), creating a vicious cycle of cause and effect. Unless a bronchodilator is administered, asthmatics can progress into respiratory failure. Stridor lung sounds (B) are typically heard with foreign body obstructions or conditions such as croup, not asthma. Destruction of the alveolar walls (C) is seen in emphysema, not asthma. Bronchiectasis is a condition that causes thickening of the bronchi and bronchial walls (E), making it harder to breathe.

### 2. B

The patient may have aspirated a foreign object, causing the airway blockage. Choice (A) is not correct because you *are* 911, although you may want additional help or an ALS intercept. Rolling over the patient and administering 5 back blows (D) is a potential action once you have examined the airway. The blind finger sweep (C) has been removed from AHA standards.

### 3. A, C, E

Exhalation is a passive process that involves relaxation of the diaphragm (E) to its normal domelike shape. This causes the space in the chest cavity to decrease, which in turn increases the pressure inside the chest (C), allowing air to exit the thoracic cavity (A). During inhalation, blood pressure normally drops (D) by 10–15 mm Hg and the intercostal muscles contract (B), making these answers incorrect.

### 4. A

The correct answer is tip of ear to tip of nose (A). Tip of ear to corner of mouth (B) is the correct answer for an oropharyngeal airway. Corner of mouth to tip of nose (C) is not used for any airway device and neither is corner of mouth to temple (D).

### 5. C

Facial trauma (C) contraindicates use of a nasopharyngeal airway due to the possibility of an opening into the cranium that would allow the device to penetrate into that compartment and complicate the fracture. Apnea (A) is the absence of breathing, which would indicate use of an airway adjunct to assist with ventilations. Seizure (B) often indicates the use of an NPA, rather than an OPA, due to teeth clenching. Pulse oximetry saturation ($SpO_2$) <90% (D) is an indication that oxygen perfusion is needed.

### 6. C

Turning the bevel toward the nasal septum is good practice and the most comfortable way to insert the NPA, especially in a conscious patient. The desired end result is the tip of the NPA lying bevel down toward the rear of the nasopharynx. The other answers are simply incorrect. The anatomical statement that the right nostril is the straighter one (A) is false. You must always properly size your equipment (B), and you must always use a water-soluble lubricant to insert the NPA, not silicone spray (D) (and never saliva!).

**7.  A, C, F**

Your patient is in significant respiratory distress, as evidenced by the tripod position and pursed-lips breathing. Despite the use of home oxygen, this scenario is describing an exacerbated case of emphysema, and the patient would be best treated now with a higher level of oxygen via non-rebreather mask (A). Depending on your protocols, you could help administer the patient's prescribed inhaler now (C) or administer or ask medical control for permission to do so. This is also a priority patient who would benefit from transport sooner rather than later (F). However, increasing the nasal cannula rate to 6 LPM is not the best next step (B); remember that a nasal cannula delivers a maximum of 40% oxygen, while a non-rebreather mask will deliver almost 100%. You could take a second set of vitals (D) en route to the hospital, where the patient will receive more definitive care, so this is not the best next step. Since the patient is conscious at this time, a bag-valve mask (E) would be more challenging to use than a non-rebreather, which allows the patient to maintain her own airway.

**8.  D**

The key to the answer choices is the pulse oximetry reading of 72%, which indicates severe hypoxia. Two puffs of inhaled albuterol (A) is an insufficient treatment for the level of distress the patient is currently experiencing, and albuterol by nebulizer mask (B) is typically administered only at the ALS scope of practice. This leaves two types of oxygen delivery. A rate of 6 liters per minute (C) will help raise this patient's oxygen saturation but not as quickly as 15 liters per minute.

**9.  C**

You would use an oropharyngeal airway (OPA) and then a bag-valve mask (BVM), choice (C). The EMT's first step is to provide artificial ventilation to this patient. Once you have manually opened the airway, use an OPA to assist in maintaining the airway, and then ventilate with a BVM using supplemental oxygen. There is no indication here for the use of suction (B) or an NPA (A and D).

**10.  A**

Rales are a fine, crackling sound caused by fluid in the alveoli. This breath sound is usually an indication of pulmonary edema, most often caused by congestive heart failure. Rhonchi (B) are snoring-type sounds, stridor (C) is a high-pitched sound coming from the upper airway, and wheezing (D) consists of lower-pitched sounds coming from the bronchi being constricted.

**11.  D**

Lack of resistance when squeezing the bag means that the air is going somewhere else. Equipment failure (B), such as a leak in the bag or mask, is a possibility but not likely. The percentages of oxygen (A) and preoxygenation (C), although important to the patient's condition, have nothing to do with the physical ventilation of the lungs.

**12.  B**

The key to answering this question is to rule out trauma. The woman with diabetes who became unresponsive in her driveway (A) hasn't driven yet, so the chance of injury is not significant. Likewise, the teen seized while in his bed (C), which is a soft area. The diner who choked on food (D) did not fall but was lowered to the floor by someone. By contrast, we can't rule out trauma for the homeless person found alone and unresponsive (B) in an outdoor setting; thus, for safety, the jaw-thrust maneuver should be used in this patient.

**13.  C**

The correct size is M. D and E cylinders are for portable use, and there is no such thing as an X tank for emergency medical oxygen.

# MEDICAL EMERGENCIES

---

**LEARNING OBJECTIVES**

- Understand foundational pharmacology concepts:
  - Dosages and routes
  - Indications and contraindications
  - Mechanism of action
- List the 7 most common medications that an EMT can administer in the field according to the *National EMS Scope of Practice Model,* including dosages and routes
- List the routes of medication administration and describe how each is given
- List the 5 rights and 3 additional considerations of medication administration
- Recognize pathophysiology and understand EMS treatments for common medical emergencies:
  - Cardiovascular emergencies
  - Altered mental status, strokes, and TIAs
  - Shock and sepsis
  - Diabetic emergencies
  - Seizures
  - Allergic reaction emergencies
  - Poisoning and overdose
  - Environmental emergencies
  - Behavioral emergencies
  - Obstetric and gynecological (OB-GYN) emergencies

---

In the practice of prehospital emergency medicine, the EMT will come across many, varied medical emergencies involving one or more body systems. The EMT will also be responsible for recognizing when and how to administer various medications and when to call for ALS if a call goes beyond their scope of practice. This chapter reviews the steps to be taken by an EMT-Basic on a call responding to several types of medical emergencies commonly seen in EMS and tested on the NREMT.

Note that respiratory emergencies are not addressed in this chapter. Please refer back to chapter 5 for a more in-depth look at airway and related emergencies.

# Pharmacology

An EMT may be instructed to administer medication to a patient in the field. Therefore, it is important to understand what these medications are, how they work, for what medical conditions they are administered (indications), and under which circumstances they should *not* be administered (contraindications).

You must always be guided by the local protocols regarding drug administration since these protocols vary widely by location.

According to the latest *National EMS Scope of Practice Model*, there are 9 medications that an EMT can administer in the field. The 7 most common are listed in the following table.

**Table 6.1** Most Common Medications that EMTs Can Deliver

| MEDICATION | DOSAGE | ROUTE |
|---|---|---|
| Oxygen | 1–25 liters per minute (LPM) depending on route and oxygen regulator used*<br><br>*Regulators with a range of 2–15 LPM are common and may be more familiar to the EMT | • Nasal cannula (NC): 2–6 LPM<br>• Non-rebreather (NRB): 10–25 LPM<br>• Bag-valve mask (BVM): 2–15 LPM<br>• Venturi may be adjusted individually to patient<br>• CPAP: typically preset to 10 LPM start, but follow directions or training by your service |
| Oral glucose | 10–50 grams | • Buccal route preferred<br>• Typically given in a predosed (10–15 g) tube; must be opened and delivered to a conscious patient who is able to protect their own airway |
| Epinephrine | Adults: 0.3 mg<br><br>Pediatrics: 0.15 mg | • Given by intramuscular (IM) route in outer lateral thigh<br>• Typically given via auto-injector; some states allow EMTs to draw from a vial using a syringe |
| Aspirin (ASA) | Tablets, available in 325 mg or 81 mg | • Oral tablet; must be nonenteric coated if chewed instead of swallowed<br>• 325 mg: give 1 tablet<br>• 81 mg: give 4 tablets |
| Opioid antagonists (naloxone) | Available in 2 mg/mL or 0.4 mg/mL | • Intranasal (IN): 2 mg/mL prefilled syringe, with 1 mL delivered per nostril<br>• Intramuscular (IM): 0.4 mg/mL, typically drawn up from a 1 mL vial (allowed only in some states) |

*(Continued)*

**Table 6.1** Most Common Medications that EMTs Can Deliver (*Continued*)

| MEDICATION | DOSAGE | ROUTE |
|---|---|---|
| Bronchodilators (e.g., albuterol, ipratropium) | Dosage depends on patient's prescription | • Generally encountered in metered-dose inhalers (MDIs)<br>• Typically given 1–2 puffs per administration; read prescription<br>• Patient may use a "spacer" (specialized tube that allows aerosolized particles to remain airborne longer), common in pediatric and geriatric populations |
| Nitroglycerin (nitro) | 0.4 mg (1/150 grain) | • Oral dissolving tablet: place under tongue and let dissolve; do not chew, crush, or swallow<br>• Spray: lift tongue and deliver sublingually 1 spray at a time<br>• Topical paste*: measure out a length of paste against the paper scale for dosage (included in the package), and then spread the whole unit across the skin (*allowed only in some states) |

As an EMT, you would also do well to familiarize yourself with the more common prescription medications, because they can provide clues to potential problems. Such clues are especially helpful for situations where a patient is found alone and unresponsive. By locating a patient's prescription (in a bag, etc.), you can get an idea of the type of medical condition you are dealing with and whether it is acute or chronic.

**Antidotes for chemical/hazardous materials exposure, activated charcoal, and glucagon** are also available at the BLS level nationally. However, some states do not allow EMTs to administer them, so these therapies may not be tested on the exam. All EMTs should know which medications are allowed within their scope of practice.

Medications may be administered to the patient in a variety of ways.

**Table 6.2** Medication Routes

| ROUTE | SHORTHAND WRITTEN FORM | HOW GIVEN | FORMS MEDICATIONS MAY COME IN |
|---|---|---|---|
| Injection | Intramuscular (IM) or subcutaneous (Sub-Q) | • IM: insert needle catheter at 90° angle into a muscle such as buttocks or deltoid muscle<br>• Sub-Q: inject needle catheter into the layer of fatty tissue between skin and muscle | Liquid in prefilled syringes that may be manual or auto-injectors |
| Inhalation/aerosolized (nebulizer administration by EMT allowed only in some states) | INH | Depress the prescribed inhaler/canister, which releases airborne droplets into the patient's mouth and airway | • Suspensions<br>• Gases<br>• Liquids<br>• Aerosols |
| Oral | PO | Place medication into patient's mouth; some are meant to be swallowed, and others are meant to melt onto the tongue | • Tablets<br>• Capsules |
| Buccal | BUC | Place medication into patient's mouth between teeth and cheek tissue | • Gels<br>• Liquids |
| Sublingual | SL | Place medication underneath patient's tongue | • Tablets<br>• Sprays |
| Rectal (allowed by EMT only in some states) | REC | Place medication into the rectum | • Suppositories<br>• Gels |

### KEY TAKEAWAY

Accredited programs are responsible for teaching the National Standard Curriculum, not just the state protocols in which the course is located. This is why the EMT may see medication questions on the NREMT exam that do not apply to their particular state's allowances.

## Medication Rights

Medication errors harm an estimated 1.5 million people per year. As health care providers, EMTs are included as one of the causes for this alarming statistic.

Many EMS systems allow the EMT to administer medication that is already prescribed for a particular patient, such as asthma medication administered by metered-dose inhaler (e.g., albuterol, metaproterenol, ipratropium), nitroglycerin for angina, and epinephrine for anaphylaxis.

When administering medication, the EMT must know the "medication rights" of drug therapy. Many programs still teach the "5 rights," as follows. Additional considerations that you should keep in mind are also listed (in *italics*):

- Is this the right **medication**?
- Is this the right **patient**? (especially important for prescriptions)
- Is this the right **route** of administration?
- Is this the right **dosage**?
- Is this the right **date**? (expiration date has not passed)
- *Is this the right time to take the medication?* (important for scheduled doses such as insulin)
- *Is this the right response to the medication?* (look for allergic reactions or adverse reactions)
- *Is this right reason for the medication?* (e.g., glucose auto-injector versus epinephrine auto-injector for a patient with diabetes who is experiencing an allergic reaction emergency)

When medication is administered, note the date and time, and document them in your run report. After the drug administration, reassess the patient for changes in condition, including vital signs.

## Cardiovascular Emergencies

One of the most common emergency calls is for chest pain. Chest pain has many possible causes, from musculoskeletal issues to cardiovascular issues or even cardiac arrest. Good assessment skills are key, because it is up to the EMT to differentiate among the various possible causes and administer the proper treatment.

Heart issues can be broken down into 3 categories:

- Is it an **electrical** problem?
- Is it a **circulatory** problem?
- Is it a **structural** problem?

## Electrical Problems

Electrical problem*s* stem from the heart's electrical pathways not functioning correctly or at all. Some terms to know when speaking about electrical issues are as follows:

- **Arrhythmia/dysrhythmia**—irregular rate or rhythm
- **Tachycardia**—fast heart rate
- **Bradycardia**—slow heart rate
- **Asystole**—no electrical impulses produced ("flatline")
- **Fibrillation** (atrial or ventricular)—the heart is "shaking" but there is no squeezing of the blood into other parts of the heart

Both knowledge of all of the heart rhythms and ability to interpret them on an EKG are outside the national scope of practice for EMTs. However, you should be able to recognize that an arrhythmia/dysrhythmia will result in various medical conditions, which range from chronic diseases (e.g., atrial fibrillation) to sudden cardiac arrest (SCA). Ventricular fibrillation is considered a lethal rhythm.

## Circulatory Problems

Circulatory problems deal with issues that arise from the vessels supplying or leaving the heart or from the fluid that flows within the heart itself.

**Table 6.3** Common Circulatory Problems

| CIRCULATORY PROBLEM | DEVELOPMENT AND PROGRESSION |
|---|---|
| Hypertension (HTN) | • Develops when steady pressure on vessel walls weakens them over time<br>• As vessel weakens, it becomes more susceptible to buildup of deposits; these may eventually break off and travel to the heart or brain, potentially causing myocardial infarction (heart attack) or stroke<br>• Weakened vessels can also fail outright, causing aneurysm |
| Coronary artery disease (CAD) | • Develops when the major blood vessels supplying the heart (the coronary arteries) become damaged or diseased<br>• Impaired vessels accumulate plaque deposits and become inflamed<br>• Vessels narrow, preventing adequate blood flow and resulting in angina (pain), shortness of breath, or complete blockage and myocardial infarction (MI) |
| Arteriosclerosis/atherosclerosis ("hardening of the arteries") | • Develops when blood flow is restricted, causing the arterial walls (normally soft and flexible) to stiffen<br>• Impaired arteries accumulate buildup of plaques<br>• Symptoms vary depending on which artery is affected; lifestyle changes (smoking cessation, weight loss, healthier diet) may relieve or reverse symptoms |

*(Continued)*

**Table 6.3** Common Circulatory Problems (*Continued*)

| CIRCULATORY PROBLEM | DEVELOPMENT AND PROGRESSION |
|---|---|
| Angina pectoris | • Type of chest pain that develops from reduced blood flow to the heart<br>• Typically unexpected, so be sure to ask OPQRST questions thoroughly<br>• Stable angina: goes away with medication or rest<br>• Unstable angina: does not typically go away with rest or medication and may signal that a heart attack is about to occur |
| Myocardial infarction (MI) | • Develops when plaque buildup has completely occluded (blocked) one of the heart's vessels, causing hypoxia and buildup of toxins in the surrounding heart tissue<br>• Unless treated quickly, can result in cardiac arrest; if caught in time, stents may be used to keep arteries open long term |
| Hypoperfusion syndrome (shock) | • Develops when circulation to the various organs of the body is inadequate due to low fluid volume (hypovolemia) or inadequate pumping of the heart (such as congestive heart failure [CHF])<br>• Can lead to electrical problems and arrhythmias<br>• Look for traumatic causes vs. medical causes, and treat accordingly |
| Acute coronary syndrome (ACS) | • Develops when blood flow to the heart is suddenly reduced; associated with a range of conditions<br>• Typically results in either MI or alteration of the blood flow (temporary or permanent) that may create unstable angina<br>• Often increases patient's risk for stroke and heart attack in the future |

## Structural Problems

Structural problems stem from damage to the heart itself. This can be a result of a traumatic injury or developments such as:

- **Congestive heart failure (CHF)**—the left or right ventricle is weakened to the point that it no longer has the strength to pump blood properly to the lungs or the body:

  - Common causes—diabetes, HTN, and CAD

  - Signs and symptoms—fluid buildup in the lungs, edema (swelling) in the extremities, tiredness, and shortness of breath

- **Cardiac tamponade**—an acute condition in which blood or fluids fill the pericardial sac surrounding the heart itself; places extreme pressure on the heart and prevents ventricles from expanding fully (if not released, can prevent the heart from beating entirely):

  - Classic symptoms (Beck triad)—hypotension, muffled heart sounds, and jugular vein distention (JVD)

  - Other symptoms—restlessness, anxiety, clammy extremities, and tachycardia

- **Pericardial effusion**—similar to cardiac tamponade but with a slower buildup of fluids

## Treatment (Emergency Care)

EMTs are not able to definitively diagnose and treat the various cardiac conditions listed above. However, they must be able to differentiate between the various possibilities in the field so that they can have a working diagnosis (and eventual treatment).

If you come upon a cardiac-compromised patient, you must be alert that this is an ALS situation and requires either an intercept or rapid transport to an emergency department. With the patient's best interests in mind, you must decide which of these two options to execute, based upon the time each will require. The longer that definitive treatment (either medical or surgical) is delayed, the more damage that can occur to the heart tissue.

Emergency care of the suspected cardiac compromise falls into two categories:

- **No pulse?** Move on to possible defibrillation with an AED and CPR.
- **Pulse present?** Move on to the initial assessment, focused history, and physical exam.

Obtain baseline vital signs, including pulse oximetry, and apply oxygen as appropriate. Also consider giving cardiac medications if indicated.

The OPQRST series of questions is important in the proper assessment of chest pain and will be communicated to the emergency department so that personnel there may properly triage the patient. Especially important is the description of the *quality* of the pain and whether it is stationary versus radiating. Remember: time is tissue in a heart attack (myocardial infarction). By performing an adequate focused exam and relaying a complete picture to the triage nurse, the EMT saves time at the triage desk, permitting faster processing to a definitive level of care that can minimize the damage to the patient's heart.

### Medication

Current studies have shown that aspirin, taken daily as a prophylactic or given at the onset of chest pain, dramatically improves a patient's chances of survival. Consequently, many local protocols now call for the EMT to administer aspirin to chest pain patients, providing they have not already taken one.

Many times, the patient has already had a prior episode and has been prescribed nitroglycerin (NTG) tablets or spray to treat sudden-onset chest pain. If your local protocol allows you to administer NTG or to assist the patient in administering it, check with your medical control and follow all directions.

Be sure to ask if the patient has **taken any erectile dysfunction medication in the last 24–48 hours**, as that could cause an unsafe drop in blood pressure when given with NTG. Ask all patients this question, including females.

NTG is a powerful vasodilator that is placed sublingually. It is rapidly absorbed and causes the arteries to dilate. Side effects may include a drop in blood pressure and headache.

Before giving NGT, be sure that the patient's systolic blood pressure is higher than 100 mm Hg since a drop in blood pressure may result in hypotension that can lead to hypoxia. After NGT administration, continue to monitor the effect of the drug by taking additional blood pressure readings.

If the chest pain is alleviated with NTG, the physician may suspect that the cause of the chest pain is not myocardial infarction but angina.

## CPR and Automated External Defibrillators

Although not every chest pain patient is going to lapse into cardiac arrest, it can and does happen. Continued assessment is important in these cases. If the patient does suddenly go into cardiac arrest, you must be prepared to respond immediately.

Always travel with the devices you would need to do CPR: the automated external defibrillator (AED), a bag-valve mask, OPAs, and suctioning equipment:

- An AED is a computer-driven device that analyzes a patient's cardiac rhythm and determines whether a countershock is advised.
- The purpose of this countershock is to reestablish a perfusing rhythm. Current research indicates that if the patient's heart is in ventricular tachycardia or ventricular fibrillation, a shock delivered as soon as possible after the condition occurs could convert the irregular rhythms to a rhythm that would once again generate a pulse.
- An exception is if the patient is in an asystole rhythm, which will cause the AED to state, "No shock advised. Continue CPR if necessary." This type of heart rhythm will respond only to high-quality CPR and cardiac medication administered by ALS providers or hospital personnel. Depending on how long the patient has been in this rhythm, they may never recover; they may die despite the EMT's best efforts.

The AED does not take the place of CPR but, rather, is an adjunct to CPR. As of this printing, the AHA suggests the following sequence for use of the AED and CPR for an adult patient:

**Table 6.4** How to Use an AED (Adults Only)

| STEP NUMBER | DIRECTION |
|---|---|
| 1 | Determine if the scene is safe and that appropriate infection control precautions are in place. |
| 2 | If CPR in progress, stop it and verify that the patient has no pulse and is not breathing. |
| 3 | Have your partner continue CPR while you prepare and attach the AED pads in the correct placement as indicated by the pictures. Listen and follow the prompts as indicated. **Do not touch** the patient during the analyze cycle. |
| 4 | If the AED states, "Shock advised," continue with chest compressions while the AED charges. When the light or sound is made alerting that the machine is charged, **all personnel** (including whomever is on airway) must stand clear while the shock button is depressed. Immediately resume compressions. |
| 5 | If the AED states, "No shock advised. Begin CPR if necessary," perform a pulse and breathing check. If these are absent, immediately resume chest compressions. |
| 6 | Use the following guidelines for chest compressions: <br><br> • Perform at a rate of 100–120/minute using 2 hands <br> • Compress at least 2-2.4 inches (5-6 cm) in depth <br> • Keep your elbows and arms locked with shoulders located directly over the patient's body |
| 7 | Continue providing compressions and breaths in a 30:2 ratio until either ALS arrives or you have made the decision to rapidly transport to avoid delay on scene |
| 8 | If the AED has restored the pulse, check the patient continually for a pulse. If the pulse disappears, repeat the CPR/AED steps. |

Some EMS systems are performing what is called **cardiocerebral resuscitation**, or CCR. Unlike CPR, the CCR technique provides *no rescue breaths* in the first 5–10 minutes after cardiac arrest. Instead, the focus is on performing continuous chest compressions at a rate of 100–120/min. CCR has shown positive results in resuscitation in some studies. As always, however, the EMT must follow the local protocols.

## Discontinuing CPR and Biological Death

The goal of CPR is a return of spontaneous circulation (ROSC), in which a pulse comes back and the person experiencing cardiac arrest recovers. Sometimes, however, a patient will not achieve ROSC despite the EMT's best efforts.

**Stop doing CPR** in the following situations:

- Patient obtains and maintains ROSC
- Verified and legal DNR (do not resuscitate) order has been produced
- Physician has ordered discontinuation of CPR
- Signs of obvious biological death are present:
  - Decapitation of the head
  - Rigor mortis/rigidity of body
  - Lividity (blue bruise-like coloring) in the trunk of body or extremities
  - Decomposition of the entire body
  - Burns that damage the person beyond recognition and no pulse or breathing

Certain EMS systems allow for their providers to initiate a "field termination" after meeting criteria laid out by their protocols. Other systems require a physician to order cessation of efforts done.

Regarding the **do not resuscitate (DNR) order**, each state has its own rules on what makes a DNR valid or not. Typically, they all follow some general rules:

- A physician must physically sign the paper.
- The patient's full legal name must be included.
- It must be dated; some papers will have expiration dates to rediscuss options.

Some states may also require the following:

- DNR must be on a specific form (which may or may not be colored)
- Paper must be produced within 2 minutes before resuscitation efforts commence
- Some may only withhold compressions but will allow artificial ventilation efforts
- Provide a photograph of the patient for additional verification against the name on the form

As always, be familiar with your system's protocols and standards.

# Altered Mental Status and Strokes

## Altered Mental Status

Altered mental status (AMS), also called altered level of consciousness (ALOC), is an umbrella term for any type of behavior that is abnormal from the patient's baseline mental function. Causes vary widely and range from cerebral hemorrhage to trauma, drug overdose, and many disease processes.

The EMT's goal is to determine the root cause of the AMS and try to fix the presenting symptoms. The only way to find the root cause is to do a proper and thorough assessment.

AMS patients are generally not alert and oriented. Thus, they are unable to provide the EMT with very reliable information. In a patient who is somewhat conscious, AMS makes it difficult to communicate. For instance, the patient may struggle to describe signs and symptoms. A patient with AMS may give vague answers; they may know that something is wrong but be unable to pinpoint exactly what that "something" is.

Available bystanders, especially those who know the patient, can provide very useful information by doing the following:

- Verifying that the information given by the patient is correct
- Attesting to the patient's baseline mental status
- Giving details that can "fill in the blanks" about the situation

Keep in mind that AMS may be just one of multiple problems going on at once. Don't let a distracting injury or illness deter you from finding out why the injury/illness occurred in the first place. Consider these examples:

- Suppose you give a presumed hypoglycemic patient oral glucose in the proper dosage, but she does not respond as you would expect (which would be to wake up and become alert and oriented). Now suppose you do a complete neurological check, noting left arm drift. Now you would suspect a stroke in addition to the hypoglycemic event.
- Suppose you are dispatched to a fall victim who has an open femur fracture. You may be tempted to deal with just the injury. If you did,  though, you would not find out that the fall was caused by a stroke whose symptoms came on suddenly.

Doing a thorough assessment can catch issues that might otherwise be dismissed. This is especially true with repeat 911 callers, even though EMS providers may be tempted to shortcut an assessment because "they were fine the last few times we came."

A helpful mnemonic to remember the potential causes of AMS is **AEIOU-TIPS**:

- **A**—alcohol
- **E**—epilepsy *(seizures)*
- **I**—insulin *(diabetic issues?)*
- **O**—overdose *(too much of a drug?)*
- **U**—underdose/uremia *(too little or no dose of a drug? toxin buildup from renal disease?)*
- **T**—toxins/trauma/temperature
- **I**—infection *(sepsis? pneumonia? urinary tract infection?)*
- **P**—psychosis/poisoning *(carbon monoxide? pesticides?)*
- **S**—stroke

Every patient should receive a complete assessment to help guide their treatment plan. Using the AEIOU-TIPS as a checklist of potential causes will help the EMT to determine what plan to follow or if ALS should be considered.

## Stroke

According to the American Stroke Association, strokes are the fifth leading cause of death and disability in the United States, killing approximately 142,000 people a year. On average, every 40 seconds, someone suffers a stroke. So it is conceivable that an EMT will be called to a scene for "stroke-like symptoms."

A stroke, also called cerebrovascular accident (CVA), is the sudden death of brain cells due to lack of oxygen. It occurs when the blood flow through an artery to the brain is blocked or ruptures. The three main types of strokes are:

- **Ischemic**—caused by a blockage in a cerebral artery
- **Hemorrhagic**—caused a blood vessel rupture, bleeds freely
- **Transient ischemic attack (TIA)**—a "ministroke," which is a warning sign that a larger stroke will occur

Whatever the cause of the stroke, the acronym **FAST** summarizes the signs and symptoms to pay attention to; these are also known as the Cincinnati Prehospital Stroke Scale (CPSS).

Pay attention to what is a normal versus an abnormal response. If the patient gives an abnormal response, it is considered a positive sign for this scale. In this context, *positive* doesn't mean "good" but, rather, that the sign or symptom is present in the patient at time of testing.

**Table 6.5** FAST Acronym to Describe Testing for Stroke-Like Symptoms

| LETTER | WHAT TO LOOK FOR |
|---|---|
| **F**: Face | Ask the patient to smile.<br><br>• Do both corners of the mouth turn upward and equally? *(normal)*<br>• Does it appear as if one side of the face is lower/unequal to the other side?<br>• Is the patient's face numb?<br><br>* Note that a condition called **Bell palsy**, a temporary or permanent paralysis of a facial nerve, may also cause facial droop. This is **not** a positive sign for stroke. |
| **A**: Arm drift | Ask the patient to raise both the arms in front of the body and hold them there for at least 5 seconds.<br><br>• Is the patient able to hold both arms up without dropping down? *(normal)*<br>• Is the patient able to lift only one arm and not the other? |
| **S**: Speech | Ask the patient to repeat back to you a simple sentence such as "The sky is blue."<br><br>• Does the patient repeat the words in the same order, without difficulty? *(normal)*<br>• Does the patient repeat the words out of order?<br>• Does the patient repeat the same words, or are they different?<br>• Does the patient repeat the sentence but really struggle?<br>• Does the patient slur the words?<br>• Is the patient unable to speak? |
| **T**: Time | Ask the patient (or bystander) the following important questions:<br><br>• When did the symptoms start?<br>• When was the last time the patient was seen without these symptoms?<br>• If this was a TIA where symptoms have resolved, how long did the symptoms last before EMS arrived and with what frequency? |

Some medical practitioners add two more letters describing additional symptoms to look out for, producing the acronym **BE FAST**. (The American Stroke Association still recommends the scale as already described, however.) These are:

- **B**—balance (have there been sudden balance issues?)
- **E**—eyes (has there been a sudden change or loss of vision in one or both eyes?)

Still other stroke scales are circulating in the medical world as well. Depending on where you practice as an EMT, you may run across them and be required to calculate with them:

- **RACE**—Rapid Arterial Occlusion Evaluation
- **LAMS**—Los Angeles Motor Score
- **LAPSS**—Los Angeles Prehospital Stroke Screen
- **MEND**—Miami Emergency Neurological Deficit
- **NIHSS**—National Institutes of Health Stroke Scale

Whatever scale is used, it is up to the EMT (as always) to know and understand the components that go into the stroke scale that their particular service or hospital prefers. Time is brain, so use your time with the patient wisely.

### Transient Ischemic Attack (TIA)

TIA, often called a "ministroke," is a temporary period of stroke-like symptoms. TIAs usually last only a few minutes and do not cause permanent damage; many symptoms resolve completely within 24 hours. However, they are a warning sign of an impending stroke. According to the Mayo Clinic, about 1 in 3 people who have a transient ischemic attack will eventually have a stroke. Of these, about half occur within a year after the TIA symptoms originally appeared.

The EMT who is called to a scene for stroke-like symptoms may arrive to find a patient who presents with no deficits, though the patient (or a bystander) describes stroke symptoms that resolved prior to arrival. While this leaves the EMT with little to test, that is not an excuse to sign a refusal and leave. Rather, do a proper assessment and thorough questioning. Better yet, try to convince the patient to transport to the hospital for further assessment, which patients may be reluctant to do if they believe they are now asymptomatic. Though it may not happen that day or that week, having a TIA strongly indicates that a CVA is coming.

## Shock and Sepsis

### The Many Forms of Shock

Shock is best defined as inadequate perfusion and blood flow to the body's peripheral tissues, which leads to cellular and tissue hypoxia if not corrected. Perfusion, or the act of delivering oxygenated red blood cells to tissues and organs, requires intact cardiovascular and respiratory systems. If there is a breakdown within either system, shock will occur.

This table examines four broad categories of shock resulting from problems with the body's pump, vessel, or fluids.

**Table 6.6** Types of Shock

| TYPE OF SHOCK | DESCRIPTION AND EXAMPLES |
|---|---|
| Distributive | Fluid problem caused by vasodilation and increased/decreased movement of fluids (typically blood):<br><br>• Anaphylaxis—widespread, allergen-triggered vasodilation and movement of fluid out of the blood and into the tissues<br>• Neurogenic—sudden loss of the sympathetic nervous system signals to the smooth muscle in vessel walls, which leads to a drop in vascular resistance and hypotension<br>• Sepsis—widespread infection that travels via the blood throughout the body |
| Hypovolemic | Fluid problem marked by loss of adequate volumes to keep the heart beating properly:<br><br>• Blood from trauma (internal or external)<br>• Blood from nontraumatic injuries (ulcers, GI bleed)<br>• Excessive vomiting<br>• Burns and fluid shifts<br>• Diarrhea<br>• Excessive perspiration (sweating) |
| Cardiogenic | Pump problem caused by heartbeat malfunction or cessation, such as:<br><br>• Myocardial infarction<br>• Trauma, such as myocardial contusion<br>• Metabolic disorders that cause arrhythmias<br>• Pulmonary embolism located in the pulmonary vessels leading from the heart |
| Obstructive | Vessel and pump problem caused by obstruction of the normal flow of blood:<br><br>• Cardiac tamponade—prevents blood from entering the heart<br>• Pneumothorax—increased pressure within the thoracic cavity blocks the flow of blood<br>• Pulmonary embolism—blockage in the pulmonary vessels impeding blood flow back into the heart<br>• Local plaque buildup or plug from another location that lodges in a cardiac vessel, blocking normal blood flow |

As shock continues over time, it progresses through a sequence of stages.

**Table 6.7** Stages of Shock

| STAGE OF SHOCK | DESCRIPTION AND SIGNS/SYMPTOMS |
|---|---|
| Stage 1 (compensated) | The body first senses something is wrong and attempts to self-correct:<br><br>• Heart starts to beat faster<br>• Blood vessels constrict (vasoconstriction), directing circulating blood to the heart and brain<br>• Respiratory rate increases to bring in more oxygen<br><br>The patient with compensated shock may or may not be symptomatic. With quick recognition and aggressive treatment, this stage can often be reversed. |
| Stage 2 (decompensated) | The natural compensation mechanisms begin to fail:<br><br>• Blood pressure falls (systolic of 90 mm Hg or lower in adults)<br>• Peripheral pulses are weak, thready, or absent<br>• Mental status decreases<br>• Breathing becomes irregular (tachycardia and tachypnea)<br>• Skin color changes (becomes pallid, ashy, or cyanotic)<br><br>Reversing this stage is not impossible, but treatment must be aggressive. |
| Stage 3 (irreversible) | Poor perfusion has existed long enough to cause permanent damage to the body's organs and tissues. Cellular death is occurring systemically, and death is the ultimate conclusion. |

## Sepsis (The "Silent Shock")

Sepsis is a cascade of inappropriate immune responses to the presence of an infection in the blood. It can lead to tissue damage, organ failure, amputations, and death.

---

Sepsis is the third-leading cause of death in the United States. Over 1.5 million cases occur per year, with nearly 270,000 deaths. Of all hospital deaths in the United States, 1 in 3 is caused by sepsis.

---

This means that you must be aware of the signs and symptoms of sepsis, as you may very well come into contact with patients experiencing this progressive condition on the job as an EMT. It is especially prevalent in nursing homes and in patients who already have compromised immune systems. However, anyone may develop sepsis; it is not specific to any certain demographic.

### Sepsis Severity

The following table shows the diagnostic criteria for tiers of sepsis in order of increasing severity. While the criteria for each tier include laboratory values for blood work, these are generally unavailable in the prehospital setting. In practice, BLS vital signs are the only clues available for EMTs to identify sepsis.

**Table 6.8** Levels of Sepsis Severity

| TIERED LEVEL | CRITERIA |
|---|---|
| Systemic inflammation response syndrome (SIRS) | 2 or more are required to be considered positive:<br>• Heart rate (HR) >90 per minute<br>• Temperature >100.4°F (38.0°C) or <96.8°F (36°C)<br>• Respiratory rate (RR) >20 per minute |
| SIRS + Source of infection = Sepsis | Any sign of infection (external or internal):<br>• Does the patient have any wounds?<br>• Does the patient have pneumonia or another previously diagnosed bacterial infection?<br>• Is the patient currently taking antibiotics, and if so, for what purpose? |
| Severe sepsis | Sepsis + 1 or more of the following:<br>• Systolic blood pressure <90 mm Hg or a drop >40 mm Hg<br>• Organ dysfunction<br>• Hypoperfusion (shock) symptoms |
| Septic shock | Severe sepsis + persistent hypotension despite adequate fluid resuscitation*<br><br>(*This level of treatment is done by ALS or hospital personnel) |

### qSOFA Sepsis Scoring

Some EMS systems are now having prehospital providers generate a predictive sepsis score. The quickSOFA, or qSOFA, is a numerical identifier for patients with suspected infection who are at greater risk for sepsis with a potentially poor outcome outside the intensive care unit (ICU).

The qSOFA was designed for rapid use by prehospital providers such as EMTs. In-hospital clinicians evaluate a patient's risk of developing sepsis using the Sequential Organ Failure Assessment score (SOFA) score, a lengthy and highly detailed scoring system that involves multiple bloodwork results and lab tests. In the prehospital setting, the qSOFA scores a patient's sepsis risk using a much shorter list of criteria, shown in the table.

**Table 6.9** qSOFA criteria

| CRITERIA | POINTS |
|---|---|
| Low blood pressure (systolic <100 mm Hg) | 1 |
| Elevated respiratory rate ( >22 breaths per min) | 1 |
| Altered mental status (Glasgow Coma Scale <15) | 1 |

Adapted from https://qsofa.org/what.php

The qSOFA score ranges from 0–3 points. A score of 2 or more qSOFA points near the onset of infection is associated with a greater risk of death or prolonged care in ICU.

EMS plays a vital role in delivering crucial information that will ultimately streamline the process of definitive patient care, leading to better overall outcomes.

### KEY TAKEAWAY

Many EMS systems have now included a "sepsis alert" system in the prehospital radio report. It is similar to calling in your regular radio report, but you would add that you believe your patient meets sepsis criteria or that you have reasonable suspicion of it. Sepsis alerts are statistically proven to result in faster blood testing for the patient along with specific treatments aimed at stopping or slowing the sepsis cascade.

## Diabetes, Seizures, and Allergies

### Diabetes

Diabetes mellitus (DM) is a disease of the endocrine system that inhibits the body's ability to metabolize sugar. The organ that is responsible for insulin production is the pancreas, specifically in the islets of Langerhans cells. If these cells are impaired or damaged, insulin production will be affected.

Patients may or may not be on chronic medications that are either delivered by injection or in tablet or capsule format. Many patients who check their own blood glucose levels (BGL) using a glucometer on a daily basis are knowledgeable about their condition and can answer questions for the EMT.

The normal range of blood sugar is 80–120 mg/dL, although the range in patients with chronic diabetes may be much wider before physical symptoms occur.

Depending on the textbook used or medical authority cited, students may see different **"normal ranges" for blood sugar**. For example:

- 70–100 mg/dL (according to the World Health Organization)
- 80–130 mg/dL (according to the American Diabetic Association)

Because of these differences, it is common to see a "normal range" that is in the middle—i.e., 80–120 mg/dL, as used in this book. On the exam, abnormal values will be far enough outside all of these limits to be clearly abnormal, regardless of which "normal range" might be used.

The following table describes the various types of diabetes.

**Table 6.10** Types of Diabetes

| TYPE OF DIABETES | KEY FACTS |
|---|---|
| Type 1 (juvenile diabetes or insulin-dependent diabetes mellitus [IDDM]) | • Less common (5–10% of patients with diabetes)<br>• Typically diagnosed in adolescence but can appear at any age<br>• Results from the pancreas producing little to no insulin<br>• Requires lifelong medication management by daily injections of insulin or by utilizing an insulin pump |
| Type 2 (adult-onset or insulin-resistant diabetes) | • More common<br>• Chronic condition that affects the way the body processes blood sugar<br>• Body produces insufficient amounts of insulin or resists insulin<br>• May be "cured" or effectively managed by making lifestyle changes such as healthier diet and exercise<br>• Patients may take pills or capsules, rather than injectable insulin |
| Gestational diabetes | • Diagnosed during pregnancy and may resolve after delivery<br>• Some women may take insulin, but not all<br>• Often causes baby to be extra large<br>• Patients are more prone to hypertension or hypoglycemic events<br>• Patients are at higher risk of developing type 2 diabetes later in life |
| Prediabetes | • Blood sugar level is higher than it should be but not high enough for the doctor to diagnose type 2 diabetes<br>• All ages and genders can be affected<br>• Lifestyle changes can reverse or halt progression<br>• Patients are typically asymptomatic<br>• One possible sign is darkened skin on certain parts of the body, such as the neck, armpits, elbows, knees, and knuckles |

### Hypoglycemia

Hypoglycemia presents when blood sugar levels drop below 70–80 mg/dL. This is most often caused by taking the prescribed dosage of insulin and not following up with the regular ingestion of food as prescribed, causing the blood sugar to drop. On the other hand, the patient may have missed an insulin dosage or have not eaten a meal recently. Some additional causes could be vomiting, unusual exercise, and ingestion of alcohol. Any of these can cause the patient to either behave strangely or suddenly become unconscious.

Treatment at the BLS level includes oral glucose, oxygen, shock management, and rapid transport if symptoms do not improve or the patient is unresponsive/unconscious. Follow your local protocols as indicated.

Signs and symptoms of hypoglycemia include:

- Shakiness/dizziness
- Irritability, anxiety, nervousness, combativeness
- Hunger
- Headache
- Slurred words/altered mental status/confusion
- Muscle weakness
- Blurred vision
- Staggered gait
- Clammy or diaphoretic skin
- Convulsions or seizures

---

#### KEY TAKEAWAY

**Patients may wear a MedicAlert bracelet or other medical jewelry** that identifies them as having diabetes. Actively look for identifiers of this type when doing an assessment of the patient. Benefits of locating any medical jewelry include:

- Saving time
- Helping you develop a treatment plan more rapidly
- Helping you advocate on the patient's behalf, since law enforcement personnel or other bystanders may not understand the symptoms of hypoglycemia

---

Treatment is as follows:

- Most state protocols will allow the EMT to administer oral **glucose** to patients who present with symptoms of hypoglycemia and are conscious. If the symptoms are the result of hypoglycemia, the patient will usually respond very quickly to the oral sugar.
- Some state protocols will allow the EMT to administer **glucagon** via intramuscular injection. Glucagon is a protein that causes sugar stored in the liver to be released into the bloodstream (and consequently is ineffective in patients with chronic liver disease, such as cirrhosis or hepatitis).

---

Not all states allow **glucagon administration** at the BLS level, and it is not included in the EMT National Standard Curriculum. However, as each state is independent in making its own protocols, this may be allowed as indicated.

---

### Hyperglycemia

Defined as high blood sugar, hyperglycemia doesn't cause symptoms until glucose values are significantly elevated—usually above 180–200 mg/dL. Some glucometers will just state "HIGH" and, depending on the manufacturer, that could indicate levels of 400–600 mg/dL.

Treatment at the BLS level includes shock management, oxygen if indicated, and rapid transport if symptoms do not improve or become worse. ALS intervention may also be indicated for airway and cardiac management. Follow your local protocols as indicated.

Signs and symptoms of hyperglycemia include:

- Frequent thirst (polydipsia)
- Frequent urination (polyuria)
- Increased hunger (polyphagia)
- A fruity odor on the breath (ketone production)
- Shortness of breath or tachypnea

The longer blood sugar levels stay high, the more serious the symptoms become. High blood sugar levels can lead to conditions such as diabetic ketoacidosis (DKA).

## Glucometer Usage

Many states now allow basic EMS units to carry portable glucometers that enable the EMT to gauge the blood glucose level (BGL) accurately. This may be especially important to the treating physician, as it will give a baseline blood sugar reading prior to any intervention by EMS.

Patients may also have their own glucometers, and you can use their reading to compare to your own results. Be aware that different manufacturers have different reading thresholds, so there may be slight variances in numerical results.

To check the BGL level, follow these steps:

1. Gather your materials: glucometer, collecting strips, lancet, alcohol prep pad, gauze pad, and adhesive bandage.
2. Insert the collection strip into the glucometer, and make sure that the machine is ready to collect the blood, typically shown with a blood drop icon.
3. Select the finger you will use to collect blood; clean the fingertip with the alcohol prep pad for at least 15 seconds.
4. Remove the safety mechanism of the lancet so that the needle is ready to deploy.
5. While holding the finger still, press the lancet (needle side down) onto the fleshy part of the underside or lateral side of the finger, deploying the needle.
6. Wipe away the first drop of blood with the gauze pad.
7. Gently squeeze the finger to produce fresh blood, and place the collecting strip directly into the blood drop; make sure the blood is drawn up completely into the strip and the glucometer indicates it is reading the results.
8. Place an adhesive bandage onto the finger, and read the glucometer results; record them in your documentation.
9. Throw away any trash produced, and place the used lancet into the sharps container.

## Seizures

Seizures, or involuntary muscular activity, may have many different causes, such as high fevers, hypoglycemia, head injuries, or brain diseases, including epilepsy. Any age or gender may experience a seizure, and the EMT may be called to an event in progress or the aftereffects of one.

Seizure activity falls into two main categories—generalized onset and focal onset. Generalized onset affects both sides of the brain or groups of cells on both sides of the brain at the same time. Focal onset can start in one area or group of cells in one side of the brain.

Keep in mind that as neuroscience progresses, there may be more categories or types of seizures being named or refined into categories. The following table attempts to list the more common type of seizure activity the EMT may be called to assist with.

**Table 6.11** Types of Seizure by Category

| SEIZURE CATEGORY | TYPES OF SEIZURE |
|---|---|
| Generalized onset seizure | • Absence (formerly known as petit mal)<br>• Tonic-clonic (formerly known as grand mal)<br>• Atonic (no shaking, only muscle weakness)<br>• Febrile (caused by high fever, typically in children)<br>• Status epilepticus |
| Focal onset seizure | • Simple focal (also known as simple partial)<br>• Complex focal (also known as a complex partial)<br>• Myoclonic (sudden movements lasting less than a few seconds at a time) |

**Absence seizure** causes rapid blinking or a few seconds of staring into space. Typically, the person may not even know they have had seizure activity, which is noticed by bystanders first. A person may have multiple episodes in a day.

**Tonic-clonic seizure** (the type most familiar to people) has two phases: In the tonic portion, the body becomes rigid. In the clonic portion, there is uncontrollable jerking motion. Episodes may last a few seconds or several minutes. A person may finish one seizure and have another one shortly afterward.

**Prolonged seizure** (known as status epilepticus) is a true medical emergency since patients will begin to develop a lack of oxygen to the brain that could result in brain damage or brain death. This condition is defined as a continuous seizure lasting >30 minutes or 2 or more seizures without full recovery of consciousness between any of them. This is why it is vitally important to ask the patient or bystanders how long the seizure activity has lasted and record their answers.

Most seizures are of short duration, and the active portion of the seizure has usually subsided by the time EMS arrives on the scene. Seizures are followed by a period of unconsciousness or semiconsciousness referred to as the **postictal phase**. In this phase, the patient may be confused, possibly combative, or take longer to answer questions than what is typically considered baseline for them. Be patient as this phase can last from 5–30 minutes or longer depending on the person.

Treatment of the seizure patient is shown in the table.

**Table 6.12** BLS Seizure Treatment

| PHASE | BLS TREATMENT |
|---|---|
| Actively seizing | • Request ALS, as they have medications to help control seizures<br>• Move the patient to a safe area or clear away any objects nearby, especially near the head (that the patient could strike)<br>• Have suction ready, as the airway may become compromised<br>• Give the patient high-flow oxygen via NRB, from 12–15 LPM, to help with increased consumption by the brain<br>• Do not attempt to stick anything in or remove (prior) objects from the patient's mouth<br>• If this is not a chronic problem for the patient, you may have to provide emotional support for family members or bystanders, who may never have witnessed a seizure and so are very confused; it can be very scary for them, and they may need reassurance about what is happening<br>• Be prepared for recurrence<br>• Make the decision to stay on scene vs. transport, especially if ALS is farther away than the hospital |
| Postictal | • Be prepared to ventilate or clear the airway if necessary<br>• If the patient remains confused >20 minutes after a seizure, consider another cause of AMS and call ALS if indicated<br>• Ask how long each seizure lasted, how many they had, and what were they doing before the seizure happened<br>• Administer oxygen via NRB at 12–15 LPM if you haven't already done so |

Transport of the seizure patient follows the usual pattern of assuring a patent airway and placing the patient on their side (recumbent) in the event of vomiting. If the EMT cannot rule out the possibility of trauma, then the patient is secured with a cervical collar, head blocks, and a spine board to guard against spinal cord injury. The patient is then transported supine and the entire board is rolled in the event of vomiting.

Remember that seizures may be caused by head trauma, and a GCS score would be appropriate in this scenario.

## Allergic Reaction

An allergic reaction is an exaggerated immune system response by the body to a substance. The most common substances that cause allergies are insect bites/stings, nuts, shellfish, medications, and certain plants. However, any substance can be an allergen, depending on the body's response to it.

A possible allergic reaction (anaphylaxis) should be suspected if the patient reports tingling and heat in the face, mouth, or extremities; severe itching; visible hives; flushed skin; and/or swelling to the extremities. The main concern is to ensure that the airway does not swell shut and prevent the patient from breathing; therefore, dispatches to possible allergic reactions are always treated as priority calls.

Other symptoms of anaphylaxis may include:

- Chest tightness and pressure
- Prolonged, uncontrolled coughing
- Tachypnea
- Dyspnea
- Hoarseness, stridor, audible wheezing
- Rapid pulse rate
- Low blood pressure (as the body attempts to regulate its response to the allergen)

If the reactions include altered mental status, then hypoxia and hypoperfusion may be severe, and immediate treatment is indicated.

---

Anaphylaxis often begins as dyspnea. So airway management is the most important step in management of possible anaphylaxis.

---

After you perform an initial assessment and treat any necessary conditions, proceed to the focused assessment. There you must be alert to any history of past allergic reactions, the events that immediately preceded the symptoms that prompted the call to the EMS system, and whether those events were related to past allergic reactions.

Food allergies may be particularly insidious in this regard. For example, a person with a severe allergy to nuts will avoid nuts, but nut by-products may be used in the processing of other foods and may cause a surprise reaction.

Treatment is, first, a complete focused assessment, baseline vital signs, and the administration of oxygen. If the patient is having difficulty breathing, epinephrine is indicated. If the patient is not symptomatic and is breathing adequately, you may see if there is a visible injection site. If you do, scraping away the stinger is indicated and can be done using a credit card or similar item. Be careful not to use tweezers when trying to remove a stinger as they could inadvertently squeeze a venom sac that may still be attached to the end of the stinger.

If epinephrine is indicated, it will reverse the effects of severe anaphylaxis long enough to transport the patient to a medical facility. It constricts the blood vessels and increases the heart rate to help raise the blood pressure and combat hypoperfusion syndrome. Remember to do the following:

- See if the patient is carrying an epinephrine syringe. If yes, the patient should have been instructed in its usage and administration route, perhaps even administering it prior to the EMT's arrival.
  - Some jurisdictions allow the EMT to administer an epinephrine syringe after consulting medical control if the patient has not already done so or has had no relief with the first injection.
  - Check the "5 rights" before administering.

- After administration, reassess the patient and note any changes in their condition.
  - If the patient had trouble breathing and airway swelling earlier, and if both have responded to the epinephrine, that usually confirms the assessment of anaphylaxis.
- Advise the receiving facility of the outcome of your intervention.

## Poisoning and Overdose

A poison is defined as any substance that produces harmful physiological or psychological effects to the body. According to the National Safety Council, poisoning is responsible for approximately 10% of all emergency department admissions in the United States. Overdose is when serious physiological and psychological effects occur from the overuse or misuse of any substance by exceeding safe dosages. The substance may be a legal substance, such as alcohol, or an illegal substance, such as cocaine or heroin.

The stereotypical poisoning case is that of the child who gets into the cleaning supplies beneath the sink, a relatively infrequent EMS dispatch. In reality, most EMTs deal with a large number of calls involving either alcohol overdose or the use of illegal drugs.

Poisons may enter the body in a variety of ways:

- **Ingestion** is when the substance is taken by mouth, such as drinking a toxic substance or taking pills.
- **Inhalation** is when the substance is inhaled into the lungs, such as breathing in poisons like carbon monoxide from car exhaust in a closed space or snorting cocaine.
- **Injection** involves placing the substance directly into the bloodstream using a hypodermic syringe, as with injecting heroin.
- **Absorption** occurs when toxins enter the body by contact with the skin, such as with poison ivy or pesticide poisoning.

Signs and symptoms of poisoning vary depending on the poison and how the body reacts to it. The EMT must be prepared to intervene if there is a sudden change in the patient's condition and to perform basic life support functions as needed. If good scene and patient assessments are done, the EMT may know what the specific poison is and be in a better position to begin treatment while en route to the emergency department.

A resource that is available to both the public and medical professionals, including EMS, is poison control. There are national numbers as well as state-run hotlines. They are available 24 hours a day, 7 days a week and can help guide treatment for both ALS and BLS providers alike.

## Scene Assessment

The EMT should be proactive in trying to determine why the patient is presenting with specific symptoms, as that knowledge may well be the difference between a successful outcome and sudden patient death:

- If you arrive at the scene of a woman down, unconscious in her bed, with bradypnea, bradycardia, pale, diaphoretic, and unresponsive, she could be the victim of a number of medical problems.

- If you notice an empty pill bottle of Percocet next to the bed, you may suspect an opioid overdose and should notify the receiving facility of this finding, which will expedite treatment in the ER.

Without that initial assessment, the receiving facility would have to perform a wide range of initial tests and could potentially lose critical time.

If you are unsure of a medication name, use reference material or do a quick online search on your cell phone to identify the drug. Be sure to use a medically oriented, verified source and not just any popular website.

Another part of a complete assessment is to bring to the receiving facility any identifying containers or labels. These may contain the chemical information necessary for treatment as well as indicate the amount of the poison ingested by the patient.

## Treatment of Poisoning

Treatment of suspected poisoning will follow the usual protocol of assessing and treating the basic life support functions. If the poison is known, basic protocols may allow treatments in the prehospital setting with proper medical control:

- Activated charcoal (oral administration), depending on the poison and the amount of time since ingestion:
  - Activated charcoal is ground charcoal in a suspension of water, forming an aqueous slurry
  - May cause vomiting but is otherwise benign
- Naloxone (or Narcan), an opioid-reversal (antagonist) medication (used routinely in EMS):
  - Can be delivered as intranasal (IN) or intramuscular (IM) by BLS
  - Dosage for IN: 2 mg/mL (1 mg per nostril)
  - Dosage for IM: 0.4 mg/0.4 mL in lateral thigh
  - Protocol will dictate how many, if any, repeat dosages can be given by the EMT

If the patient is actively vomiting (or has previously done so), this is more problematic if the poison is caustic, corrosive, or a petroleum product. These poisons will cause more damage to the esophageal passage as they come back up and thus are better treated by being neutralized in the stomach. Petroleum products may also cause problems in the lungs if their vapors are aspirated.

**Syrup of ipecac**, which is still sold in pharmacies today, is not used in EMS routinely and is not included in the National Standard Curriculum for EMTs as a standard medication administered.

Emergency care for poisoning and overdose involves good basic life support: maintaining an airway, adequate oxygen perfusion, and circulatory support if necessary. A complete initial assessment followed by a comprehensive focused assessment is crucial to good prehospital care. As always, scene safety is crucial. Be aware of the following:

- In the case of bee sting, if the bees are still swarming, the scene is not safe and should not be entered unless the EMT is wearing suitable protective equipment. If the EMT is safe, the patient must be removed as expeditiously as possible from the unsafe condition.

- In the case of carbon monoxide poisoning, the EMT must be aware of the lethality of the odorless gas in a closed space. If the scene is safe, the EMT can transport the poisoned individual to a receiving facility with a hyperbaric chamber, a device helpful in treating carbon monoxide poisoning.

## Environmental Emergencies

In order to function properly, the human body consistently maintains an average internal temperature of ~98.6°F (37°C).

Note that the key word in the previous sentence is *average*. Some people may normally run a slightly lower or slightly higher internal temperature as their baseline; a person slightly outside the average may be either asymptomatic or in distress. However, for diagnostic purposes, most medical professionals use 98.6°F (37°C) as the starting point.

When writing or reading temperatures, if you are not already aware, F is shorthand for Fahrenheit while C is shorthand for Celsius. The United States is one of the few countries in the world that uses Fahrenheit as its standard of measurement. So if you come across something written in Celsius, you may have to convert it in the field.

Core temperatures are considered the most accurate. This is achieved by measuring internally with a rectal thermometer. Rest assured, however, that most EMS systems do not use these types of thermometers; rather, oral, tympanic (ear), or axillary (armpit) options are more commonly used.

In a hot or cold emergency, energy may be transferred in a variety of ways.

**Table 6.13** Pathways of Heat Energy Transfer

| TYPE OF ENERGY TRANSFER | KEY FACTS |
|---|---|
| Radiation | • Heat is given off into an area or object that has a lower temperature than the radiating object<br><br>Example: a person standing outdoors in subfreezing temperatures radiates heat to the surrounding cold atmosphere, primarily through the extremities |
| Convection | • Heat or energy is transferred through a fluid (gas or liquid) from high temperature to low temperature by molecular movement<br><br>Example: when blood circulates, heat is generated by the cells in the body and then transferred to air or water that is flowing over the skin (which explains why we will feel chilly if a cool wind blows over our arms when we are sweating) |
| Conduction | • Heat is passed through a colder object by direct contact<br><br>Example: water conducts heat 240 times faster than air, which is why a person immersed in cold water is subject to rapid hypothermia |
| Evaporation | • Liquid absorbs surrounding energy and changes into a gas, reducing the temperature of the surface that it escapes<br>• A type of latent heat transfer<br><br>Example: the process of perspiring (sweating) is one of the regulatory mechanisms the body uses to maintain normal temperature |
| Condensation | • Gas condenses to form liquid droplets, releasing heat energy<br>• A type of latent heat transfer<br><br>Example: steam condenses on skin, releasing heat and causing a steam burn (scalding) |

## Hypothermia

Hypothermia (heat loss) is a loss of body temperature. It is a commonly seen situation in emergency medicine. The EMT might respond to a patient in a cold environment without suitable clothing or someone who has been rapidly immersed into cold water. Especially susceptible to this condition are the extremely young and the extremely old.

There are three levels of hypothermia a patient can experience:

- **Mild**—core temperature 90–95°F (32–35°C)
- **Moderate**—core temperature 82–90°F (28–32°C)
- **Severe**—core temperature below 82°F (28°C)

**Figure 6.1** Transfer of Heat Energy

Studies have shown that exposed flesh will freeze in <1 minute at −70°F (−56.7°C). Although this temperature is not common in the continental United States, that has the same effect as −20°F (−28.9°C) + a wind of 25-30 mph, which is a common winter condition in the northern United States.

Gradual hypothermia progresses through five stages:

- **Stage 1**—the body shivers as it attempts to raise its core temperature by the activity
- **Stage 2**—mental apathy and loss of motor functions begin to occur
- **Stage 3**—decreased level of responsiveness; freezing of the extremities
- **Stage 4**—vital signs begin to decrease and slow
- **Stage 5**—death

Assessment of hypothermia by the EMT includes the following:

- Feel the patient's torso or abdomen, which will be the best indicator for a low core body temperature.
- If it feels cold to the touch, check verbal and motor responses, and note whether they are normal or impaired (and if so, to what degree).
- If shivering is present, the patient may be in stage 1. If shivering is absent, the patient may already be in stage 2 or 3.
- As hypothermia progresses, skin color will initially be red, then pale, and finally cyanotic or black. The skin will also become stiff and hard in the advanced stages.

Treatment of hypothermia starts with removing the patient from the cold environment and removing any wet clothing:

- Warm the patient gradually with blankets and warm-water bottles or hot packs to the groin, axillary, and cervical regions.
- Raise the ambient temperature of the truck as the patient is transported.
- Give supplemental oxygen at the highest level that the patient can tolerate.

Localized cold injuries, or frostbite, begin in the extremities and in any areas with poor circulation. The skin initially turns white and progresses to a waxy appearance as the injury progresses. The affected area feels frozen and rigid upon palpation, and swelling and blisters may be present. Treatment includes:

- Gradually rewarming the extremity (use a warm-water bath if there is a long or delayed transport)
- Be aware that the patient will complain of severe pain as the injured extremity begins to thaw
- To minimize long-term damage of the extremity, splinting may be needed.

## Hyperthermia

Hyperthermia is abnormally high body temperature. Heat gained exceeds heat lost, which can lead to a potentially fatal increase in the core body temperature. Specific types of hyperthermia are shown in the table.

**Table 6.14** Heat Emergencies

| TYPE OF HYPERTHERMIA | KEY FACTS AND TREATMENT |
|---|---|
| Heat cramps | • Muscle cramps caused by excessive body heat, which are not always due to strenuous activity<br>• Usually the first indicator of hyperthermia<br>• Treat by cooling the patient gradually |
| Heat exhaustion | • General weakness accompanied by warm skin and profuse sweating<br>• To transport, remove to a cooler environment and place in a semi-Fowler position<br>• Treat by cooling the patient gradually and increasing the air-conditioning |
| Heatstroke | • Severe hyperthermia caused by a failure of the body's cooling mechanism<br>• **Onset of altered mental status** (main difference between heat exhaustion and heatstroke)<br>• Skin might be hot + dry or hot + sweaty<br>• Treated by cooling the patient aggressively with cold, wet towels or ice packs to the groin, axillary, and cervical regions (done en route to the emergency department, i.e., do not delay transport) |

## Water Emergencies

Water emergencies present their own unique set of challenges to the EMT. Scene safety is always paramount, with the following guidelines:

- No rescue should ever be attempted that is beyond your skill level.
- First, try to throw an object or a flotation device to the victim.
- On open waters, attempt to use a boat if one is available.
- As a last resort, swimming out to a victim who is drowning should be undertaken only by a suitably trained rescuer.

As with any situation where the mechanism of injury is unknown, assume that the victim has suffered a traumatic injury and take the suitable spinal precautions. If the victim is breathing and has a pulse, consider placement on a spine board while still in the water. Note the following:

- A victim who has been immersed in cold water and who presents with no breathing or pulse should be given CPR immediately, as the mammalian diving reflex may have taken effect.

- A victim who has been in the water for less than 1 hour should receive resuscitation efforts. (In cold weather, patients have been resuscitated up to 2 hours after being submerged.)

If there is a problem ventilating a patient due to abdominal distension, the patient should be placed left lateral recumbent and gentle pressure should be applied to the abdomen to relieve the distension. Suction should be ready to assist in clearing the airway if fluid is vomited by this maneuver.

---

All mammals, including humans, have the **mammalian diving reflex**. The body has an innate physiological response to submersion in cold water. It selectively shuts down parts of the body, conserving oxygen while maintaining homeostasis within the body.

---

### Drowning Emergencies

According to the World Health Organization (WHO), drowning is the third leading cause of unintentional injury-related deaths worldwide, accounting for 7% of all injury-related deaths. Children, people who have increased contact with water, and males statistically are the most at risk for drowning incidents.

Studies suggest that the higher drowning rates among males are due to increased exposure to water and riskier behavior such as swimming alone, drinking alcohol before or during water activities, and boating accidents.

Children, on the other hand, typically have drowning emergencies due to either lack of supervision or accidental falls into a body of water. In fact, statistics show that drowning is the leading cause of death in children ages 1–4, with children 5–9 not far behind.

Anywhere there is a body of water that can allow for submersion of a head or body there is a risk of having a drowning incident. This can include buckets, bathtubs, pools, lakes, or even showers!

Treatment is the same regardless of what caused the drowning: If artificial respirations are required, they must be performed with adequate tidal volume and rate. If CPR is indicated, make sure the patient is out of the body of water and is on a hard surface for compressions. Make sure the chest is wiped clean of water before using an AED. Have suction ready to go for secretions or any water that may come up. If traumatic injuries are present, manage them appropriately. Finally, be prepared for hypothermia and shock management.

## Diving Emergencies

Although not always a common call, diving emergencies must be thoroughly explored by asking good assessment questions such as:

- "How long did it take the diver to ascend to the surface, and did the diver stop along the way?"
- "How deep and long was the dive?"
- "How long was it before the diver showed signs or symptoms?"
- "What type of breathing gas was the diver using?"

Types of emergencies that divers, trained veterans, or beginners alike can experience are described in the table.

**Table 6.15** Diving Emergencies and Systems Affected

| AFFECTED SYSTEM | ISSUES THAT CAN ARISE |
|---|---|
| Temperature | <ul><li>Needs to be regulated; certain types of clothing or protective gear can help or hinder this</li><li>In cold water, the body could automatically gasp for breath, which could escalate into hyperventilation and drowning</li><li>Heat loss and gain, plus dehydration can occur</li></ul> |
| Cardiac | <ul><li>Immersion into water (especially cold water) can cause arrhythmias leading to syncope or death</li><li>Nervousness or fright may cause tachypnea or tachycardia, especially if the diver is inexperienced</li></ul> |
| Respiratory | <ul><li>In cold-water temperatures, the body could automatically gasp for breath, which could escalate into hyperventilation and drowning</li><li>Expanding air due to pressure changes may rupture the lung and cause a pneumothorax<ul><li>Subcutaneous emphysema can result from air that escapes</li><li>Air emboli may travel to or form in the brain, causing syncope or stroke-like symptoms</li></ul></li><li>Pressure changes can cause injury to ears and sinuses</li></ul> |
| Musculoskeletal | <ul><li>Nitrogen can be forced into or released from tissues, depending on descent or ascent ("the bends"); the result is pain and death if not corrected</li><li>Traumatic injuries can occur if struck by objects or animals underwater</li></ul> |

Treatment includes thorough questioning, removing the patient from the environment using safety or possible spinal precautions, disconnecting equipment that will be in the provider's way, providing oxygen as necessary and indicated, and transport to the hospital.

Some divers may require the use a hyperbaric chamber that can safely reduce the pressure inside their body in a controlled manner, but not all hospitals have this capability. Refer to your local protocols for guidance and potential identification of such facilities.

## Bites and Stings

Bites and stings are treated as both wounds and possible injection poisonings. In addition, there is always the possibility of an allergic reaction.

Never attempt to "suck" out any venom with your mouth or the patient's. A tourniquet or pressure bandage above or below could help stop spread of the venom. The EMT may also wish to draw a circle around the bite using a pen or marker. Doing this can help determine if swelling or skin redness is growing by comparing the circle drawn to where the outside edges of the swelling or redness are located while en route. Transport to the most appropriate hospital or, if available in your service area, to a hospital that has an envenomation specialist on staff.

If bleeding is associated with the wound, control the bleeding as necessary using sterile gauze and bandages. Always remember to check and reassess pulse, motor function, and sensory abilities when bandaging any wounds.

If appropriate and indicated by local protocol, consider the usage of epinephrine and oxygen if respiratory symptoms are present.

Unless specifically directed by local protocol, do not attempt to collect or capture the animal that caused the bite or sting. This could result in injury to the EMT, not to mention there is no place to dispose of the animal, especially if it is still alive, in the hospital. Contact animal control or similar services to perform this task if necessary.

Keep good documentation, however, of the type of animal that caused the injury as this could be helpful information in treatment decisions at the hospital as well as in your own run report.

## Height and Climbing Emergencies

Activities such as climbing at elevations may involve emergencies requiring EMS assistance:

- Thermal emergency (hyperthermia/hypothermia), especially if wearing inappropriate clothing for the activity pursuing
- Musculoskeletal trauma, such as a twisted ankle, broken hand, shoulder dislocation, head injury, or spinal damage, if falling from a height
- Dehydration due to thermal emergency but also due to overexertion
- Exhaustion and/or confusion if the patient has gotten lost

Height matters with respect to documentation and also as a clue to the type of injury the person has suffered. Consider the following guidelines:

- Report ground-level falls as zero (0) feet.
- If the patient has fallen from a natural object or ladder, use the distance from lowest part of the body to the ground/surface. For instance, if the patient fell from the 5-inch step of a ladder, the fall was 5 inches. If the patient fell from a 12-foot tree onto the grass, the fall was 12 feet.

- Look for injury patterns that are not obvious visual injuries. With falls from heights, even if landing on the feet, energy can transfer from the feet, up the spine, and into other parts of the body, causing damage. Internal bones can become fractured as well. Use spinal precautions as directed by local protocols.

# Behavioral Emergencies

When an emergency doesn't fall into the category of a police situation or fire emergency, the default agency called is EMS. That includes what's called "behavioral emergencies," i.e., situations involving patients with psychiatric or emotional emergencies.

In the early days of EMS, there was very little training for patients with psychiatric or emotional problems even though EMS was the lead agency called. As a result, many EMS treatment protocols were developed over time, "after the fact."

The National Standard Curriculum mandates that the EMT be able to define "behavior" and "behavioral emergency":

- **Behavior** is defined as the "manner in which a person acts or performs; any or all activities of a person, including physical and mental activity."
- **Behavioral emergency** is defined as "a situation in which the patient exhibits abnormal behavior within a given situation that is unacceptable or intolerable to the patient, family, or community." Causes include:
  - Extremes of emotion, leading to violence or other inappropriate behavior.
  - A psychological or physical condition such as lack of oxygen or low blood sugar in diabetes.

Some behaviors are obviously unacceptable or intolerable. Threatening to commit suicide or threatening to violently assault another person are clear examples. These may be conscious, rational decisions, or they may be brought on by certain medical conditions in otherwise healthy individuals:

- Low blood sugar
- Anoxia
- Inadequate blood perfusion to the brain
- Head trauma
- Mind-altering substance
- Psychosis
- Excessive heat/cold

The key words in the definition of behavioral emergency are "unacceptable" or "intolerable." This is often a subjective determination. A person walking down the street naked and singing may be acceptable in a nudist camp but in any metropolitan area would likely be arrested or require EMS intervention.

Be aware of the standards of behavior in the community in which you practice.

The good news is that most behavioral emergency calls are usually nonviolent. A patient may have a panic attack, with a sudden irrational fear, or may be crying and unable to stop. However, some patients with mental illness may become violent, so you must be prepared to react quickly to ensure a safe environment for all, leading to the proper treatment of the patient.

## Common Psychological Crises

EMS may encounter several common psychological crises on the job. Any of these crises may pose a danger to the patient (increased risk of bodily harm due to risky or suicidal behavior) or to bystanders and responding EMTs.

**Table 6.16** Common Behavioral Emergencies

| PSYCHOLOGICAL ISSUE | DEFINITION AND MANIFESTATIONS |
|---|---|
| Anxiety or panic disorder | Agitation or unreasonable fear of current or future events <br><br>• Tachypnea; tachycardia; numbness/tingling of the extremities <br>• Mistrust of the provider <br>• Low oxygen saturation levels if hyperventilating |
| Phobia(s) | Irrational fear of (specific) things, places, or situations <br><br>• Hallucinations (auditory or visual) <br>• Tachypnea, tachycardia <br>• Mistrust of the provider or bystanders |
| Depression | Deep feelings of sadness, worthlessness, and discouragement with no sign of any relief <br><br>• Flat affect (monotone voice or animation of body) <br>• Suicidal thoughts <br>• Risky behavior such as use of illegal drugs, excessive alcohol consumption or self-harm, i.e., cutting or burning their skin <br>• Lack of desire to eat, drink, or do daily activities of living such as showering or cleaning <br>• Noncompliance with medication |

*(Continued)*

**Table 6.16** Common Behavioral Emergencies (*Continued*)

| PSYCHOLOGICAL ISSUE | DEFINITION AND MANIFESTATIONS |
|---|---|
| Bipolar disorder | Mood of extreme euphoria alternating with extreme depression (stages may last a few minutes to months at a time)<br><br>• Risky behaviors seen with depression (above)<br>• Suicidal or homicidal thoughts<br>• Elevated vital signs if in a manic episode<br>• Noncompliance with medication used as mood stabilizers |
| Paranoia | Chronic and deep fear and mistrust of everyone and everything<br><br>• Mistrust of the provider<br>• Elevated vital signs if anxious or agitated<br>• Confusion or disjointed speech<br>• Auditory or visual hallucinations |
| Schizophrenia | Chronic and severe mental disorder that affects how a person thinks, feels, and behaves<br><br>• Delusions/hallucinations; disorganized speech or behavior; blunted or flat affect; thought disorders (unusual or dysfunctional ways of thinking); catatonia<br>• Poor "executive functioning" skills, i.e., the ability to understand information and use it to make decisions<br>• Noncompliance with prescribed medication |
| Suicidal and homicidal thoughts | Thoughts to harm oneself or others, with or without a clear plan to do so; may or may not be an underlying mental illness<br><br>• Flat affect or speech patterns<br>• Refusal to be transported (especially if someone else called 911)<br>• A collection of items that could be used to harm: guns, excess of pills (prescription or not), ropes, knives<br>• Depression or agitated mood |
| Excited delirium | An acute state of agitation and confusion typically caused by illicit stimulant drug usage or underlying mental illness; often first experienced in prehospital setting<br><br>• Sudden onset<br>• Bizarre and/or aggressive behavior; shouting or verbal agitation<br>• Paranoia or panic<br>• Violence toward others<br>• Unexpected and strong physical strength<br>• Hyperthermia, even up to 102°F (38.9°C) or higher |

As part of securing the scene and doing patient assessment, be alert for patients who pace nervously, shout, threaten others, curse, throw objects, or stand grimacing with clenched fists. A patient exhibiting any of these signs should be presumed capable of a sudden violent attack. If a behavioral problem is ever suspected on one of your calls, police support should be available.

## Suicidal Behavior

This category of behavioral emergencies requires special mention. The EMT may be called out for "suicidal idealizations" or an unknown behavioral emergency that turns out to be a suicide attempt. Some patients are very honest and seek assistance, in which case your empathy and care can be of enormous help. Other patients, such as a severely depressed person, might decline medical intervention (which is their right unless they are impaired).

That said, a patient who is at an increased risk for suicide is presumed to "not have the capacity to refuse medical treatment." In other words:

- If the patient states something like, "I want to kill myself," you must insist on transport (i.e., you must not allow the patient to refuse transport) to a medical facility.

- If a patient makes a vague reference to not wanting to be here anymore or something like, "Nobody would miss me anyway," you must decide whether the patient is actually at risk for a suicide attempt:

  - Ask clarifying questions to determine the true reason that 911 was called, either by the patient or by a bystander.

  - If the patient has made suicidal comments, it is often helpful to repeat back the statement and ask if that is true or not. Do so with the idea of verifying information, not with judgment or hostility in your voice and body language.

- Indicators of an increased risk of suicide, and thus in determining if a patient cannot refuse transport, include the following:

  - Age >40 and single/widowed/divorced

  - History of alcohol abuse, illegal drug use

  - History of depression, especially if not medicated or receiving professional treatment

  - Individuals who have a defined lethal plan of action that they verbalize

  - Unusual gathering of articles that can cause death, i.e., guns, pills, ropes

  - Previous history of suicide attempts/behaviors

  - Recently diagnosed serious illness

  - Recent loss of a loved one or relationship troubles

  - Recent arrest or imprisonment

  - Loss of job or financial security

As you assess a patient with any of these risk factors, be sure to present a calm yet authoritative demeanor:

- Maintain eye contact, and speak in a measured, calm tone.

- If the patient questions you, answer honestly yet in a way that is noninflammatory. Rather than come across as "disagreeing" with the patient, try an approach that presents more positive alternatives, such as the concern of the patient's family.

- If the patient is delusional or hallucinating, assure them that the symptoms are not real.

Finally, be sure to properly document the patient's statements (even if they change) and report to hospital personnel.

# Restraints

Behavioral calls are normally longer in duration than others, as the EMT often has to get the patient to cooperate in transportation to the medical facility. Yet in spite of all of the EMT's best efforts, it is sometimes necessary to restrain a patient forcibly.

Local protocols vary in the use of restraints. Some jurisdictions limit the application of restraints to police, some allow EMS to restrain patients with medical control approval, and others allow EMS to restrain if it can document a clear threat. Local protocols should always be followed since the alternative may be a charge against the EMT for assault, battery, and/or false imprisonment.

Most services allow the use of soft restraints and have migrated away from the usage of leather or vinyl restraints. It is very rare for EMS services to allow the usage of handcuffs or zip ties, as that is often only handled by police officers.

Police may sometimes deliver patients to EMS with their wrists secured behind their backs with handcuffs and their ankles in leg irons secured to the handcuffs. Police will routinely subdue violent patients with this technique in a prone position. If this patient is then delivered into EMS care, the EMT must immediately place the patient on their side in a lateral recumbent position to preclude asphyxia. The use of metal restraints (handcuffs and leg irons) is discouraged by current EMS standards due to the danger of violent patients causing damage to their tendons and ligaments as they struggle against the restraints. These restraints, however, with their ease of use and application, are often much safer to apply than leather and vinyl ones. A patient in metal restraints should be shifted to softer restraints once a sufficient number of personnel are available to accomplish this change safely.

If EMS is authorized to restrain a violent patient, then ideally, a minimum of five people are necessary for the safe application of soft restraints, one for each limb and one to apply the restraints. As it is not always possible for this number of people to be on scene initially, consider calling for additional assistance before attempting a restraint maneuver. Never attempt to restrain a patient without having a clear plan and ensuring that every member of the team has verified they are clear on their roles. If this is not done, the situation is a sure recipe for disaster and can result in harm to the patient as well as the EMS crew.

A patient should never be restrained in a prone position with ankles drawn up, the so-called "hog-tie." Many deaths due to asphyxia have been documented of patients in this type of restraint.

Securing a patient to a backboard requires the following steps:

1. With a person holding on each limb, the patient is forced into a supine position on a backboard.
2. Restraint cuffs are placed on each ankle and then secured to prevent kicking.
3. A strap is used to secure the patient's legs just above the knees.
4. Another strap is used across the chest just below the armpits.
5. A restraint cuff is applied to each wrist, and the arms are crossed over the chest and restrained to the backboard.

Alternatively, you could restrain the wrists with the nondominant hand (if known) secured along the side of the body and the dominant hand secured to the top of the backboard above the patient's head:

- The advantages to this method are that the patient's torso is clear. If chest compressions suddenly have to be performed, the EMT can observe the patient's diaphragm for signs of respiratory distress, and the patient's arm is available for an IV if one becomes necessary.
- The disadvantages are that the patient is less secure than with the arms crossed over the chest since the arms would help to maintain the supine position.

Respiratory function and distal circulation should be constantly checked, as the patient could quickly become impaired because of the restraints.

Another option is to secure the patient onto the stretcher mattress frame using the stretcher frame (not arm rail) as an anchoring point. Place restraint cuffs on each ankle and secure to prevent kicking. A restraint cuff is then applied to each wrist and secured to the stretcher frame as well. Any number of knots could be used to secure restraints that will minimize harm to the patient while allowing you to manage any safety concerns effectively.

To reiterate, local medical protocols must always be followed. Behavioral emergencies, because of their medical and legal complexities, must be thoroughly documented, both as to observation of the patient and EMS interactions. Any medical control permissions must be documented completely as to the individual giving permission for specific actions and the time of permission. Since complaints against EMTs are common in these situations, it is important that the names of witnesses, assisting EMT, and police officers are also well documented.

If a situation becomes unsafe, you must evacuate, call for additional help, and replan. Do not place yourself in serious danger trying to restrain someone.

## Obstetric and Gynecological Emergencies

Childbirth is a natural process, and the EMT's role is one of support as well as recognition of abnormal situations should they present. As with medical emergencies and trauma, the EMT must be aware of the special anatomy and physiology of the pregnant female and her unborn child.

### Pregnancy and Childbirth

The unborn child (fetus) lives in the uterus, or womb, of the mother.

- Once a female's ovum (egg) is fertilized by a male's sperm, it begins to grow and divide into multiple cells and implants itself in the wall of the uterus, where it will be nourished.
- Gestation usually lasts approximately 40 weeks from the time of ovum fertilization.

- The opening of the uterus into the birth canal, or vagina, is called the cervix. This opening is blocked by a mucus plug during pregnancy; the mucus plug is discharged as labor begins and the cervix begins to dilate in preparation of delivery of the fetus.

In addition to the fetus, the uterus contains the placenta and other structures that mediate between the fetus and the mother's body.

- The placenta is the organ through which the fetus receives nourishment and to which the fetus is connected by the umbilical cord.
- A sac of amniotic fluid (bag of waters) surrounds the fetus while in utero to cushion and protect the fetus.

Usually the amniotic sac ruptures on its own; "breaking water" is often the precursor of active labor. Occasionally, though, the sac will deliver unruptured with the baby. In this case, the EMT must tear the amniotic sac to allow the baby to breathe.

The perineum is the external surface of the pelvic floor, an area of skin that extends from the anus to the scrotum (in males) or the vulva (in females). This tissue commonly tears during delivery of a baby. In a hospital setting, an obstetrician or a midwife may cut the perineum between the vagina and anus before crowning occurs to expedite delivery. (Crowning is the point in labor when the baby's head is consistently visible in the birth canal.) This procedure is called an episiotomy; the perineum is then stitched after birth to facilitate healing.

### Labor

Labor is the process of delivering a baby. It is defined as beginning with the first pronounced uterine contraction and terminating with the delivery of the placenta. Labor is divided into three stages:

- The first stage of labor occurs as contractions begin and may last from a few minutes to many hours. The contractions can be palpated on the mother's abdomen. These contractions cause the cervix to dilate in preparation for the baby's expulsion from the uterus.
- The second stage of labor is reached when the cervix is fully dilated and the baby's head begins to enter the birth canal. It is at this stage that the EMT should be able to observe the baby's head during the contraction. This stage culminates with the delivery of the baby.
- The third stage of labor is the delivery of the placenta.

The first part of the baby that is visible is referred to as the **presenting part** and is usually the baby's head. If any other part of the baby presents first, this is referred to as a **breech delivery**.

Each EMS unit should carry an obstetrical kit, ideally at least two. These kits may be preassembled, or standard prepackaged kits may be purchased. Each kit, at minimum should include:

- Surgical scissors or scalpel
- Two hemostats or cord clamps
- A bulb syringe
- Sterile towels
- 2 × 10 gauze sponges
- Sterile gloves
- Sterile baby blanket
- Sanitary napkins
- Biohazard plastic bag

## Obstetrical Assessment

Assessment of a patient in labor is the same as any other medical assessment but with several additions. It is useful to know which pregnancy this is for the mother. A first pregnancy will usually have a longer labor period than a fourth or fifth pregnancy.

Document a patient in labor as follows:

- **Para** is the number of live births the mother has had.
- **Gravida** is the number of times the mother has been pregnant.
- If a woman has been pregnant 3 times, with 2 miscarriages and 1 live birth, it would be written as **P1 G3**.

While this may be considered private or uncomfortable information for the EMT to ask, the patient or a bystander should also be asked if her prior pregnancies have ended in live births or miscarriages, whether the live births were vaginal deliveries or cesarean sections, and whether there were any specific complications with her prior births. Some women may deny that they are pregnant due to social stigma or other concerns, and you may have to rely on your own observations about whether an obstetrical emergency exists. If the patient is in active labor, you must ask how far apart the contractions are and how long they last. The longer the contractions last and the more frequently they occur, the more likely that delivery is imminent.

## Miscarriage/Abortion

The EMT must be aware of the predelivery emergency conditions that may be encountered. The first is spontaneous abortion, or miscarriage. A miscarriage is when the products of conception are delivered early in the pregnancy. This will usually be dispatched as "female vaginal bleeding" or "female hemorrhaging." The assessment and care of the patient will be the same as for any patient with severe hemorrhaging. If the products of conception are available, they should be placed into a plastic bag and transported to the hospital out of the sight of the mother for the obstetrician to evaluate.

A miscarriage is an emotionally traumatic event for both the mother and the family, and prehospital care for the emotional trauma is as important as the physical care. The EMT must be supportive and encouraging, just as they would be if a patient's loved one had died. The pain of loss should not be minimized by the EMT because the loss is not a fully developed human being. Statements like "You can always have another child" are minimizing statements and may not even be true. Support is often best given by conveying your concern and sense of loss to the mother.

Some women may also elect to have a scheduled medical abortion, which can be either surgical or through various medications prescribed by a medical professional. It may involve a process called a dilation and curettage (D&C), which is a procedure to remove tissue from inside the uterus. This can lead to hemorrhaging directly after or for a few days after the procedure has been done. There are also times when a woman may not have had a sterile procedure done, in which case there may be internal damage that requires bleeding control as well as infection worries to consider. Regardless of how the procedure was done, there is often abdominal pain or tenderness after the procedure and EMS may be summoned. It is not up to the EMT to judge a woman's decision to have an abortion, no matter their own personal beliefs. The EMT is there to provide appropriate medical care and delivery to the proper medical facility.

In the case of hypovolemic shock, or low blood volume, due to hemorrhage, the EMT must be prepared for an expedited transport or to call ALS for backup if they are closer than a facility. Shock management includes keeping the patient warm, providing oxygen, managing the bleeding, and constantly assessing vital signs.

Keep in mind there may also be a need for psychological support. Regardless of why or how the mother has lost a child, it is still a loss or an upsetting situation for the female patient. Be empathetic, and document as factually as possible. Be an advocate for your patient always.

## Complications in Pregnancy

While many pregnancies are often uneventful and uncomplicated, some complications may develop acutely or slowly over time, resulting in EMS being needed. The following table lists some of the more common emergencies the EMT may encounter.

**Table 6.17** Pregnancy Complications

| COMPLICATION | KEY IDEAS |
|---|---|
| Ectopic pregnancy | • Egg is fertilized outside the uterus<br>• Most commonly these fertilizations happen in the fallopian tubes, but rarely they may also happen in the abdominal tissue<br>• Are nonviable, meaning that the pregnancy will not result in a live birth<br>• Bleeding from ectopic pregnancy causes 10% of all pregnancy-related deaths, and it's the leading cause of first-trimester maternal death<br>• If the patient was hopeful for a pregnancy, there is an element of psychological support that will need to be provided as well |

*(Continued)*

**Table 6.17** Pregnancy Complications (*Continued*)

| COMPLICATION | KEY IDEAS |
|---|---|
| Seizure (medical emergency, regardless of the cause) | • Has various causes, e.g., hypoglycemia, epilepsy, anoxia, and eclampsia; a thorough assessment should identify the underlying reason<br>• Transport patient left lateral recumbent to allow for the best possible blood flow and avoid constricting the inferior vena cava |
| Preeclampsia and eclampsia | • Characterized by high blood pressure and signs of damage to another organ system; if left untreated, can result in seizures<br>• Usually begins after 20 weeks of pregnancy in women whose blood pressure had been normal (below 140/90 mm Hg)<br>• Hypertension may develop slowly over time, or it may have a sudden onset<br>• Sudden weight gain and edema, particularly in face and hands, can be an early indicator but is not always accurate<br>• Other symptoms can include:<br>  — Severe headache<br>  — Nausea and vomiting<br>  — Shortness of breath<br>  — Decreased urine output and excess protein in urine<br>  — Upper abdominal pain |
| Supine hypotensive syndrome | • Compression of the inferior vena cava and aorta by the fetus, leading to decreased venous return and resulting in hypoperfusion in the supine (upward) position<br>• Loss of consciousness and even maternal and/or fetal death can occur<br>• Symptoms (typically seen 3–10 minutes after lying down) can include:<br>  — Tachycardia<br>  — Diaphoresis<br>  — Nausea/vomiting<br>  — Weakness/dizziness/light-headedness<br>  — Pallor |
| Abruptio placenta | • Partial or complete separation of the placenta from the inner wall of the uterus before delivery<br>• Can decrease or block the baby's supply of oxygen and nutrients<br>• Causes heavy bleeding in the mother—internally and/or externally<br>• Symptoms include abdominal and back pain<br>• Most likely to occur in the last trimester of pregnancy, often close to the due date |
| Placenta previa | • Placenta lies lower in the uterus than the usual position and partially or completely covers the cervix<br>• Typically occurs in the third trimester<br>• More common in women who have had multiple births or a previous cesarean section (C-section) birth<br>• Most common symptom is painless vaginal bleeding; premature contractions may occur<br>• If diagnosed, typical treatment is bedrest for the mother |

*(Continued)*

**Table 6.17** Pregnancy Complications (*Continued*)

| COMPLICATION | KEY IDEAS |
| --- | --- |
| Vaginal bleeding (serious, regardless of whether accompanied by abdominal pain) | • Can be controlled by application of sanitary napkins to the external vagina<br>• Manage shock symptoms if present<br>• Transport should be expedited if bleeding is heavy or uncontrolled |
| Traumatic injury | • Treat like any other trauma victim, with special attention to the abdomen and vagina for signs of bleeding<br>• If spinal immobilization is indicated, place the patient on spine board, with pillows underneath the right side so board tilts to the left; if spinal immobilization is not indicated, transport the patient on her left side<br>• Remember that you have 2 patients, the mother and the child; so reassess frequently |

## Emergency Procedures for Delivery

If the call is for a patient in normal first-stage labor and delivery does not appear to be imminent based upon the primary assessment, the EMT must complete the secondary assessment and determine if there is enough time to transport the patient safely to the hospital or if it would be safer to deliver the baby at the current location. This decision should be made in consultation with medical control, which will want to know specific symptoms and vital signs.

If the baby is crowning and delivery is imminent, the EMT should open the emergency obstetrics kit and prepare for delivery. Proper body substance isolation (BSI) precautions include sterile gloves, mask, gown, and eye protection. The procedures are as follows:

- The mother should lie on her back in a semi-Fowler position, propped up with pillows and with her knees drawn up and spread apart. Elevate the mother's buttocks with blankets or pillows.

- Create a sterile field around the vagina using paper barriers or towels. Do not touch the mother's vagina except during delivery if necessary to maintain the baby's airway and, even then, only when your partner is present.

- As the baby's head is delivered, apply gentle pressure on the skull to prevent explosive delivery, avoiding the baby's fontanel, or soft spot.

- If the amniotic sac is still intact, puncture it and pull it away from the baby's mouth and nose as they appear.

- As the baby's head is delivered, check that the umbilical cord is not wrapped around the neck. If it is, try to unwrap it. If that is not possible, clamp the cord and cut it between the clamps.

- After the head is delivered, support the head with one hand and suction the mouth and nose two or three times with the bulb syringe. Next:
  - Turn the baby so the shoulders are horizontal instead of vertical as this will help the rest of the body to slide out.
  - The torso and the rest of the body will usually be delivered with the next contraction.
  - As the feet are delivered, grab the feet with one hand and wipe the blood and mucus from the mouth and nose with sterile gauze.
- If the baby is breathing normally, wrap the baby in a warm blanket, being sure to cover the baby's head to minimize heat loss. Place the baby on its side, the head slightly lower than the trunk. The baby should be level with the mother's vagina until the cord is cut.
- When the baby is stable (if the cord was not already cut due to being wrapped around the baby's neck), clamp the cord 3–4 inches from the baby. Wait for the cord's pulsations to cease, then cut it between the clamps.
- If the baby and the mother are stable, the EMT should prepare to deliver the placenta:
  - As the uterus contracts, the EMT should urge the mother to push and expel the placenta.
  - Once the placenta is delivered, place the placenta into the plastic bag and transport it along with the baby and mother to the hospital.
  - The obstetrician will want to examine the placenta to be sure that all of it was expelled.
- Place two sanitary napkins over the vagina, and have the mother close her legs. Have the mother massage her uterus through her abdomen to assist in the control of bleeding.
- If the mother begins to exhibit signs of shock (pale and diaphoretic), administer oxygen via non-rebreather and expedite transport.

## Apgar Score

Patient assessment of a neonate (newborn baby) includes the Apgar score (introduced in 1952 by Virginia Apgar, MD), which should be performed at 1 minute postpartum and 5 minutes postpartum. This index gives an excellent overall summary of the baby's condition and will alert the receiving hospital to the actual condition. The Apgar score evaluates 5 criteria corresponding to the letters of the name: appearance, pulse, grimace, activity, and respirations.

It is a good idea to have this scorecard posted on the action wall of the truck. Each item receives 0, 1, or 2 points. The maximum score is 10 points, and the minimum is 0.

**Table 6.18** Apgar Score

| SIGN | 0 POINTS | 1 POINT | 2 POINTS |
| --- | --- | --- | --- |
| Appearance | Baby is cyanotic or pale | Baby's torso is pink, but extremities are bluish | Baby's extremities are pink |
| Pulse | No pulse | Heart rate <100 per min | Heart rate >100 per min |
| Grimace (tested by flicking baby's feet) | No response | Slight facial grimace | Baby grimaces, coughs, sneezes, or cries |
| Activity | No movement / limp | Some flexion of extremities | Baby is actively moving |
| Respiration | No respiration | Slow and irregular breathing / weak cry | Good respiration / strong cry |

The number of personnel available may dictate that this assessment not be done. For example, a finding of no respirations should lead the EMT to begin respiratory assistance and not to be recording assessment findings.

Apgar scoring is as follows:

- **7–10 points**: neonate is in good condition
- **4–6 points**: neonate is moderately depressed, and stimulation and oxygen are indicated
- **0–3 points**: neonate requires aggressive resuscitation, including positive ventilation and chest compressions

## Abnormal Delivery

Abnormal delivery situations are rare but still are a concern to the EMT. Some situations requiring EMT intervention are as follows:

- **Prolapsed cord** is a condition in which the cord presents from the vagina before the head of the baby is delivered. This presents a serious emergency for the viability of the fetus. Treatment for this condition, in addition to normal assessment and oxygenation for the mother, includes positioning the mother with the head lower than the level of the buttocks to reduce pressure on the birth canal and fetus. If the cord is still pulsating, insert a gloved hand into the vagina and push the presenting part of the fetus away from the cord to prevent the pressure of the neonate from cutting off the flow of blood through the cord. Transport immediately, and continue to monitor the pulsation of the cord.

- **Breech presentation** is the name for any part of the fetus other than the head presenting through the birth canal first. This requires immediate transport upon recognition. The mother should be placed on high-flow oxygen and transported in a head-down position with her pelvis elevated.

- **Meconium aspiration** occurs when a neonate, due to distress during labor, defecates into the amniotic fluid and then aspirates this fluid as it begins to breathe. The presence of meconium is detectable when the amniotic fluid is greenish or yellowish brown instead of clear. If meconium is detected, the EMT should aspirate the oropharynx before trying to stimulate spontaneous respirations.
- **Premature birth** occurs before the full 37-week gestation period and poses an especially high risk of hypothermia to an infant. The baby must be kept warm (especially the crown of the head), so the neonate can retain heat. Early premature infants—less than 30 weeks—also usually require manual resuscitation.

## Gynecological Emergencies

Gynecological emergencies also present special considerations, especially for male EMTs who may be sensitive or embarrassed by treating female genitalia. Severe vaginal bleeding is treated in the same way as any other internal hemorrhage, with oxygen and immediate transport.

Special sensitivity is required in dealing with women who have been sexually assaulted. It is always preferable to have a female EMT be the primary caregiver if possible, as the victim may be fearful of any male at this time, especially those in uniform who are projecting an image of power:

- The primary EMT should take a thoughtful, nonjudgmental approach with victims of sexual assault. The key words are sensitivity, support, and professionalism.
- Aside from taking the normal trauma assessment protocols, preserve all evidence for possible criminal prosecution.
- Discourage the patient from showering, bathing, or voiding if possible.
- A good practice is to open the stretcher bed sheet fully and allow the patient to wrap herself if wanted. This can provide a "cocoon" feeling that may not only make her feel safe and enclosed but also allow any blood, hair, etc., to collect on the sheet as the hospital or police offers may use it as more evidence.
- Visual examination of the genitalia should be conducted only if profuse bleeding is present.
- Depending on your state, as a medical practitioner you may be required to report any sexual assault that you learn has occurred.

# Practice Set

1. Which of the following medications can cause hypotension?

    A. Nitroglycerin

    B. Aspirin

    C. Oxygen

    D. Epinephrine

2. What is the dosage for nitroglycerin in the spray or tablet form?

    A. 0.2 mg

    B. 0.4 mg

    C. 1 mg

    D. 4 mg

3. Which of the following is the correct dosage and administration route of epinephrine for an adult to be delivered by EMTs?

    A. 0.15 mg; IM

    B. 0.15 mg; IN

    C. 0.3 mg; IM

    D. 0.3 mg; IN

4. You respond to a call for difficulty breathing. When arriving on scene, you find a male in his sixties breathing rapidly and sitting in tripod position. His color is bluish, and he is sweaty and cool to the touch. You perform your initial assessment, which is unremarkable, and his vital signs are all within normal range except for his respiratory rate, which is 22. What is your first therapy of choice to treat this patient?

    A. Epinephrine

    B. Albuterol

    C. Nitroglycerin

    D. Oxygen

5. Nitroglycerin (nitro) has multiple mechanisms of action to relieve a patient's chest pain. Which of the following are mechanisms of action for nitroglycerin? Select the 3 answer options that are correct.

    A. Vasodilation

    B. Bradycardia

    C. Tachycardia

    D. Decreased cardiac workload

    E. Increased blood flow

    F. Increased preload

6. Which of the following signs and symptoms is indicative of inadequate air exchange?

    A. Breath sounds clear in all fields

    B. Chest rises and falls with each breath

    C. Respiratory rate 12–20 per minute

    D. Altered mental status

7.  You arrive on the scene of a call for difficulty breathing. You enter the kitchen, and you see a 70-year-old male seated at the table, leaning forward. He is having severe trouble breathing, his skin is bluish gray, and he is sweaty. You hear a gurgling sound as he tries to inhale. As you ask him questions, he tries to respond between gasps, but his answers are not comprehensible. He is clutching his chest and appears to be in severe pain. His wife advises you that he had a heart attack last year and takes nitroglycerin, hydrochlorothiazide, and digitalis. The chest pains began as he finished supper. The patient took two NTG tablets, but the pain has continued to get worse. His vital signs are BP 180/120 mm Hg, pulse 120, respiratory rate 28, pulse oximetry 82%. What is your next intervention?

    A.  Load and go

    B.  Oxygen 15 LPM via non-rebreather

    C.  Contact medical control for NTG 1:150 sublingually

    D.  Apply the AED and analyze his cardiac rhythm

8.  You have made the load-and-go decision on the patient in question 7 and removed him immediately to the truck after applying the oxygen mask at high flow. As you begin your focused exam en route to the hospital, you notice your patient is now unconscious and has stopped breathing, and you cannot palpate a carotid pulse. You instruct your partner to begin ventilating the patient with a BVM and OPA and hook up the AED to the patient. You ask the driver to stop while you analyze the patient with the AED. The AED reads "no shock advised." Which of the following statements is correct as your next action?

    A.  Deliver 2 breaths using BVM, then start compressions.

    B.  Contact medical control for permission to administer NTG 0.4 mg sublingually.

    C.  Continue transport with no further intervention.

    D.  Begin chest compressions for 2 minutes and then reanalyze with the AED.

9.  You are dispatched to a call for a man down. You arrive on scene and find a male in his seventies lying on his back on the front lawn. There are no bystanders or family members present. He is cyanotic, pulseless, and apneic. He is cool to the touch, and when you try to move his limbs and jaw, they are rigid and do not move. You pull his shirt up and notice that the anterior portion of his torso is pale and the posterior is black-and-blue, with a definitive line between the two areas. Which of the following conditions should you suspect?

    A.  Cardiac arrest

    B.  Myocardial infarction

    C.  Apnea secondary to COPD

    D.  Biological death

10. You are dispatched to a residence for a male patient with a possible myocardial infarction. Prior to administering him nitroglycerin, which of the following medications should you ask the patient if he has taken?

    A. Tylenol

    B. Lasix

    C. Viagra

    D. Prilosec

11. Which of the following best describes the condition atherosclerosis?

    A. Hardening of the arteries

    B. Chest pain that goes away with rest

    C. Buildup of plaque in the arteries

    D. Plaque that traveled to the brain

12. Your patient is a 34-year-old woman who has a history of being sick for the last 2 weeks "but it's not getting better and it's getting harder to breathe. I also don't have a lot of energy. My doctor gave me some antibiotics, but I don't think they're working" Out of the following symptoms, according to the SIRS criteria, which would NOT contribute to her likelihood of developing sepsis from a prolonged infection?

    A. Systolic blood pressure of 76 mm Hg

    B. Respiratory rate of 32

    C. Heart rate of 86

    D. Temperature of 95.2°F

13. Ventricular fibrillation is a condition affecting which system of the heart?

    A. Electrical

    B. Circulatory

    C. Mechanical

    D. All of the above

14. Out of the following patients, which is at the lowest risk of developing sepsis?

    A. 82-year-old male who is recovering from abdominal surgery

    B. 19-year-old male who broke his wrist in a skateboard crash

    C. 2-year-old female who developed pneumonia in her lungs bilaterally

    D. 23-year-old female with a permanent gastrostomy tube

15. You arrive on the scene of an unknown medical call to a residence. The husband advises that he went to check on his wife and found her unresponsive. He directs you to the bedroom, where there is a female lying supine, pale, and cyanotic in bed. She does not appear to be breathing and has no carotid pulse. What must you do before beginning CPR?

    A. Call medical control.

    B. Place her onto a hard surface.

    C. Hook up your AED and shock as advised.

    D. Request an ALS intercept.

16. You are dispatched to a college dorm room for a report of a man down. You respond emergently, arrive on scene with suitable protective equipment, and have determined that the scene is safe. You find an 18-year-old male lying on his back, unconscious, and not responsive to any stimuli. He has an airway and is making snoring sounds at a regular rate. As you are checking his breathing, you notice that his breath has a fruity odor. His carotid pulse is strong, rapid, and regular. His girlfriend is also in the room and is hysterical as she tells you they were sitting talking when he suddenly collapsed. What question do you want to ask the girlfriend next?

    A. "Does he have any allergies?"

    B. "Does he have diabetes?"

    C. "Does he often lose consciousness?"

    D. "Does he take any medications on a regular basis?"

17. What type of stroke is caused by a burst vessel in the brain that causes bleeding?

    A. TIA

    B. Infarction

    C. Hemorrhagic

    D. Ischemic

18. Which of the following conditions may cause a seizure?

    A. High body temperature

    B. Head injury

    C. Epilepsy

    D. All of the above

19. A 21-year-old homeless male presents with altered mental status, drooling, and moderate respiratory distress. There are no bystanders, and you do not see any obvious illicit drug paraphernalia surrounding him. What should you do as you treat this patient? Select the 4 answer options that are correct.

    A. Deliver 0.4 mg IN of naloxone.

    B. Administer high-flow oxygen.

    C. Proceed with the assumption that this patient is under the influence of drugs, despite no obvious signs.

    D. Examine the oropharynx.

    E. Begin to use the BVM at 10–12 breaths per minute.

    F. Suction the oropharynx.

    G. Take a thorough medical history, including questions about recent exposures to infectious disease.

20. You are dispatched to a restaurant for a report of difficulty breathing. You respond emergently wearing appropriate protective equipment, and there are no scene safety concerns. You are directed to a table where a male and a female are seated. The female has her hand to her throat and appears to be in respiratory distress. She is moving air with difficulty, and her male companion is upset. She is unable to answer your questions, and her companion knows of no medical history, medications, or allergies. He advises that she had just eaten a shrimp cocktail when the symptoms suddenly developed. The patient is pale and diaphoretic, with a rapid pulse. The police officer who searched her pocketbook for her driver's license hands you an EpiPen that he found in the pocketbook. What should you do at this point?

    A. Administer the EpiPen to the lateral thigh.

    B. Have your partner call medical control while you prepare to ventilate the patient.

    C. Administer oxygen via nasal cannula at 10 liters per minute.

    D. Place the patient onto a stretcher and transport priority to the nearest medical facility.

21. You are on duty in your station when an adult male comes running in. He is pale, diaphoretic, and short of breath. He keeps stammering the word "bee" and is pointing to his arm, where you notice a large welt. He is unable to respond to your questions and is beginning to lose consciousness. What condition do you suspect?

    A. Anaphylaxis

    B. Diabetes

    C. Myocardial infarction

    D. Epilepsy

22. You are dispatched to a residence for a possible overdose. You arrive on the scene and find that police have secured the scene. You are wearing appropriate protective apparel. The husband advises that his wife has been despondent and he fears she may have overdosed on her prescription tranquilizers. He states that she has been drinking all day and is now semiconscious. In the bedroom you find a female in her fifties who appears to be sleeping. She is supine, making snoring sounds, and has a slow pulse. She responds when you call her name but will not answer any questions. Her gaze is unfocused, and her pupils are dilated and do not respond to light. There is an empty bottle of clonazepam next to the bed that was refilled yesterday and contained 30 tablets, 1 mg each. There is also an empty fifth of gin, and her breath smells of alcohol. Her husband states that she entered the bedroom 15 minutes before he called 911. Her vital signs are 100/60, respirations 12, and pulse 55. What is your next course of action?

    A. Transport the patient.

    B. Contact medical control.

    C. Administer 0.2 mg naloxone IN.

    D. Administer 50 mg of activated charcoal.

23. You are dispatched to meet the police at a residence with no other information available. You arrive on scene, and police lead you to a person seated in his car, which is parked in his garage. The officer tells you that when they arrived, the garage door was closed and the car was running. Police have shut off the engine and left the doors open. You enter the garage and observe a male seated behind the wheel of a car. He is unconscious and not responding to any stimuli. He is cyanotic, with slow, shallow respirations and a weak, thready pulse. What should you suspect as the cause of his unconsciousness?

    A. Heart attack

    B. Seizure

    C. Stroke

    D. Carbon monoxide poisoning

24. In the scenario in question 23, as you arrive and meet with the police officer, what determination should you have initially made with the information the officer has given you?

    A. This is a load and go.

    B. This is a crime scene that must be preserved.

    C. The scene is unsafe.

    D. This call needs an advanced life support unit.

25. In the scenario in question 23, you find the victim has been extricated to the front lawn by police prior to EMS arrival. You have performed your assessments, and the vital signs are blood pressure 110/80 mm Hg, pulse 50, respirations 12 and shallow, and pulse oximeter shows that his oxygen saturation is 98%. What should be your next intervention?

    A. Do nothing.

    B. Administer 15 LPM oxygen.

    C. Call ALS.

    D. Administer 6 LPM oxygen via nasal cannula.

26. In the scenario in question 25, which piece of specialized equipment might influence your choice of destination hospital?

    A. Heart-lung machine

    B. Hyperbaric chamber

    C. CPAP machine

    D. Positive pressure ventilators

27. What body temperature is considered to be moderately hypothermic?

    A. 81°F

    B. 89°F

    C. 91°F

    D. 93°F

28. You arrive on the scene of a motor vehicle accident on a cold, snowy evening. The outside temperature is 0°F. You observe a person lying in the snow next to a wrecked car. Police are on scene, and you are wearing appropriate protective gear. The patient is a 35-year-old male, semiconscious and breathing rapidly, with a weak, thready pulse. You detect the odor of alcohol on his breath. As you palpate his torso, beneath his shirt you notice he is cold to the touch but is not shivering. His hands and feet feel cold and rigid. Which stage of hypothermia do you suspect?

    A. Mild stage

    B. Moderate stage

    C. Severe stage

    D. Frostbite stage

29. In the scenario in question 28, you find two additional patients who have been ejected from the car and who present with the same symptoms. One is a 78-year-old female, and the other is a 32-year-old female. Which of the following should you treat first?

    A. 35-year-old male

    B. 78-year-old female

    C. 32-year-old female

    D. None; treatment should occur at the receiving facility

30. In the scenario in question 29, you have removed the 78-year-old female to your truck and have begun transport. In addition to her lethargy, her vital signs are beginning to drop. You notice that her right hand, which was not gloved, now appears whitish and waxy. Which of the following treatments would be appropriate for this patient?

    A. Warm packs under her arms, beneath her neck, and between her legs

    B. Warm water bath for her right hand

    C. Oxygen

    D. All of the above

31. You are standing by a summer road race and are summoned to a runner who has fallen. The patient is an 18-year-old female who is lying underneath a tree, clutching her right leg. She is breathing rapidly and is flushed. Her skin is hot and dry. Which of the following conditions do you suspect and should treat first?

    A. Heat cramps

    B. Heat exhaustion

    C. Heatstroke

    D. Heat conduction

32. You are en route back to the station from the hospital when you observe a person in the water 30 feet from a lakeshore in apparent distress. You notify your dispatcher and stand on the shore. The person is flailing their arms and yelling, "Help!" Your own swimming ability is limited, and your partner cannot swim at all. What should be your next course of action?

    A. Dive in and swim to the victim as quickly as possible.

    B. Attempt to throw the victim the rescue rope from the truck.

    C. Drive back to the station and get a boat.

    D. Buddy swim with your partner to the victim.

33. You are dispatched to a residence for an unknown-type medical call. An adult female tells you she was working in her garden when she felt a stinging sensation on the back of her left arm. She is conscious, alert, and oriented 3 three with normal respirations and pulse. She has no significant medical history and no known allergies. You examine her left arm and see a bright-red area 5 inches in diameter with a white spot in the center and a small black speck in the center of the white spot. What is your next course of action?

    A. Contact medical control.

    B. Administer epinephrine via auto-injector.

    C. Scrape the black speck off with a credit card.

    D. Administer oxygen 10 liters per minute via non-rebreather mask.

34. You are dispatched to a residence for a woman in labor. You arrive on scene, having taken the usual precautions, and observe a female in her early thirties lying on the couch in the living room. She advises you that this is her third pregnancy, her bag of waters ruptured 30 minutes ago, and her pains are increasing in intensity and are currently 3 minutes apart. Which of the following should be your next move?

    A. Place her onto the stretcher and respond emergently to the nearest maternity unit.

    B. Tie her legs together to prevent premature birth and expedite transport.

    C. Remove her underwear, and at the next contraction, examine the birth canal for signs of crowning.

    D. Insert your gloved hand into the birth canal and see if you can feel the baby's head.

35. In the scenario in question 34, you take vital signs and prepare for transport. The mother suddenly tells you she is having a contraction, and you observe the top of the baby's head as her labia separate. What should you now do?

    A. Place her onto the stretcher and respond emergently to the nearest maternity unit.

    B. Open the obstetrical kit and prepare for delivery.

    C. Administer 15 LPM oxygen to the mother.

    D. Call ALS because this is a higher-level call.

36. In the scenario in question 34, instead of the top of the baby's head, you see the baby's arm protruding from the mother's vagina. What should you now prepare to do?

    A. Place her onto the stretcher and respond emergently to the nearest hospital that has maternity capabilities.

    B. Open the obstetrical kit and prepare for delivery.

    C. Pull gently on the arm to facilitate delivery.

    D. Wait for the next contraction and see if the condition rectifies itself.

37. You are dispatched along with police to an unknown-type medical call. You arrive simultaneously with the police and observe a large male trying to throw a refrigerator at his wife. You assist police in wrestling the man to a prone position, and the police handcuff his wrists behind his back as he continues to struggle and curse. His wife advises you that he has no medical problems, takes no medication, and has no history of any psychological problems. She indicates he was behaving normally until she asked if he would like a cup of tea, at which point he suddenly became violent and assaulted her. The police place him under arrest and begin to walk him to the squad car. What is your role as the medical provider?

    A. Assist the police in subduing and arresting the man.

    B. Intervene and insist on transporting him via ambulance to the hospital.

    C. Go back in service, as this call is now a police matter.

    D. Remove the man's restraints, place him onto your stretcher, and transport.

38. In the scenario in question 37, how should this patient be restrained by EMS?

    A. Leave him in handcuffs and use leg irons to secure his ankles to his wrists in a prone position.

    B. Place him in a supine position on a backboard and secure his limbs with soft restraints.

    C. Place him a supine position on a backboard with his hands cuffed behind his back, place another backboard on top of him, and secure the backboards together with handcuffs.

    D. Remove his metal restraints, wrap him in a blanket, and secure him to the stretcher with soft restraints.

39. You are dispatched to a college dorm for a possible diabetic emergency. You respond emergently and arrive on scene. As you walk down the hallway, you observe a female whom you have previously treated for hypoglycemia secondary to diabetes talking and humming to herself. She is walking near the edge of a high balcony. Her roommates tell you that she has been behaving strangely all morning. What should be your next move?

    A. Tackle and restrain her.

    B. Administer 15 mg oral glucose.

    C. Request police assistance.

    D. Take her by the arm and gently sit her in a chair for a more thorough evaluation.

40. In the scenario in question 39, your evaluation reveals that the patient's answers are incoherent and inappropriate; her blood pressure is 120/80 mm Hg, pulse is 72, and respirations are 12. Her blood glucose is 76. She does not refuse to be transported and allows you to lead her to the truck, where you place her in a semi-Fowler position and secure her to the stretcher with the normal straps. She now tries to unfasten the straps and pushes your arm away. What should you do?

    A. Restrain her arms with soft restraints.

    B. Handcuff her hands to the middle strap.

    C. Call for police assistance.

    D. Contact medical control for permission to restrain.

## Answer Key

| | | | | | | | | | |
|---|---|---|---|---|---|---|---|---|---|
| 1. | **A** | 9. | **D** | 17. | **C** | 25. | **B** | 33. | **C** |
| 2. | **B** | 10. | **C** | 18. | **D** | 26. | **B** | 34. | **C** |
| 3. | **C** | 11. | **C** | 19. | **B, D, F, G** | 27. | **B** | 35. | **B** |
| 4. | **D** | 12. | **C** | 20. | **A** | 28. | **C** | 36. | **A** |
| 5. | **A, D, E** | 13. | **D** | 21. | **A** | 29. | **B** | 37. | **B** |
| 6. | **D** | 14. | **B** | 22. | **A** | 30. | **D** | 38. | **B** |
| 7. | **B** | 15. | **B** | 23. | **D** | 31. | **C** | 39. | **C** |
| 8. | **D** | 16. | **B** | 24. | **C** | 32. | **B** | 40. | **D** |

## Answers and Explanations

**1.  A**

Nitroglycerin can cause hypotension because it causes the vessels to vasodilate (open).

**2.  B**

The correct answer is 0.4 mg (B). If you are unsure of the dosages, please refer back to the pharmacology section and table.

**3.  C**

The correct answer is 0.3 mg IM (C). Remember that IM stands for intramuscular while IN stands for intranasal. 0.15 mg is the pediatric dosage for epinephrine, while 0.3 mg is the adult dosage. Epinephrine is delivered IM on the mid-lateral thigh, most commonly through an auto-injector pen.

**4.  D**

This patient is presenting signs of hypoxia, and nearly all state protocols allow the EMT to administer oxygen (D) for immediate relief. Epinephrine (A) would be indicated for an allergic reaction, albuterol (B) for an airway obstruction, and nitroglycerin (C) for chest pain. Be aware that albuterol may be indicated if the dyspnea is being caused by constricted bronchioles, but permission must first be obtained from medical control following a detailed assessment. Oxygen is always the first drug of choice in these situations.

**5.  A, D, E**

Nitroglycerin has a dilation effect on vessels (A) that causes pooling of the blood in the peripheral arteries. This, in turn, decreases the effort the heart has to work (D). Because of the larger vessel area, the blood more readily flows around a potential blockage (E), thus helping relieve some of the patient's chest pain. The other answers have to do with the heart rate (either slower [B] or faster [C]) or an increased amount of blood that enters into the heart (F).

**6.  D**

Altered mental status (D) may be caused by insufficient oxygen supply to the brain. The other answer options are all indicative of normal respiratory pattern.

**7.  B**

This patient is having severe difficulty breathing, and his pulse oximetry and skin color indicate hypoxia. This is a moderately difficult question, as all of the other answers could also be considered correct actions over the course of time. However, the question asks what your *next* intervention is, and this would be to try and relieve the hypoxia with supplemental oxygen therapy.

**8. D**

The current protocols require chest compressions before breaths in the C-A-B sequence. Thus administering breaths before starting compressions (A) is incorrect. Seeking authorization to administer NTG (B) is incorrect because the patient's problem at this time has progressed from chest pain to cardiac arrest. Protocols require CPR for this patient until ordered to discontinue by a physician, so (C) is also incorrect.

**9. D**

This patient exhibits the signs and symptoms of rigor mortis and postmortem lividity, which will allow you in most jurisdictions to not perform CPR and turn this case over to law enforcement for investigation of sudden death. The cause of the sudden death may have been any of the other answers.

**10. C**

It is important to ask the patient if he has taken Viagra (sildenafil citrate) within the last 24 hours. If he has, nitroglycerin is contraindicated because it can cause a sudden and severe drop in blood pressure.

**11. C**

The correct answer is buildup of plaque (C). Hardening of the arteries (A) is often the result of atherosclerosis, but they are two separate conditions. (B) describes angina, while (D) describes what can happen during a stroke.

**12. C**

The correct answer is heart rate of 86 (C) as SIRS criteria state that a heart rate above 90 would be a positive finding and the question asked for which one was NOT a contributing factor. Respiratory rate and temperature given are within the SIRS criteria, and systolic blood pressure is referenced under the qSOFA score, not the SIRS criteria.

**13. D**

Ventricular fibrillation occurs when the electrical system of the heart no longer energizes the heart to pump properly and instead just vibrates (fibrillates) the cardiac muscle. (D) is correct because although it is an electrical problem overall, if the electricity is out, the pump (the heart) stops working (mechanical) and the circulation stops as well. Ventricular fibrillation is considered a lethal rhythm and needs to be corrected by an electrical charge (AED or manual defibrillation).

**14. B**

The patient with a broken wrist is at lowest risk of sepsis (B) due to the low probability of infection provided the wrist heals correctly and the patient takes care of it. The other patients have surgical openings or an infection already present, all of which can progress to sepsis.

**15. B**

The chest compressions of CPR are most effective if the patient is lying on a hard, flat surface. CPR done on a mattress is not as effective since there is not enough pressure created in the thoracic cavity to compress the heart and initiate the pumping action. It is not necessary for an EMT to contact medical control (A) to begin CPR. An ALS intercept (D) should be requested but not at the expense of time for beginning CPR.

**16. B**

You should be considering diabetes because of the fruity odor of this patient's breath, which could be indicative of hypoglycemia. The key word in the question is "next." It is always important to fully read each question and each answer to find the choice that is *most* appropriate.

**17. C**

The correct answer is (C), and the key word is hemorrhage, which means bleeding. Infarction (B) typically refers to a heart attack, not a stroke, and is the body's reaction to a lack of perfusion. This closely relates to ischemia, which can be caused by a blockage in a vessel and describes (D).

**18. D**

Any of the answer choices may cause a seizure.

**19. B, D, F, G**

It is easy to assume that many homeless people are drug addicts, and it is tempting to apply that assumption to this patient (C) and administer naloxone (A). No matter how many addicted patients you may have seen or heard about, however, you must consider each patient case individually. Your patient in this question appears to be having a legitimate medical emergency, and most likely he is experiencing altered mental status due to the respiratory distress. You should administer high-flow oxygen (B) and must also check the oropharynx (D) for a possible foreign body obstruction, which could also be causing the respiratory distress and altered mental status. Suctioning the airway (F) and taking a thorough medical history (G) will help identify the correct treatment path as well.

**20. A**

This patient is suffering an acute allergic reaction to shellfish and needs epinephrine immediately. The EMT does not need to contact medical control (B) to administer the EpiPen according to the *National EMS Scope of Practice Model*. Supplemental oxygen (C) will help the hypoxia but needs to be given by non-rebreather mask at 10–15 LPM. Quick transport (D) may not be sufficient if the airway is closing quickly.

**21. A**

The patient is probably having an allergic (anaphylactic) reaction to a bee sting, as evidenced by his symptoms and his repeating the word "bee." A diabetic emergency would cause him to lose consciousness, a myocardial infarction (heart attack) is usually accompanied by chest pains, and epilepsy is a condition that causes seizures followed by loss of consciousness.

**22. A**

This patient should be transported immediately. Answer choice (B) should be done while en route. Naloxone (C) is used for opioid drugs, which clonazepam is not; 0.2 mg is also not the correct dosage. (D) may be indicated in some systems but is not indicated on a national level in the scope of practice for EMTs.

**23. D**

Circumstances would indicate that a running car in a closed garage emitting carbon monoxide, a poison, has caused this condition, although the others cannot be ruled out initially.

**24. C**

EMS personnel should not enter this environment without proper respiratory protection, such as a self-contained breathing apparatus. To do so invites possible carbon monoxide poisoning, which delays proper care to the initial patient and complicates the entire rescue by adding to the total number of victims who must be treated. Answer choices (A) and (B) might be correct if the scene were safe. Regarding (D), there is nothing in this scenario that would indicate the intervention of an ALS unit.

**25. B**

This patient is severely hypoxic as indicated by his physical appearance, and high-flow oxygen therapy is indicated. The high pulse oximeter is grossly misleading in carbon monoxide poisoning, as it can give a false high reading due to the presence of carbon monoxide in the red blood cells. Thus it cannot be relied on in this case.

**26. B**

The hyperbaric chamber, in which outside oxygen pressure is increased, has proven effective in the treatment of carbon monoxide poisoning. This decision may be made by protocol or medical control. However, if you are given the choice between two hospital emergency departments, in this scenario you should go to the hospital with the hyperbaric chamber. Answer choice (A) is normal equipment for any hospital with a full operating suite and would not be necessary for treating carbon monoxide poisoning. Answer choice (D) is standard equipment in any hospital emergency department, and answer choice (C) is located in most ambulances as a piece of standard equipment.

**27. B**

Moderate hypothermia is between 82–90°F (27.8–32.2°C), which makes all the answer options incorrect except for (B).

**28. C**

The absence of shivering means the patient has moved beyond the mild stage. Moderate hypothermia is marked by increasing mental apathy and loss of motor function, but the severe stage is when the extremities begin to freeze. While frostbite is present in the severe stage, it is only a symptom, not a whole stage of events, so the correct answer is (C).

**29. B**

The older adult (78-year-old passenger) is more at risk for increasing hypothermia due to her age.

**30. D**

The patient is in fourth-stage hypothermia and needs to be warmed. In addition, she has symptoms of frostbite to her right hand that can be treated en route with a warm water bath. Oxygen is indicated for this patient due to her increasing lethargy.

**31. C**

Answer choices (A) and (B) may seem correct. While reading the options, though, you must be able to identify that heatstroke is the most serious condition and the one you should be concerned about. This patient has a high core temperature, and her body's heat-regulating mechanisms are not working. So she must be cooled with cold packs to the axillary, cervical, and groin areas.

**32. B**

Never undertake a rescue unless you are confident in your abilities to perform the necessary activity. Since neither you nor your partner is trained in water rescue techniques, you should not attempt to swim to the patient. If you have an object to throw to the victim, this is your best course of action. Leaving the scene to go and get a boat could be considered abandonment of the patient. Since your partner cannot swim, a buddy swim is not a possibility nor does it solve the problem of being able to approach and assist the victim.

**33. C**

The patient's symptoms are consistent with a bee sting, and she is giving no evidence at this time of anaphylaxis. You should, however, continue to monitor the patient and urge her to go to the emergency department for a more definitive diagnosis.

**34. C**

The correct next step is to look for crowning. Answer choice (A) is incorrect since you have not yet performed an adequate assessment. Answer choice (B) is never correct as it will endanger both the baby and the mother. (D) is also incorrect since the only time you place your gloved hand into the birth canal is to assist in maintaining the baby's airway or to loosen the cord if it is wrapped around the baby's neck.

**35. B**

The correct next action is to prepare for delivery. (A) is incorrect since with the baby crowning, delivery is now imminent, and you are probably better off in the living room than in the back of the truck. (C) is not going to do any harm but is not really indicated at this time. (D) is not true, as simple, uncomplicated births are a BLS-level skill nationwide.

**36. A**

The correct answer this time is to respond emergently to the nearest hospital that has maternity capabilities. This is a breech delivery that places the baby at great risk for asphyxia and the mother at risk for delivery complications. The baby either has to be repositioned for a normal vaginal delivery, which is beyond the scope of EMS training, or has to be delivered by cesarean section, which is a hospital procedure. You will also want to support the mother with high-flow oxygen and continue to monitor the delivery. You may also have to provide airway support to the baby by inserting your hand into the birth canal.

**37. B**

This patient's violent outburst has no apparent cause, and he must be medically evaluated. EMS will always assist police, providing it can be done safely and with a minimum amount of risk to the EMTs. Remember that the police carry weapons and are trained in dealing with violent individuals, whereas EMS is not. (C) is incorrect since it could be considered abandonment of a seriously ill patient. (D) is incorrect because removing handcuffs would render this man a danger to the EMTs as well as any bystanders.

**38. B**

The patient should be placed in a supine position on a backboard with limbs secured with leather or vinyl cuffs. This position gives the EMT the best position to continually evaluate the patient and treat any problems as they occur. Answer choice (A) is incorrect since this patient is at an increased risk for restraint asphyxia. (C) is incorrect because the handcuffs will be forced into the small of his back; also, you will be unable to see the patient or intervene if serious conditions develop. (D) is incorrect because the patient may easily withdraw his limbs and then assault the EMTs.

**39. C**

The patient's behavior is abnormal and should be considered risky. After you have requested police to respond, you may then take her gently by the arm and escort her to a place where you can evaluate her more thoroughly. (A) is incorrect because her behavior is not violent at this time and she has not demonstrated a clear threat to you, bystanders, or herself. (B) is incorrect because you have not done a thorough examination to determine hypoglycemia. Just because she has had this condition in the past does not mean that this is the case at this time.

**40. D**

In some jurisdictions, it may be permissible to restrain without medical control. Still, to prevent a future charge of assault, battery, or false imprisonment, it is more prudent to seek medical control. The need to restrain is demonstrated by the patient's attempts to escape from the stretcher. This patient's answers to questions indicate that she is somehow impaired, and she must be transported to a medical facility for evaluation. Once permission from medical control is obtained, she should be restrained with the least amount of force and restraint necessary. Consequently, her wrists could be restrained to the sides of the stretcher, rather than her arms (A), since she is not kicking or punching violently. Handcuffs (B) should not routinely be used by EMS. Police assistance (C) is unnecessary for this nonviolent patient.

# CHAPTER 7

# TRAUMA EMERGENCIES

**LEARNING OBJECTIVES**

- Define the "golden hour" of trauma emergencies
- Recognize the pathophysiology of and understand EMS treatments for:
  — Bleeding and shock
  — Soft tissue injuries and burns
  — Injuries to the musculoskeletal system
  — Injuries to the head and spine
  — Injuries to the eyes, face, and neck
  — Injuries to the chest, abdomen, and genitalia

## The Science of Trauma

Before you arrive on the scene of a 911 call, it is important to understand the mechanisms of how injuries work. The rapid assessment of any serious injury is critical to success in patient management.

The assessment of a serious injury starts with an understanding of kinematics and velocity.

### Kinematics

Kinematics refers to looking at a trauma scene and attempting to determine what injuries might have resulted from the incident that took place. Certain injury patterns occur with certain mechanisms of injury (MOI), such as:

- Whiplash of a driver as a result of a rear- or front-end motor vehicle accident
- Abdominal injury, fractured extremities, or head injury of a pedestrian as a result of being struck by a vehicle while walking
- Spinal injury to cervical or lumbar sections of a diver as a result of diving headfirst into a shallow swimming pool

Similarly, low-energy weapons such as knives have a different injury severity than a high-energy weapon such as a gun.

**Kinetic energy** is the energy of a moving object. **Kinematics** is the evaluation of the accident scene to identify potential injuries that may have occurred as a result of the moving forces.

You must also look at the actual force or impact sustained by the body and soft tissues, so ask yourself the following questions:

- Was it a **soft or hard object** that struck the body?
- At what **velocity (speed)** did the object strike the person?
- Was it **one object or multiple objects** that struck the person?
- What is the **person's weight or body mass versus the weight or mass of the object struck**?

Having an understanding of how these scientific principles are at play can help predict injury patterns. In the field, this will help you determine the most appropriate facility for the given patient, i.e., level 1 versus level 3 trauma center.

## Prioritization of Patients

With trauma emergencies, the goal is to get the patient to the trauma surgery center within **60 minutes of the injury**, i.e., the "**golden hour**." Research has shown that serious trauma patients have a much higher survival rate when surgical intervention is started within that time frame.

Thus, the EMT must calculate the amount of time for the following:

- Time between the patient's injury and EMS notification
- Time spent in responding
- Time on scene assessing and treating immediate injuries
- Time required to transport the patient to the trauma center

After taking all of those factors into consideration, the EMT should determine a treatment plan, extrication process (if needed), immobilization technique, and proper facility to transport to.

## Trauma Center Levels

Determining what level of trauma center to transport to depends on not only the severity of the injury but also what capabilities the hospital has and if it specializes in adult or pediatric medicine. In general, there are four levels of trauma centers. The EMT must be familiar with what hospitals are located in their coverage area.

As an EMT, it is your job to identify the patient's level of trauma and transport to an appropriate nearby facility. In mass casualty incidents, such as bombings, it is also important not to overwhelm one particular hospital.

**Table 7.1** Trauma Levels

| TRAUMA LEVEL | CAPABILITIES |
|---|---|
| Level 1 (highest level of trauma care certification) | **Can provide total care, from prevention through rehabilitation**<br><br>• 24-hour in-house coverage by general surgeons<br>• Prompt availability of specialties such as orthopedic surgery, neurosurgery, anesthesiology, emergency medicine, radiology, internal medicine, plastic surgery, oral and maxillofacial, pediatric, and critical care |
| Level 2 | **Can initiate definitive care for all injured patients**<br><br>• 24-hour immediate coverage by general surgeons but not necessarily in-house<br>• Specialties include orthopedic surgery, neurosurgery, anesthesiology, emergency medicine, radiology, and critical care<br>• Cardiac surgery and hemodialysis may be referred out to a level 1 facility |
| Level 3 | **Can provide prompt assessment and stabilization of patients but will refer out to higher level of care hospitals**<br><br>• 24-hour immediate coverage by emergency medicine physicians<br>• Prompt availability of general surgeons and anesthesiologists but not necessarily in-house<br>• Provides backup care for rural and community hospitals |
| Level 4 | **Can provide advanced trauma life support (ATLS) prior to transfer of patients to a higher-level trauma center**<br><br>• Basic emergency department facilities and 24-hour laboratory coverage<br>• Trauma nurse(s) and physicians available upon patient arrival<br>• May provide surgery and critical care services if available |

Adapted from **amtrauma.org**

## Common Types of Trauma

The most common type of trauma seen by EMS is the motor vehicle accident (MVA), also called motor vehicle collision (MVC). Falls are the second most common trauma dispatch.

### Motor Vehicle Accident

Multiple forces are at work when an MVA happens. Knowing the patterns will help you interpret injuries that might not be visible with the naked eye. Being familiar with these patterns will also help clarify why a particular injury may be presenting with certain symptoms.

Speed matters. If a moving vehicle strikes an immovable object such as a tree (versus a moving car), the vehicle decelerates from its forward speed to zero. However, the driver and passengers continue moving forward at the original rate of speed, striking the interior parts of the vehicle.

If a driver is not restrained by a seat belt and the vehicle is moving at 50 miles per hour, the individual will strike the steering wheel with the chest, abdomen, and pelvis. The driver's head may continue upward into the windshield, which is constructed of double-thickness glass lined with a plastic sheet. Depending on how the vehicle is struck, the driver could have injuries in all planes of movement: lateral, rotational, anterior, and posterior. At the scene of an MVA:

- Approach the patient from the front of the vehicle if possible to avoid cervical rotation.

- Communicate with the patient and ask them to hold as still as possible and not turn their head.

- Inform the patient ahead of time if your partner will be taking C-spine precautions from behind the head so the patient does not inadvertently rotate the head to see what is happening.

Injury patterns can be predicted or anticipated depending on how the vehicle was struck.

There are five types of collision: frontal, broadside (T-bone), rollover, rotational, and rear-end.

A **frontal** collision between two moving vehicles is referred to as a **head-on collision**, and the force of impact is the total of both speeds. Suppose there is a head-on crash of two vehicles each doing 30 miles per hour. That is the equivalent of a single vehicle striking a tree or wall at 60 miles per hour. Watch for injuries such as "down and under" or "up and over," which could include the following type of injuries:

- **Down and under**—occupant continues to move downward into the seat toward the dashboard and steering column:
  - The chest and lower extremities are often the first point of contact after striking the steering wheel or gas/brake pedals
  - Look for lower-extremities injuries such as the knee striking the dashboard, dislocated knees and hips, and fractures to the femur and/or tibia
- **Up and over**—occupant continues in a forward motion, which then carries the body up and over the steering wheel:
  - The head is often the first point of contact, colliding with the windshield
  - Look for "starring" or "bull's-eye" patterns in the glass, which would suggest that there are cranial and spinal injuries from impact

A **broadside** (or **T-bone**) crash is a crash in which a vehicle either strikes an object sideways or is struck by another vehicle from the side. In this type of collision, there is usually more than one patient on scene, so you may need to call for additional units. Depending on whether there is "intrusion" into the vehicle (e.g., a door is pushed inward and unable to be opened), extended extrication efforts may need to be done by properly trained personnel.

Common injuries seen in broadside crashes include:

- **Head/neck injury**, such as whiplash from hyperextension or head strike to the window/door/other occupant
- **Chest injury**:
  - Rapid compression of the thoracic wall and resulting fractured ribs on the side that was hit in collision
  - Pulmonary contusion
  - Aortic injuries, e.g., dissection, which is life-threatening
  - Compressed and/or fractured clavicles
  - Compression fracture due to sudden tightening of the seat belt against the chest wall
- **Abdominal/pelvic injury**—internal organs may have been lacerated or burst; intrusion can compress and fracture the pelvis and dislocate the femur
- **Entrapped limbs**—this may cause compression and crush injuries

A **rollover** accident can be visually distracting but doesn't always cause major injuries, which can be surprising for the EMS provider. Sometimes the occupants will self-extricate or even be ejected from the vehicle from the sheer velocity of the spinning vehicle. Those accidents that do require careful extraction by emergency personnel can cause injuries of all kinds and in all planes. Never attempt to move a patient from an unstable vehicle, and be aware of scene safety at all times. Be aware of the following possibilities:

- **Shearing injury** can occur in the form of internal organs moving and tearing at their points of attachment, e.g., the aorta or liver
- **Fracture(s)** can occur in any angle, depending on what the patient strikes while inside the vehicle
- **Crush injury**, where the vehicle comes to rest and crushes the patient at any point on the body, is especially serious if the patient was ejected as the vehicle rolled over and was crushed by the weight of the car

A **rotational** accident is when one corner of a vehicle strikes another vehicle or object, for example, when a car "clips" another car but they don't fully crash. The corner of the vehicle striking the object will come to a standstill while the rest of the vehicle will spin until the momentum dissipates and the vehicle finally comes to a full stop. This means that the patient inside will continue to move around and may have injuries seen in both frontal and lateral impact collisions.

A **rear-end** accident is where a vehicle strikes another vehicle from behind. This can be done at either slow or fast speeds and can involve more than two vehicles in a chain reaction. Remember that the faster a car is traveling, the more force will be exerted on all passengers, no matter which vehicle is theirs; so be prepared for multiple patients. Take spinal precautions as indicated. Common injuries include:

- **Head/neck**—whiplash is a common complaint from one or both drivers or occupants due to a rapid back-and-forth movement of the cervical spine. They may also have facial or head injuries from striking the windshield or headrest of the seat.
- **Chest/back**—these injuries are caused by strikes to the steering wheel, seat belt restraints locking, and airbag deployment.
- **Extremities**—watch for direct and indirect forces acting on the upper and lower extremities. For example, if someone slammed on the brakes, they may have ankle or leg fractures. If they reached out with outstretched arms to prevent from going forward, they may have arm fractures or dislocations.

Airbag deployments in any type of accident should be noted: whether or not the airbags actually deployed, which ones have deployed, and how many deployed. Be aware that patients may complain of facial pain from the force of airbags deploying. They may also complain of respiratory issues due to the sudden force to their chest or by inhaling the chemicals used to inflate the airbag.

### KEY TAKEAWAY

If a patient self-extricates from an MVA and is found walking around prior to EMS arrival, that does not always mean the individual is fine. Adrenaline and shock have a way of masking injuries that are very serious. Therefore, it is imperative that anyone involved in an MVA have a physical and neurological exam—not only from a patient care perspective but also from a legal one.

### Falls and Penetration Injuries

Again, the EMT must understand how the fall occurred in order to perform a correct assessment. For example, a person who jumps from a second-floor window and lands on their feet will be at risk for serious leg and spinal injuries, while a person who falls from the same window and lands face forward will be more at risk for internal organ damage.

If full spinal immobilization is indicated, then do so. However, some falls result in only localized injuries and do not require a full spine board. Different types of splinting are reviewed later on in the chapter.

Penetration injuries from sharp objects and firearms are a specialty all their own. Fortunately, our skin is designed with multiple layers to protect underlying organs and structures. However, depending on the size, force, and material, the skin can protect from only so much. Treatment of penetrating injuries varies depending on the object that caused the issue, but in general, the following guidelines should be observed:

- If the object is blocking the airway, remove it carefully and manage any bleeding or suction needed and ventilate if necessary.
- If the object is still inside the skin, do not remove it as it could be acting as a type of internal tourniquet. If removed in the field, bleeding may be uncontrollable.
- Stabilize the object with gauze and bulky dressings, and secure it firmly. Make sure to assess and reassess for pulse, motor, and sensation function.
- Attempt to control any bleeding that is found.

Penetrating injuries can be very distracting, but what matters most is what lies beneath and how the patient is presenting. Be prepared to manage shock symptoms and airway issues if they arise and to transport rapidly if needed.

## Bleeding and Shock

### External Bleeding

The average adult human has approximately 5–6 liters of blood in circulation. If blood is lost as a result of a traumatic injury, the result may be a condition called **hypoperfusion syndrome**, or traumatic shock. This condition is defined as the inadequate circulation of blood through an organ.

The sudden loss of 1 liter of blood from an average adult is considered significant as it affects the circulatory system's ability to perfuse the organs. If blood loss continues, this can lead to devastating results. If a person has less than 2.5 liters of blood circulating, death is almost certain, if they are not dead already. Be aware of the following:

- **Gross hemorrhage** identifies blood that can be seen to the naked eye and its growing volume. For example, if an uncontrolled femoral artery bleed is not stopped, the person will exsanguinate (bleed out) and most likely die due to the amount of blood volume lost.
- **Occult hemorrhage** is blood that cannot be seen to the naked eye. It is usually confirmed with lab tests done upon arrival at the hospital, i.e., not done in the prehospital field.

There are three types of external bleeding:

- **Arterial bleeding** occurs when an artery is lacerated and the blood spurts from the wound. This blood is bright red because it is oxygen rich. Arterial bleeding is more difficult to control than venous or capillary bleeding because it is at a higher pressure.
- **Venous bleeding**, which is dark purplish in color because it is oxygen poor, flows normally or even slowly oozes rather than spurts from a wound.
- **Capillary bleeding** is usually minor and dark red in color, and it often clots on its own without outside intervention.

Before the EMT considers the medical care of external bleeding, you must be sure to be wearing the proper protective equipment to assure your own safety. Depending on the amount of blood involved, that means some or all of the following: disposable gloves, masks, eye protection, and gowns.

### Emergency Care of External Bleeding

A patient with a severe amount of bleeding may demand that the EMT immediately stop the loss of blood, but the EMT must always first secure the airway. Remember: a patient without an airway will arrive at the ER dead.

**Table 7.2** Types of Bleed and Steps to Take

| TYPE OF BLEED | STEPS TO TAKE |
|---|---|
| Arterial bleeding | Spurting blood, typically in rhythm with pulse. Can cause massive hemorrhage in a very short amount of time. Life-threatening.<br><br>1. Immediately apply direct pressure to wound.<br>2. Prepare and use tourniquet (see section below).<br>3. Immediately transport and provide supplemental oxygen as necessary. |
| Open venous wound (not head or nose) | Goal is to constrict the blood flow from the ruptured vessels and promote clotting.<br><br>1. Take a sterile dressing, and apply direct pressure to the wound using a gloved hand.<br>2. If patient is awake and able to follow commands, you can ask them to hold direct pressure.<br>3. Elevate wound above the head and torso to help slow the flow of blood and control the bleeding.<br>4. Add additional gauze on top of gauze bled through if necessary, but be prepared to take more aggressive measures if necessary.<br>5. Splinting using an air pressure/vacuum splint or traction splint may also help to control bleeding caused by broken bones by applying consistent pressure.<br><br>* If direct pressure or splinting fails to work, pressure to an extremity artery between the heart and the wound may facilitate clotting. Pressure points are located where:<br><br>• Brachial artery crosses the humerus.<br>• Radial artery crosses the wrist.<br>• Femoral artery crosses the femur. |
| Epistaxis | Medical terminology for "bloody nose."<br><br>1. Have patient sit up and lean forward (leaning backward can cause aspiration).<br>2. Apply pressure at the bridge of the nose.<br>3. Be prepared if blood has trickled down the back of patient's throat (may feel urge to cough or vomit); proper eye protection may lessen the risk to the provider. |

*(Continued)*

**Table 7.2** Types of Bleed and Steps to Take (*Continued*)

| TYPE OF BLEED | STEPS TO TAKE |
|---|---|
| Ear and nose (not spontaneous epistaxis) | May be the result of trauma to the skull and should not be controlled by direct pressure.<br><br>1. Check for indications of underlying skull fractures—spongy feeling when palpating, obvious bone shards, Battle sign of bruising behind the ears, or deformities.<br><br>2. Check for cerebrospinal fluid (CSF) leakage or blood leaking from ears; cover with gauze and tape to "catch" the fluid.<br><br>3. Assess and calculate a GCS score—reassess every 5–10 minutes depending on severity of patient. |
| Capillary bleeding | Typically very easy to control and may already have stopped bleeding prior to EMS arrival.<br><br>1. Identify all areas of bleeding, and expose wound to make sure there is not a deeper bleed occurring.<br><br>2. If wound has not already begun to clot, provide direct pressure on wound until bleeding stops.<br><br>3. Place and secure bandage if necessary. |

**Tourniquets**

A **tourniquet** is the most efficient way to control arterial bleeding in an extremity. A tourniquet is a bandage at least 4 inches wide placed between the heart and approximately 2 inches above the wound. When applied and tightened, it will stop all blood flow to the wound distal to the device:

- Consequences may include nerve and tissue damage secondary to the stoppage of oxygenated blood flow to the tissues and cells beyond the application point

- If done correctly, can be in place for up to 2 hours without causing irreversible tissue or nerve damage

- Receiving facility should be advised immediately that the tourniquet has been applied; "TQ" should be written on the patient's forehead or other visible location, especially in a mass casualty situation

Tourniquets have become required equipment on both BLS and ALS units nationwide. While most services utilize commercial tourniquets such as C-A-T, SOF, Israeli bandages, or SWAT-T, it is also possible to improvise and make tourniquets if necessary.

To make a tourniquet:

- Use a wide bandage (never rope or wire that could cut into the tissue and cause necrosis)

- Tie the bandage with a half hitch, and place a stick or bandage scissors on top of the knot; then complete the knot by tying an opposite half hitch to complete a square knot

- Twist the stick or scissors to tighten the bandage until the bleeding stops, and then secure the stick or scissors with another bandage
- A quick tourniquet that can be improvised is the use of the blood pressure cuff (monitor for air loss)

Regardless of whether it is a commercial or an improvised unit, once applied, the EMT should never loosen a tourniquet. Doing so could result in severe shock as blood rushes from the brain to fill the injured extremity.

Remember: Never apply a tourniquet directly over a joint. Familiarize yourself with all of your service's equipment because a true emergency is NOT the time to stop and read directions on the package. Remember that all bleeding eventually stops, but the amount of blood loss it takes to get to that point can and should be managed appropriately before it results in loss of life.

### Hemostatic Agents

A hemostatic agent is a type of substance that is used to control injured blood vessels, typically arteries due to their hard to control nature when lacerated. It is also known as antihemorrhagic agent, and it works by contracting tissue to seal injured blood vessels.

Originally used mainly in the military, studies have shown that hemostatic agents have a usage in the prehospital field as well. They come in different commercially available formats to help EMS professionals, such as:

- Impregnated gauze
- Free-flowing powder
- Granule packets

Not all units nationwide carry hemostatic agents. So it is up to the EMT to be properly trained in their usage if they are present on the truck.

## Internal Bleeding

Internal bleeding is more problematic for the EMT since it is not always apparent yet may lead to severe hypovolemic shock and death. This is especially true when internal organs in the torso have been ruptured due to severe trauma such as an automobile accident or fall. Blunt force trauma can also be caused by blast injuries.

Suspicion of serious internal bleeding may be deduced from the mechanism of injury and the signs and symptoms that the EMT finds when performing the trauma assessment. These signs and symptoms include:

- Pain, tenderness, swelling, or discoloration of the suspected site
- Bleeding from the mouth, rectum, vagina, or other body orifices
- Blood in vomit, urine, or stool
- Tenderness, rigidity, and distension of the abdomen

Treatment of internal bleeding treats the hypoperfusion syndrome that results. Suspicion of internal bleeding raises the priority of the transport, and the "golden hour" becomes much more critical in these types of cases. Transport to the proper facility rapidly, ideally one with surgical capabilities.

## Emergency Care of Shock

As the body's own mechanisms attempt to heal and compensate for a traumatic injury, these systems may be overwhelmed. Serious harm may occur as a result.

**Hemorrhagic shock** occurs when the volume of blood becomes insufficient to provide oxygen and nutrients to the cells or remove waste products from the cells. This condition may lead to serious organ damage or death.

The EMT must also be aware of the signs and symptoms of hypovolemic shock, which include:

- Anxiety or altered mental status
- General weakness or dizziness
- Tachypnea and tachycardia
- Cool, pale, and clammy skin
- Delayed capillary refill—i.e., >2 seconds
- Nausea and vomiting
- Dilated pupils that are sluggish in response to light

### KEY TAKEAWAY

Note: The classic sign of hypovolemic shock is dropping blood pressure. This is considered a late sign, and measures for treatment should be begun before it develops. In the case of pediatric patients, since they have a lower blood volume than adults, a dropping blood pressure may indicate that they are close to death, and aggressive treatment is necessary.

Treatment for hypoperfusion syndrome includes the following:

- Maintain the airway, ventilating if necessary
- Administer high-flow oxygen
- Control external bleeding
- Elevate the lower extremities 8–12 inches
- Splint any suspected fractures
- Prevent heat loss by covering the patient with blankets
- Expedite transport to a trauma center if indicated

If your protocols allow, and with the approval of medical control, consider application of a pneumatic anti-shock garment called a PASG. *(Note: Very few agencies still use these devices.)*

## Soft Tissue Injuries and Burns

### Soft Tissue Injuries

Soft tissue injuries are injuries to skin, muscle, tendons, and/or ligaments. In other words, these are not direct fractures to bone or injuries to internal organs. However, soft tissue injuries are not always isolated, i.e., they may occur alongside bone fractures or underlying internal damage.

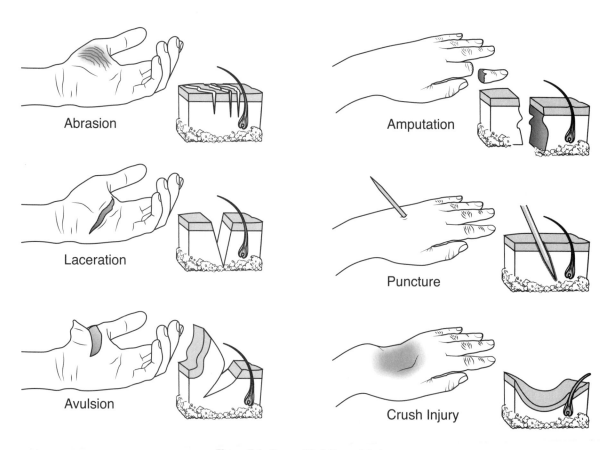

**Figure 7.1** Types of Soft Tissue Injuries

Recall that the skin has 3 layers: the outermost **epidermis**; the **dermis**, which contains the oil glands and hair follicles; and the **subcutaneous layer**, which contains fatty deposits and helps to provide cushioning and/or temporary protection.

The degree of soft tissue injury is directly related to the number of skin layers involved:

- For a burn, you need to know which layers of skin have been affected to determine the depth and severity.
- For a laceration or avulsion, you need to know the depth of skin layers that have been injured. A superficial abrasion is confined to the top layer of skin, while an avulsion may go all the way down to the subcutaneous layer.

Treatment protocols necessitate that the EMT can recognize these as well.

## Closed Injuries

A closed injury is damage in which the epidermis remains intact and there is no external bleeding. There are three types of closed injury:

- In a **contusion**, the cells and smaller blood vessels are damaged below the epidermis from some type of trauma and blood pools in the tissues causing a purplish discoloration. This area is often swollen and painful to the touch.
- A **hematoma** involves laceration of a larger blood vessel, either an artery or a vein, and results in a large pool of blood beneath the epidermal layer.
- A **crush injury** is a closed tissue injury that may cause internal organ rupture; the accompanying bleeding may be so severe as to cause hypoperfusion syndrome (shock).

Emergency medical care for these types of injuries involves appropriate body substance isolation (BSI), airway and ventilatory support, treatment for shock, and rapid transport. If the injury involves an extremity, splinting the extremity is often helpful for both treatment of hypovolemia and pain management. Since these types of injuries cannot be well managed in the prehospital setting, rapid transport to a trauma center is always indicated, remembering the "golden hour."

## Open Injuries

Open injuries are open wounds with external bleeding.

**Table 7.3** Open Soft Tissue Wounds

| OPEN WOUND TYPE | CHARACTERISTICS | PATIENT MANAGEMENT |
|---|---|---|
| Abrasion | • Epidermal layer damaged by shearing or scraping<br>• Very painful, though superficial injury<br>• Causes minimal blood loss<br>• Because of the larger area involved, more prone to infection than smaller-area wounds | Consider using sterile gauze and tape to secure, if the minimal bleeding persists |

*(Continued)*

**Table 7.3** Open Soft Tissue Wounds (*Continued*)

| OPEN WOUND TYPE | CHARACTERISTICS | PATIENT MANAGEMENT |
| --- | --- | --- |
| Laceration | • Break in the skin, of varying depth<br>• *Linear laceration* is an incision caused by a sharp object, while *irregular laceration* is caused by blunt trauma<br>• Depending on depth and location, bleeding may be minor to severe<br>• The deeper the wound, the greater the danger of infection, as bacteria may have been introduced deep into the tissues by the object causing the laceration | Consider use of hemostatic agent if indicated |
| Avulsion | • Flap of skin or tissue torn off by a traumatic force<br>• Very painful<br>• Causes significant blood loss | Fold flap of skin back into original position if possible |
| Amputation | • Complete separation of a distal extremity or part from the extremity or trunk<br>• May cause minimal bleeding if it is a clean cut (rather than tearing off) | Attempt to find amputated item to transport to hospital with patient |
| Penetration/ puncture | • Deep intrusion into soft tissue by any object (e.g., bullet, knife)<br>• May cause minimal or no external bleeding, but depth of the injury may produce significant internal bleeding | • If object is still protruding from body, stabilize it with gauze and secure it with tape so it doesn't move and cause further damage during transport<br>• Search and identify all wounds (don't forget the back and sides) |
| Crush | • Crushed body part due to pressure from a heavy object<br>• May be open or closed<br>• Greater danger is to the underlying organs and tissues | • Call for additional personnel to remove crushing object if present; also consider calling ALS<br>• Depending on location and time of crush, be prepared for traumatic cardiac arrest |

Management of soft tissue injuries is as follows:

- Your first concern is to protect yourself from the dangers of blood-borne pathogens. A massive trauma scenario involving large volumes of blood loss requires more extensive precautions than a simple finger laceration. Precautions may include:
    - Full-body gown.
    - Mask.

- Eye protection.

- Gloves.

- Shoe coverings.

- Once the scene is safe and precautions have been taken, you must secure the patient's airway and provide ventilatory support. In the presence of a gross traumatic injury, some EMTs will focus on the injury site and neglect to check the airway (called a **distracting injury**). It is human nature to want to address all injuries at once, but remember that a patient without an airway will arrive at the ER dead.

- Once the airway and breathing are secure, the area of bleeding must be exposed and the rest of the body thoroughly checked for other wounds, including exit wounds:

  - For legal reasons, be careful *not* to document each wound as such in your PCR; only note that you found "multiple wounds" and describe the location and severity of each.

  - In calls where weapons were involved, police may be involved to secure the scene. There may also be a potential criminal case where you may be called to testify.

  - To clarify even further, EMTs are not trained to be ballistic experts nor are they trained as coroners. So they do not have the expertise to properly identify which wound is which—lawyers will point this out if the case goes to court.

- With an open wound, it's important to prevent further bacterial contamination. Minimize the risk of further contamination by doing the following:

  - Open packages only as items are needed.

  - Use rubbing alcohol (at least 60% strength) to clean off equipment prior to use.

- Once bleeding has been controlled, dress open wounds with dry, sterile dressings and secure with clean bandaging materials such as muslin cravats or self-securing bandaging material:

  - Remember that blood loss leads to shock and that the treatment of hypovolemic syndrome must always be a concern.

  - Refer back to the previous section on bleeding and shock management for review.

Following treatment of a severe trauma patient, it is always prudent to remain out of service until the unit has been properly decontaminated. Providers may choose at their discretion (and with approval from supervisors or dispatch) to return to the station for a shower and clothing change. Any clothing that has been exposed to blood must be considered contaminated and washed properly, in accordance with local guidelines for dealing with objects contaminated by bodily fluids.

There is no set amount of time that is "required" to be out of service when decontaminating your truck unit. Depending on the level of cleaning required, it could run from wiping down any visible blood from the doors, windows, bench seats, and equipment used (e.g., blood pressure cuff or pulse oximeter) to fully mopping the floors. Thus, you could be out of service from 10 minutes to over 60 minutes.

Whatever amount of cleaning that needs to be done, it must first be cleared with your supervisor or dispatch center. The expectation is that your unit should be back in service within a reasonable amount of time and be ready to take additional emergency calls as soon as possible.

### Special Situations and Treatments

Some wounds, due to their location on the body, present special situations and require special treatments:

- **Chest wound** accompanied by a gurgling sound and frothy blood indicates that the lung has been penetrated:
  - This could lead to a severely collapsed lung or pneumothorax (known as *sucking chest wounds*).
  - If collapse is so severe as to cause the organs in the chest to shift position, e.g., tracheal deviation (called a *tension pneumothorax*), that is a life-threatening situation requiring rapid treatment and transport.
  - Treatment is dressing with an occlusive dressing, which will block airflow into the collapsed pleural space. Always administer oxygen as the patient will almost always have compromised breathing.
- **Abdominal injury** accompanied by protruding organs (called an *evisceration injury*) is always serious. Do your best not to touch the organs or attempt to put them back inside the abdomen. Treatment is coverage of the wound with a sterile dressing, thoroughly moistened with sterile water or saline. Transport immediately.
- **Impaled object** in the body should not be removed, as it typically tourniquets the blood internally. (Exceptions include an object through the cheek, an object that would interfere with chest compressions, or an object that would interfere with transport.) Treatment is contacting medical control for advice on how to proceed, but that often includes securing the object, controlling any peripheral bleeding, and transporting.
- **Extremity amputation** is treated as any other open wound:
  - It may be partial or complete.
  - It may produce tremendous blood loss, depending on location.
  - It has a psychological component for both the EMT and the patient.
  - Treatment is immediate transport to the emergency department; if possible, locate and transport the amputated part as well for possible reattachment:
    - Wrap the amputated part in a sterile dressing and place into a plastic bag.
    - Place the plastic bag onto an ice pack to keep the bag cool; **do not place the amputated part directly on ice as it will freeze**.
    - If amputation is partial, stabilize as best as possible; **do not attempt to complete amputation**.

- **Neck injury** poses unique challenges in both securing a bandage and also making sure the airway stays patent. If there is frothy bleeding, this may indicate injury to both the airway and blood vessels in the neck. Treatment is an occlusive dressing, which will prevent an embolism from entering the circulatory system and causing cardiac/respiratory arrest.

---

An **occlusive dressing** is a sterile dressing made with nonbreathable material that covers the wound hole. It is then secured with adhesive tape either on all 4 sides or on 3 sides, leaving one side untaped as a "flutter valve" that allows excess air to escape out the fourth side ("burping"). The number of sides to tape depends on the location of the wound:

- Chest/thorax = 3-sided occlusive dressing
- Open neck wound = 3-sided occlusive dressing
- Abdominal evisceration = 4-sided occlusive dressing

Commercially premade options are available. Alternatively, there are a variety of materials you can use to make your own:

- Impregnated gauze, which is gauze thoroughly soaked in a material (e.g., petroleum, hemostatic agent) that leaves no areas for air to pass through
- Paper or plastic packaging from a gauze pad (with the gauze discarded)
- Plastic food wrap

Note that regular sterile gauze is not used because it is too breathable. Air can permeate.

Whatever material is used, place it directly over the wound and tape as many sides as the wound requires. Make sure to reassess as needed every 5–15 minutes depending on the stability of your patient.

---

## Burns

### Burn Depth

Burns are classified according to the depth of the injured tissue. Even though the current literature lists the three categories as superficial, partial thickness, and full thickness, EMT and hospital staff may still refer to these as first, second, and third degree:

- A **first-degree (superficial) burn** involves only the epidermis:
  - Characterized by a reddening of the skin and local pain
  - Example—ordinary sunburn

- A **second-degree (partial-thickness) burn** involves both the epidermis and dermis but not the underlying tissue:
  - Accompanied by intense pain and blistering of the skin
  - Skin may be bright red to white
  - Example—sunburn that has fluid-filled blisters
- A **third-degree (full-thickness) burn** involves all three layers of skin and possibly underlying muscles, bones, tissues, and organs:
  - Characterized by charred, dry, and leathery skin
  - May cause little or no pain where skin is burned if sensory nerves were damaged or destroyed
  - Peripheral areas usually have lesser-degree burns with extreme pain

### Rule of Nines

The overall survivability of a burn patient is contingent not only upon the depth/type of burn but also on the amount of skin surface (body surface area [BSA]) involved.

The **rule of nines** was developed to assist EMS in relaying to the receiving facility how much BSA is involved in the burn injury. There are 11 body areas, each of which contains approximately 9% of the body's overall area. For an adult, they are broken down as follows.

**Table 7.4** Rule of Nines

| BODY PART | % OF BODY AREA |
|---|---|
| Head and neck | 9 |
| Chest | 9 |
| Abdomen | 9 |
| Front of each leg | 9 |
| Back of each leg | 9 |
| Front and back of each leg | 18 |
| Front of each arm | 4.5 |
| Back of each arm | 4.5 |
| Front and back of each arm | 9 |
| Upper back | 9 |
| Lower back (ends at top of buttocks) | 9 |
| **Note:** The genitalia counts as 1%. | |

Suppose a patient sustains burns on their face and both arms. Each arm is 9%, for a total of 18%. The front of the head is 4.5% (half of 9%). Thus, the total BSA is 22.5%.

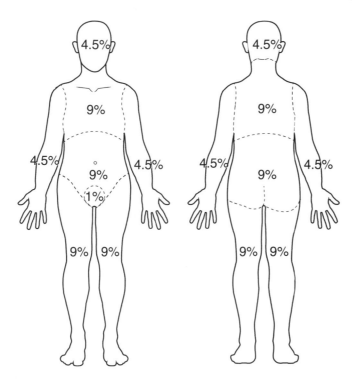

**Figure 7.2** Rule of Nines for Burn Assessment (Adult)

An alternative method for measuring burns is the **palmar method**. The patient's palm and fingers equal approximately 1% of BSA burned. It is not to be used on large surface area burns, however, where the rule of nines would be more appropriate.

---

**TEST YOURSELF 7.1**

**What percentage is this patient burned?**

A 45-year-old female has sustained some burns after a cooking accident where hot oil splashed up from the pan onto her. She has sustained burns to her hands, anterior forearms, and upper chest. What percentage of her body has been burned?

---

## Burn Severity

Burn severity is also gauged by location. Once the type of burn and the BSA affected have been determined, the EMT can determine the severity of the injury.

Burns to the face and torso are highly challenging given the patient's risk of inhaling any products of combustion, leading to possible swelling of the airway and fluid buildup in the lungs.

**Table 7.5** Severity of Burns

| SEVERITY | LOCATION, EXTENT, AND OTHER FACTORS |
|---|---|
| Minor burn | Superficial burn covering <50% of BSA |
| | Second-degree burn covering <15% of BSA |
| | Third-degree burn covering <2% of BSA |
| Moderate burn | Any third-degree burn involving 2–10% of BSA, unless it involves the hands, feet, face, genitalia, or upper chest |
| | Any second-degree burn involving 15–30% of BSA |
| | Any first-degree burn involving >50% of BSA |
| Severe burn | Any third-degree burn involving the hands, feet, face, or genitalia |
| | Any burn involving respiratory damage |
| | Third-degree burns involving >10% of BSA |
| | Second-degree burns involving >30% of BSA |
| | Any burns complicated by painful, swollen, or deformed extremities |
| | Moderate burns to pediatric and geriatric patients |
| | Any burns that encompass an entire body part, such as an arm, leg, chest, etc. |

Suppose a male patient has a sunburn that covers all of his body except the area covered by a bathing suit. EMS would identify him as having a superficial burn covering 70–80% of his BSA. That is considered a moderate burn injury, not a minor burn.

## Treatment

Treatment of burns ranges from minor wound management using sterile gauze to emergent transport to a certified burn center. Severity depends on the type, size, location, and depth of the burn. However, there are some universal steps to take no matter the type of burn inflicted.

First, stop the burning process:

- Remove any burned clothing and all jewelry.
- Pour copious amounts of water or saline onto the burned area.
- Be alert for airway compromise if there has been exposure to any products of combustion.

Second, use extreme caution to prevent any infection:

- Create as sterile an environment for the patient as possible.
- Once cooled, cover burned areas with loose, dry dressings.

- Do not ever break blisters.
- Do not ever apply ointment, lotion, or antiseptics in the emergency care setting. These products can trap excess heat, thus raising the body temperature unnecessarily.

Third, address the patient's temperature since a severe burn can affect the body's ability to regulate core temperature:

- Manage any hypothermia or dehydration.
- Give supplemental oxygen therapy as needed.

Chemical and electrical burns have additional considerations:

- Treat **chemical burns** by flushing with water or with fluids recommended for that particular chemical (try to read the label or material safety data sheet [MSDS]):
  - Brush any caustic powder off the skin before flushing.
  - Take care not to allow the runoff fluid to injure unaffected body parts.
  - Never attempt to neutralize a chemical burn using another chemical, such as applying a base to an acid burn. The resulting chemical reaction can create heat that will further burn the patient.
  - You may also ask the patient if they know the chemical name—if yes, then it may be looked up in the *Emergency Response Guidebook* (ERG). This book allows the provider to not only look up the chemical's properties but also lists first-aid responses and how far away a provider should be if there is a leak or spill.
- **Electrical burns** are a concern for the safety of the responding crew:
  - Be sure that the person is not still energized by contact with the electrical object that caused the injury; if you are unsure, do not touch the patient (for your own safety).
  - Once you have determined that the patient is safe to touch, treat the wound as you would any burn.
  - Contact with an electrical object may cause both an entrance and an exit wound as the electricity goes to ground.
  - Electrocution may cause cardiac arrhythmia, so have the AED ready to use in case the victim's heart begins to fibrillate.

## Injuries to the Musculoskeletal System

Injuries to the musculoskeletal system of the body are among the most challenging to the EMT. The principles of this type of care are important to understand since trauma patients will rarely present with a textbook example of a musculoskeletal injury. The EMT will have to improvise treatment utilizing these principles.

In order to implement a treatment plan for this type of injury, a study of the **mechanism of injury (MOI)** is necessary.

## Types of Force

The EMT National Curriculum mentions three types of force that cause injury:

- In **direct force**, the injury occurs at the point of impact. If a window falls onto someone's forearm and fractures the radius, this is an example of a direct force injury.
- In **indirect force**, the injury occurs away from the point of impact. An example of indirect force would be when a person falls and lands on their feet and the force of the landing causes the person's hip to dislocate.
- **Twisting force**, as the name implies, occurs when one part of an extremity remains stationary while another part rotates. An example of this is a sprained ankle, in which the person's ankle twisted, causing the person to stumble and possibly fall.

## Types of Bone Injury

There are two types of bone and joint injury:

- **Open** fracture, sprain, or strain—broken bone or torn tissue that has a break in the continuity of the skin
- **Closed** fracture, sprain, or strain—broken bone or torn tissue that has no break in the skin

The signs and symptoms of a bone or joint injury are the following:

- Deformity
- Pain
- Grating (bone ends or shards scraping/rubbing upon each other)
- Swelling
- Discoloration
- Exposed bone ends
- Locked joint

Emergency care is to splint the injury, apply cold to reduce swelling, and elevate the extremity to reduce the pain as well as treat for shock.

Note: Because an open fracture is a "combination injury," it requires treatment of both the broken bone/damaged joint and the accompanying wound with bleeding control and management.

## Splinting

Management of musculoskeletal injuries involves a technique known as splinting, which is the immobilization of a broken bone or damaged joint as well as any adjacent joints. A properly applied splint helps to prevent further damage to tissues irritated by the broken bone ends. Splinting also minimizes the danger that a closed injury may progress to an open injury, further complicating patient care and resulting in a much longer recovery period.

Prior to applying a splint, you must assess distal **p**ulse (or circulation), **m**otor function, and **s**ensory function (or sensation), abbreviated as **PMS** (or CMS).

Compare the injured side to the noninjured side, especially with regard to length. The splint must immobilize the area where the EMT suspects the break has occurred as well as the adjacent joints:

- Suspected midshaft tibia fracture—splint must immobilize not only the midshaft area of the bone but also the ankle joint and knee joint
- Finger dislocation—splint should wrap together the injured finger and an uninjured finger next to it as a type of "natural splint"
- Fractured forearm—splint should secure the wrist joint in place as well as the forearm to create a sturdy, straight line

Prior to application of any splint:

- Remove or **cut away clothing** to show the entire wound area. You need to see what you're working with!
- **Remove shoes and boots** in lower-extremity injuries to assess distal pulse and assure proper splinting.
- In open fractures, **control bleeding** as necessary and dress the wound with a **sterile dressing** before applying a splint.
- If an extremity is severely deformed or a distal area is cyanotic with absent pulses and sensation, the **limb must be realigned** with gentle traction prior to splinting. **Do not force** any movement; this could cause further damage or pain.

After splinting any injury, always reassess distal PMS. Then compare the new results against the initial vital signs to see if anything has changed. (If the patient had a distal pulse before splinting but now doesn't, for example, the splint may be incorrectly applied or too tight.) After comparing these PMS assessments, reapply splinting as needed.

## Types of Splints

There are many types of splints, including improvised splints used in wilderness EMS. Basically, a splint is any object that immobilizes the suspected injury and adjacent joints.

The splints most common to EMS are the **rigid board splints** (or padded board splints), which come in a variety of sizes. These boards are secured in whatever configuration is necessary with the use of cravats or straps. Variations include the vinyl splints with rigid spines that secure quickly with Velcro.

Other examples include the following:

- A **long backboard (LBB)** can immobilize the entire body.
- **Vacuum** or **air pressure splints** not only splint but also provide pressure uniformly to the extremity, which is useful in wound management as well.
- **PASG** is a type of air splint that also immobilizes the entire lower body, including the pelvis. It is also known as MAST trousers. Many systems no longer utilize this in their protocols.
- **Traction splints** provide continuous traction of the lower extremities and are often indicated by protocol for management of closed femur fractures. A traction splint helps to alleviate pain by preventing the broken bone ends from aggravating the surrounding tissue.

- **Structural aluminum malleable (SAM) splints** are lightweight aluminum strips that are enclosed in a flexible foam padding. This makes them easily moldable to various shapes to accommodate the extremities.

Finally, many ordinary objects can be adapted for splinting, such as pillows, large towels, and large magazines. However, no matter what material is used, always remember to assess and reassess PMS before and after splinting has been applied. Readjust as necessary.

## Injuries to the Head and Spine

With injuries to the head or spine, EMS should pay close attention to the mechanism of injury and should visualize what may have happened to the body of the patient:

- The **brain** is responsible for operating the multiple systems of the human body. It receives sensory information and sends electrical impulses to the organs, muscles, and tissues via the nervous system.
- The **spinal cord**, which runs from the base of the brain down the back, is the main transmission line for these actions. If it is damaged or severed as a result of trauma, these systems may be compromised. The spinal cord is surrounded and protected by the bony spinal column, which is composed of 33 bones called **vertebrae**.

Injury to the spinal cord may be caused by the following types of scenarios:

- **Spinal cord compression** due to significant force applied to the top of the head (as in a person diving head first into an empty swimming pool)
- **Spinal column and spinal cord damage** due to excessive motion (as in a sports injury)
- **Spinal column distraction** (the pulling apart of adjacent vertebrae) due to excessive stretching (as in hanging by the neck)

If you suspect spinal injury upon arrival at the scene, you will need to perform half or full immobilization utilizing a cervical collar.

### KEY TAKEAWAY

Gone are the days when every patient routinely got a backboard. Newer research has shown that indiscriminate backboarding may do more harm than good. As a result, many **EMTs are being authorized to perform "spinal clearance"** in the field. This means that if a patient does not fit certain criteria or have complaints of spinal injury, full immobilization may not be required.

Make sure that you are familiar with the local protocols of your EMS service for immobilization of patients.

## Head Injuries

Injuries to the head present a special challenge to the EMT. The scalp is extremely vascular, and any open wound there causes a large amount of bleeding. Be aware that open head wounds typically look worse than they are; clean the wound with saline and examine closely.

A closed wound from blunt force trauma may cause bleeding inside the cranial compartment, causing increased pressure inside the skull (known as **intracranial pressure [ICP]**) and complicating both breathing and circulation. Keep in mind that in addition to trauma, some medical conditions, such as stroke, may give the same signs and symptoms as head trauma.

You should suspect a brain injury when any of the following are present during the primary or focused assessment:

- Altered or decreasing mental status
- Irregular breathing
- Bleeding or bruising to the head
- Blood or fluid (cerebrospinal fluid) leaking from the ears, eyes, nose, or mouth
- Bruising around the eyes (raccoon eyes)
- Bruising behind the ears (Battle sign)
- Any neurological disability, nausea and vomiting, or pupils of different sizes with altered mental status
- Seizure activity
- "Spongy" areas noted on palpation (could be underlying fracture)

Proper treatment of suspected skull fracture or brain injury is critical:

- Expedite transport to a trauma center immediately.
- Any head injury is assumed to involve the cervical spine, so immobilize the head and spine.
- Closely monitor the patient for abrupt changes in mental status and vital signs—monitor using the GCS score.
- Control any bleeding from the head as you would with any open wound. However, do not apply pressure to an open or depressed skull wound since that would risk pushing a bone fragment into the brain or increasing the intracranial pressure.

## Spinal Injuries

As you perform the assessment, the suspicion of a spinal cord injury rises significantly if any of the following signs or symptoms are present:

- Tenderness or pain in the back or neck
- Pain when the neck or back is moved
- Intermittent pain in the spinal column or legs independent of motion or palpation

- Any open injuries to the back or neck
- Numbness, tingling, or weakness in the extremities
- Loss of sensation or motion in the extremities
- Incontinence (involuntary loss of urine or feces)

If the spinal cord injury is located in the upper cervical vertebrae, the ability to breathe or move the extremities may be compromised. You must be prepared to intervene to correct these conditions.

If a spinal injury is suspected and the patient is responsive, you must ask the patient if they have back or neck pain, if they can move their fingers and toes without pain, and if they can feel you touching their extremities.

Following inspection and palpation of the neck, back, and extremities and as part of the focused trauma assessment, ask the patient to complete two important tests to determine if there is communication from their brain to their extremities. This is achieved by asking the patient to complete the following commands and noting if there is equal strength in each extremity, if the movement causes pain, and whether or not the patient is able to complete the task:

- Ask the patient to grab your hands and squeeze as hard as they can.
- With your hands pushing gently on the soles of the patient's feet, ask the patient to push down and then point their toes toward their head.

When a spinal injury is suspected, you must immobilize the cervical spine as follows ("hold C-spine") until a cervical collar and backboard or KED can be placed:

1. Align the spinal cord in a neutral (straight) "eyes forward" position:
   - Take the head in both hands and gently align it with the spine.
   - If you suspect a cervical injury, you can also use your first and middle fingers to perform a modified jaw thrust and secure a patent airway.
2. Maintain this stabilized immobility while the patient is secured to a long backboard or KED board.
3. Check the following:
   - Does the patient have a patent airway?
   - Are they breathing?
   - Do they have a palpable carotid pulse?
   - Has major life-threatening bleeding been controlled?
4. If the answer to *all* of the preceding questions is "Yes," you can perform the remainder of the initial assessment and start to apply spinal protective equipment.

### Applying a Cervical Collar

Once the head and neck have been assessed by sight and touch, a **rigid cervical collar (C-collar)** should be applied to assist with maintaining stabilization. The C-collar must be the correct size for the patient and must be properly applied or more harm can result.

The collar must hold the head and chin up in the neutral position, without hyperextending the neck. It must touch the skin on the chest and back as well as the chin and back of the neck. To properly size a C-collar, follow these steps:

1. Obtain a lateral view of the patient's head while your partner maintains the neutral in-line position.

2. With fingers outstretched, place all fingers including your thumb next to each other with no space between.

3. Pinky finger side down, rest your outstretched hand on the base of the patient's shoulder.

4. While looking at the patient's chin, draw an imaginary straight line with your eyes.

5. Count the number of fingers it takes to meet with that imaginary straight line. For example, if your middle finger matches the line, you have three fingers worth of space to measure with on the collar.

**Figure 7.3** Measuring for Cervical Collar Height

If you are using a C-collar that is adjustable, follow the manufacturer's guidelines to find the appropriate measurement tool on the collar itself. Place your fingers in the specified space to determine the size of the collar so it matches the number of fingers you have previously measured with. Sizes will range from "no-neck" to "tall." Secure the collar in the measured selection.

If using a nonadjustable collar, the sizing process is still the same; however, you must identify which collar to use. They will be individually labeled with sizes. Because this equates to having multiple individual pieces, most systems do not utilize these, rather opting for an all-in-one adjustable collar.

Pediatric patients require the usage of smaller collars, and your service will have them available to use. The steps to apply them are mainly the same as previously described.

### Securing to a Long Backboard

When the initial assessment is complete and the c-collar has been placed, the patient is then secured to a long backboard (LBB), or **spine board**, as follows.

**Table 7.6** Securing a Patient in Full Immobilization

| STEP NUMBER | PROCEDURE |
|---|---|
| 1 | With patient laying supine, one EMT places the board next to the patient. |
| 2 | One EMT continues to hold the C-spine, while the second EMT places the C-collar. If this has already been done, move to step 3. |
| 3 | While kneeling on the opposite side of where the LBB is placed, the second EMT crosses the patient's arms over the chest (as an X) so they are safely out of the way during the logroll maneuver.<br><br>*Ideally a third provider is on scene to help with the next steps, but they can be achieved with 2 providers. |
| 4 | Whoever is holding the patient's head then confirms that everyone is ready, and on the count of 3, all providers roll the patient on their side toward the EMTs (called the "logroll maneuver"). The person holding the head rolls the head at the same time, keeping it aligned with the spine.<br><br>*Which side you roll toward doesn't matter as long as everyone does the same thing in unison. If there is an injury, however, it is advisable to roll to the uninjured side. |
| 5 | One EMT quickly assesses the posterior side of the patient, and the EMT controlling the backboard places it beneath the patient. |
| 6 | Once everyone is again in position and ready, the EMT holding the head counts to 3 and the team proceeds to roll the patient to the supine position, this time on the backboard. |
| 7 | The patient is then properly positioned on the board at the command of the EMT holding cervical stabilization; everyone must make coordinated movements to avoid excessive spinal movement. |
| 8 | The patient is then secured to the board using a minimum of 3 straps: one across the chest, one across the pelvis, and one across the legs. |
| 9 | The patient's head is then secured to the board using an approved device, usually head blocks and Velcro straps (check to see what your employer uses). |
| 10 | All distal neurological signs are checked again. The patient, now properly splinted, is placed onto the stretcher, secured with further stretcher straps, and moved to ambulance for transport. |
| *11 | *If the patient is found in a sitting position, a short spine board or intermediate transport device such as a Kendrick Extrication Device (KED) is used to remove them from the immediate area to a long backboard. |

When dealing with head or spinal injury, there are some special considerations:

- Decide whether to extricate the patient (from car, etc.) using the **time-consuming method of full spinal and head immobilization** or the more **rapid method using minimal immobilization**. The rapid method is more appropriate for unsafe situations (e.g., fire), unstable patients (e.g., not breathing), and patients who may be blocking access to a more critically injured patient.

- Decide whether to remove a sport bike or motorcycle helmet. Current protocols advise the following:

  - Remove any face guards and shields for assessment. (If at a sporting event, the team medic or coach may have a special key to deflate the pads inside.)

  - Leave the helmet on unless it is necessary to ventilate a patient or treat a severe, bleeding wound. Perform spinal stabilization with the helmet in place.

  - If removal of the helmet is necessary to prevent a potentially life-threatening condition, do it in two steps—one EMT stabilizes the head/neck, while the second EMT uses the hands to spread the helmet wide, push up, and lift off with minimal movement and strain on the head/neck.

## Injuries to the Eyes, Face, and Neck

### Eye Injuries

Injuries to the eye are almost always considered serious since they may have long-term consequences to the quality of life of a victim of trauma. In assessing trauma to the eyes, in addition to palpating for broken bones, you should use your diagnostic penlight to determine the reactivity of the pupils to light and compare the responses from each eye to the other. Also, the patient should be able to track the light with their eyes without moving the head and the tracking should be smooth for both eyes.

Often, foreign objects take up residence in the eye. Small particles of dust and other foreign matter are usually removed by flushing the eyeball with sterile water or saline. Chemicals and irritants splashed into the eyes can also be removed by flushing. This can be done in a myriad of ways:

- Have the patient splash water into both of their eyes over a bowl or other receptacle such as an emesis bin.

- Have the patient turn their head with the affected eye down laterally, and then pour sterile water down in a stream over the eyes.

- Use a nasal cannula connected to saline and placed over the bridge of the nose to irrigate both eyes:

  - Connect the NC to an IV set and a 1-liter bag of saline instead of oxygen.

  - Nasal prongs rest over the medial edge of the eye socket.

  - Open the IV set to flow and allow saline to come through.

If there is a penetrating injury to the eye, the object is not removed but secured in place with bandages and dressings. In this type of injury to the eye, both eyes are always covered so that the parallel motion of the uninjured eye does not cause the injured eye to move. In the case of an avulsed eyeball, do not attempt to replace the eye. Instead, cover the eyeball with a moist, sterile dressing and a clean paper cup, and then bandage them in place to protect the eye. Once again, cover the other eye as well.

## Face Injuries

Because of the extensive vasculature of the face and head, injuries to these areas bleed profusely. Injuries to the face are treated in the same way as other injuries, with the exception that an impaled object through the cheek may be removed by the EMT in the field in order to facilitate management of the airway. Expect profuse bleeding. Note the following:

- If there is quite a bit of blood, dampen gauze with sterile saline, attempt to clean up the blood, and look for additional wounds that were not initially visible. This also helps you identify wounds that are continuously bleeding and need to be treated.
- If an airway needs to be established and there is facial trauma, avoid placing an NPA, which could protrude into the cranial cavity.
- Check inside the mouth for bleeding and/or displaced or missing teeth and to confirm that there is a patent airway. Suction as needed.

## Neck Injuries

Injuries to the neck may involve the great vessels leading to the brain as well as injury to the airway. Bubbling and gurgling of a neck wound are indications that the injury involves the airway. This type of wound requires an occlusive dressing to prevent outside air from entering the blood vessel and causing an air embolism.

If an object penetrating the neck does not directly block the airway, *stabilize the object in place* and bandage as needed. Do not attempt to remove the object. Doing so may damage the underlying structures. The carotid artery and jugular vein are located in that area bilaterally, meaning that attempted removal can cause massive bleeding.

**Never** place a tourniquet on the neck to control bleeding. This will result in asphyxia and, most likely, death of your patient.

If you suspect cervical spine injury, an appropriately sized C-collar should be placed. Be aware that if one section of the spine is compromised, other sections may be as well.

## Injuries to the Chest, Abdomen, and Genitalia

### Chest Injuries

If the assessment of a trauma victim reveals paradoxical motion of the rib cage, combined with pain and crepitus of the ribs, that is an indication of a condition called **flail chest**, defined as 2 or more adjacent ribs fractured with 2 or more breaks per rib. Flail chest leaves part of the rib cage unattached to the chest wall. The broken or "flailed" area floats freely on the chest wall, causing **paradoxical motion** during respiration. Paradoxical motion means movements that are opposite those of normal breathing. Normally, the chest rises when a person breathes in and falls when they breathe out. In paradoxical motion, the opposite happens instead: When the patient breathes in, the chest falls, and when they exhale, it rises.

---

### KEY TAKEAWAY

A **flail chest** is a major trauma. Expedite transport to a level 1 trauma center. Treat with high-flow oxygen via non-rebreather mask. Be alert for respiratory failure, which will require assistance with ventilations.

---

A chest injury that is bubbling is called a **sucking chest wound**. It must be dressed with an 3-sided occlusive dressing to prevent air from entering the pleural space and increasing the likelihood of a pneumothorax. The fourth side is left untaped to allow "burping" of any excess air that may have accumulated in the pleural space. Possible occlusive dressings for a sucking chest wound include:

- Waterproof thin-film-type dressings
- Premade commercial bandages
- Impregnated gauze pads
- Plastic food wrap (in an emergency)

Closed chest wounds are especially dangerous, the more so when they involve the heart or the great vessels leading to and from the heart. A serious condition known as **cardiac tamponade**, caused by blunt trauma to the heart, occurs when the sac surrounding the heart (pericardium) fills with blood; this puts pressure on the heart and deprives it of the space needed to beat and refill properly.

Be especially alert for the possibility of tamponade in cardiac trauma patients who spit or cough up blood. These patients have a higher suspicion of a closed chest injury involving the heart or lungs.

No basic intervention can be done in the field. If you suspect cardiac tamponade, make this patient a load and go, and proceed straight to a hospital with surgical capability.

## Abdominal Injuries

In the abdominal cavity, there are multiple organs that are described as either hollow or solid. Damage to either type of organ will lead to issues not only with the organ itself but also with the surrounding tissues.

- **Hollow organs**, such as the bladder and stomach, contain acids that help digest or break down substances in the body:

- If these organs become ruptured and discharge digestive products into the peritoneal space, patients are at increased risk of infection of the abdominal cavity.

- For example, if the bladder is lacerated, both urine (which is acidic to a certain extent) and bacteria will be released. This acidic urine and bacteria mixture will then touch or coat other organs and tissues surrounding the bladder, causing irritation.

- Another example is the stomach, where there are acids (gastric) and broken-down food particles. If the stomach is lacerated or burst, these substances will then "float" all around the abdominal cavity and cause inflammation.

- **Solid organs**, such as the liver and spleen, are very vascular in nature, with multiple veins and arteries that populate the tissue:

  - If these organs become damaged, the result will be bleeding into the surrounding tissues. It is entirely possible for someone to exsanguinate (bleed out) into their abdominal cavity, as it is a large area that can collect blood.

  - For example, a liver laceration can be a very serious event, as it is a large organ containing multiple veins and arteries.

Regardless of the specific injury, if the naked eye can see blood or other fluid collecting in the abdominal cavity, the EMT must take note and expedite transport.

Some signs and symptoms are as follows:

- Rigidity and tenderness of the abdomen are an indication of potential fluid buildup underneath the skin.

- Leaking fluid requires immediate attention
  - If it is a yellow color, it may be urine.
  - If it is a brown color, it may be a damaged organ responsible for holding feces, such as the intestines.
  - If it is a reddish, blood-tinged color, it may be damage to a solid organ.

- If the injury has exposed the intestines and they are protruding from the wound (called an **abdominal evisceration**), do the following:
  - Drape the intestines with moist, sterile dressings.
  - Irrigate with sterile water or saline.
  - Secure the dressing on all 4 sides.
  - Transport immediately. Do not attempt to push the intestines back into the cavity.

Finally, keep in mind that pain can be felt in the abdomen in a variety of ways. Some common symptoms are described in the table.

**Table 7.7** Types of Abdominal Pain

| PAIN TYPE | KEY FACTS |
| --- | --- |
| Visceral pain | <ul><li>Dull, achy in nature</li><li>Typically intermittent</li><li>Patient may not be able to identify where pain is coming from</li></ul> |
| Parietal pain | <ul><li>Sharp, stabbing</li><li>Typically localized in nature</li><li>Patient can often directly identify where pain is coming from</li></ul> |
| Referred pain | <ul><li>Unique in that pain is felt "elsewhere in the body," i.e., not where the injury actually occurred</li><li>Has to do with afferent and efferent nerve tracks, e.g., the signals have gotten crossed on the way to and from the brain</li><li>A patient with gallbladder issues may have pain in the right shoulder, but upon inspection there is no injury to the shoulder itself</li><li>Research is not yet clear on why referred pain occurs, but EMTs need to be aware of it in the field</li></ul> |
| Tearing/ripping pain | <ul><li>Often associated with ulcers and AAAs (abdominal aortic aneurysms)</li><li>Aorta spans from the heart down into the abdominal cavity and is under high pressure at all times</li><li>If aorta has burst or lacerated, patient will experience immense level of pain and can bleed out (internally) quickly</li><li>EMT may see a pulsating mass, or patient's stomach may pulsate in time with radial or carotid pulse</li><li>Some patients live with AAA for years and are monitored to see if it grows larger or needs surgery; most often, a 911 call is made if the aneurysm has burst due to:<ul><li>Medical reason such as uncontrolled growth and breakdown of the artery tissue wall that finally bursts</li><li>Traumatic injury such as a fall or car accident</li></ul></li></ul> |

## Injuries to the Genitalia

Any injury to the genitalia in either males or females is extremely painful due to the high concentration of nerves in this area. Injuries to this area are treated in the same way as any other wound.

Some common conditions seen in the field include:

- **Testicular torsion** (males) is a condition where the testicle becomes twisted in the scrotum, causing severe pain. This injury is caused by strenuous activity and must be corrected in the emergency department. Care by the EMT involves application of an ice pack to relieve the pain and careful transport to minimize movement.

- **Sexual assault** victims require special handling by the emergency medical system since EMTs are often the first responders on site:

  - The victim should be assessed by an EMT of the same gender if possible.

  - Care should be supportive and affirming, without making unrealistic promises. Sexual assault victims are often sensitive to being touched in any way by an EMT, so it is important to keep a calm voice.

  - Remember that a patient, unless impaired or unconscious, has the right to refuse any medical procedure. So request the patient's permission to perform each and every assessment, particularly those involving the genitals.

  - Most states require medical personnel to report these events to the police, especially if the victim is a minor.

  - Be very careful to preserve any evidence of a crime, such as torn clothing and stains from blood and other fluids.

# Practice Set

1. You are dispatched to a motorcycle accident on the interstate. You respond emergently and arrive on the scene 10 minutes after being dispatched. Your patient is unconscious and unresponsive to any stimuli. Your rapid assessment shows that he is breathing with ragged breaths at a rate of 16 and has pulse 60 with pulse oximetry 94%. He is lying 80 feet from his motorcycle face down on the pavement. Your transport time to the trauma center is 30 minutes. How long do you have to assess and treat this patient on the scene?

   A. 10 minutes

   B. 20 minutes

   C. 30 minutes

   D. Enough time to properly treat all of the patient's injuries

2. What trauma center level provides the highest level of care with 24-hour, in-house availability of surgeons?

   A. Level 1

   B. Level 2

   C. Level 3

   D. Level 4

3. You are dispatched to a 2-car accident on a rural highway. You arrive on scene, and the incident commander directs you to a car that has been struck broadside by the other vehicle. There is severe damage to the driver's side of the vehicle, and the driver is lying on the front seat on her back. She is unconscious and unresponsive. She appears pale and diaphoretic with a weak, thready pulse. Her right leg is lying beneath the steering wheel at an awkward angle. She has a large scalp laceration that is bleeding purplish blood. You are wearing suitable precautions against blood-borne pathogens. Which of the following is the next correct step in management?

   A. Gently splint the right leg with a board splint.

   B. Apply a sterile dressing to the scalp laceration.

   C. Perform a rapid extrication and transport priority to the trauma center.

   D. Take cervical stabilization and open the airway using the modified jaw thrust.

4. In the scenario described in question 3, your patient has been extricated to the truck on a backboard with full cervical stabilization. The right leg has been splinted, and the head wound has been dressed. Your assessment of the head reveals nothing unremarkable. As you examine her chest, you notice a large bruise on the right side of her chest. Her blood pressure is 95/65 mm Hg. Which of the following is NOT a treatment for hypovolemic shock?

   A. Keep the backboard flat on the stretcher.

   B. Warm the patient with blankets.

   C. Elevate the head of the backboard 8–12 inches.

   D. Administer high-flow oxygen via NRB mask at 12 LPM.

5.  You are dispatched to the scene of a child who was struck by a car. Which of the following are characteristics of pediatric trauma that can mask significant internal injuries in this patient? Select the 2 answer options that are correct.

    A.  Children normally have bruises in multiple stages of healing.

    B.  There may be no obvious evidence of external trauma.

    C.  Children normally have lower pulse rates than adults.

    D.  Children's abdominal organs are better protected by the ribs.

    E.  Children have a natural higher tolerance to pain.

    F.  Compensatory mechanisms are not as well developed as in adults.

    G.  Bones normally heal faster in children than in adults.

6.  A 16-year-old female patient complains of chest pain and difficulty breathing after being kicked in the chest by a horse. Her skin is pale and diaphoretic. You observe a contusion to the right side of her anterior chest wall. Breath sounds are absent over her right lower lung. Her vital signs are pulse of 112, respiratory rate of 24, blood pressure of 92/80 mm Hg, and $SpO_2$ of 93% on room air. What condition should you expect she is experiencing?

    A.  Hemothorax

    B.  Spontaneous pneumothorax

    C.  Deep contusion

    D.  Flail chest injury

7.  Which of the following definitions best describes an avulsion?

    A.  Separation of a limb or other body part from the remainder of the body

    B.  A smooth or jagged cut caused by a sharp object of blunt force that tears the tissue

    C.  An injury that leaves a piece of skin or other tissue partially or completely torn from the body

    D.  An injury that does not break the skin but causes tissue and vascular damage under the skin

8.  You respond to a fight in progress call to assist police with a possible gunshot victim. You arrive on scene wearing suitable protective equipment, and the police have secured the scene. They direct you to a male in his midtwenties, lying supine on the ground. His shirt is full of blood; he is conscious and alert but is having trouble breathing. What should be your next move?

    A.  Apply a tourniquet to both arms to minimize extremity blood flow.

    B.  Apply an NRB mask, and administer oxygen at 12 liters per minute.

    C.  Remove his shirt and check for wounds.

    D.  Place the patient onto a backboard and transport immediately to the nearest trauma center.

9.  In the scenario in question 8, you observe a puncture wound 0.5 inches in diameter in the left chest 2 inches superior to the left nipple. It is actively bleeding bright-red, frothy blood. What is your next procedure?

    A.  Apply a sterile 4 × 4 gauze dressing to the wound.

    B.  Apply a sterile occlusive dressing.

    C.  Apply a trauma dressing.

    D.  Request an ALS intercept.

10. You respond to the scene of an MVA. You and your partner are assisting another ambulance crew with spinal immobilization for a patient with a suspected cervical spine injury. Which of the following EMTs will direct the movement of the patient?

    A. The most experienced EMT on the scene

    B. The highest-ranking EMT on the scene

    C. The EMT holding stabilization of the head

    D. The EMT who is not actively involved in patient care

11. How do you treat an amputated finger?

    A. Transport it with the patient.

    B. Secure it to the patient's hand with sterile gauze and tape.

    C. Keep it cool by placing it directly onto an ice pack.

    D. Transport it separately in a second rescue or police car to avoid traumatizing the patient.

12. Which of the following impaled objects should you remove in the field?

    A. Pencil through the cheek

    B. Fishing spear embedded in the left thigh

    C. Fence post through the abdomen

    D. Knife embedded in the chest causing a pneumothorax

13. You respond to a house explosion with fire and police. You have suitable protective equipment, and the scene is secure upon your arrival. On scene you are directed to a patient with soot on his face. The patient states rather sheepishly that he was lighting his charcoal grill and, having run out of lighter fluid, poured gasoline on the charcoal and then attempted to light it, resulting in an explosion. He is conscious and alert with superficial burns to both of his arms and hands and to his face. What is your primary concern with this patient?

    A. Hypovolemic shock

    B. Danger of infection

    C. Airway compromise

    D. Secondary explosion

14. Your patient is a 62-year-old female who suffered a steam burn from a large pressure cooker while working in a school cafeteria. You observe circumferential blistered and mottled skin on her left forearm and hand. What percentage of her total body surface area (BSA) do you estimate is burned?

    A. 4.5%

    B. 9%

    C. 13.5%

    D. 18%

15. A 12-year-old male tripped and fell onto a toy action figure, which pierced a two-inch hole in his left upper chest wall. You observe muscle tissue and bone fragments in the wound and hear bubbling sounds when he breathes. Which of the following steps should you take FIRST in the treatment of this patient?

    A. Apply an occlusive dressing.

    B. Suction the wound.

    C. Assist his ventilations with a BVM.

    D. Pack the wound with hemostatic gauze.

16. You respond to an industrial plant for an injured worker. You respond with lights and sirens, and you are wearing suitable BSI precautions. You arrive on scene and observe a male lying atop a wire, obviously unconscious. Which of the following should be your primary concern?

    A. Airway

    B. Scene safety

    C. Burn injury

    D. Cardiac arrhythmias

17. You arrive on the scene of a motorcycle accident. The police are on scene, and you are wearing suitable BSI gear. The driver is lying supine 15 feet away from his motorcycle, which is lying on its side. He is screaming in pain, and you perform your initial assessment and rapid trauma assessment. He is conscious, alert, and oriented with no injuries other than an angulated right femur that is causing him severe pain. His vitals are BP 160/100 mm Hg, pulse 120, and respirations 22. Which of the following devices should you use to splint his injury?

    A. KED

    B. Traction splint

    C. Long spine board

    D. Padded board splint

18. You respond to a soccer field for an injured player. You respond emergently and wearing suitable precautions. When you arrive on the scene, you are directed to the soccer field where an 11-year-old female is conscious, alert, and oriented, lying supine in severe pain. She is clutching her left upper arm with her right hand, and her shoulder is displaced to the anterior. Bystanders state she was in a collision with another player and fell to the ground. She did not lose consciousness, her vital signs are within normal limits, and the remainder of the assessment is unremarkable. What injury do you suspect?

    A. Broken humerus

    B. Broken radius

    C. Dislocated patella

    D. Dislocated shoulder

19. What does PMS stand for in regard to splinting an injury?

    A. Pulse, management, and sensory function

    B. Pulse, management, and swelling

    C. Pulse, motor function, and swelling

    D. Pulse, motor function, and sensory function

20. You are treating an MVA patient who was the driver in a front-end collision. In the crash, he slammed into the steering wheel, deploying the airbag. The patient complains of shortness of breath and says, "I think my ribs are broken!" On assessment, you observe unusual motion during breathing: As the patient breathes in, his chest falls instead of rising. You note visible left-side bruising over the third, fourth, and fifth ribs, and when you palpate, it causes a yelp of pain. What injury does this patient have, and what is this pattern of breathing called?

    A. Clavicle fracture; paradoxical motion

    B. Flail chest; paradoxical motion

    C. Bell chest; dyspnea

    D. Multiple rib fracture; dyspnea

21. You are dispatched to a man who fell off a ladder at his home. You arrive on the scene with suitable BSI precautions and find a male sitting on the floor with a blood-soaked trouser leg. He is conscious, alert, and oriented; has normal vital signs; and has no other injuries or loss of consciousness. You expose the leg by gently cutting the trouser leg away and observe that the fibula is broken and the superior end is exposed through the anterior side of the leg. It is still actively bleeding. What must you do BEFORE you splint the leg?

    A. Check DCAP-BTLS.

    B. Feel for pedal pulse.

    C. Apply a sterile dressing to the wound.

    D. Irrigate the wound with sterile saline.

22. In the scenario in question 21, the patient had a good pedal pulse prior to your applying the splint. Upon rechecking, it is no longer palpable and the foot is becoming cold and cyanotic. What should you do next?

    A. Request an ALS intercept.

    B. Remove the splint.

    C. Expedite the transport.

    D. Immobilize the patient on a backboard and transport rapidly.

23. You arrive on the scene of a 2-car motor vehicle accident, and the incident commander directs you to the first car, which was rear-ended by the second car. The driver is alone in the vehicle and is still wearing her seat belt. She is conscious, alert, and oriented and is complaining of neck pain and being unable to turn her head. You and your partner are wearing appropriate BSI gear, and there is no gross hemorrhage. What should be your next move?

    A. Rapidly extricate the patient onto a long back-board.

    B. Place the patient in a KED and extricate.

    C. Take manual stabilization from the rear seat and apply a cervical collar.

    D. Perform a modified jaw thrust.

24. A patient is found lying prone on the ground, unconscious with shallow breaths at 8 per minute. After performing a rapid logroll with proper cervical precautions, you find that it is difficult to manage the patient's airway without removing his full-faced motorcycle helmet. What is your next step?

    A. Remove the helmet carefully while your partner continues to hold C-spine precautions.

    B. Remove the face mask only and apply an NRB at 15 LPM.

    C. Remove the helmet while your partner hooks up a BVM to the oxygen cylinder.

    D. Perform a head-tilt, chin-lift with the helmet in place and see if his breathing improves.

25. You are dispatched to a home under construction for a man who fell off a roof. Your patient is a roofer who walked off the roof and fell approximately 20 feet to the ground. He is conscious but dazed. He has an airway, his respiratory rate is 14, and his pulse is 72. There is no gross hemorrhage or sign of any bleeding. Your partner takes manual stabilization of the head and neck while you perform a rapid trauma assessment, which is negative for any potentially broken bones. You apply a cervical collar and logroll him onto a backboard and secure him. En route to the trauma center, you expose the patient by cutting off his clothes. Your focused exam is negative; however, when you push against his feet, he complains of pain in the back of his neck. What injury should you suspect?

    A. Ruptured spleen

    B. Broken femur

    C. Fractured cervical vertebra

    D. Fractured skull

26. You respond to a local construction site for a man with an abdominal injury. After taking proper BSI precautions, you find what appear to be parts of his intestines coming out of a large laceration to his lower abdomen. He is tachypneic, anxious, and pale in color. What is your next step?

    A. Call for ALS while you attempt to calm the patient.

    B. Place the patient on an NC at 8 LPM.

    C. Cover the intestines with a moist sterile dressing and secure on 4 sides with tape.

    D. Attempt to place the intestines back inside with gloved hands and secure with a moist, sterile dressing.

THIS PAGE INTENTIONALLY LEFT BLANK

## Answer Key

| | | | | | | | | | |
|---|---|---|---|---|---|---|---|---|---|
| 1. | **A** | 7. | **C** | 13. | **C** | 19. | **D** | 25. | **C** |
| 2. | **A** | 8. | **C** | 14. | **B** | 20. | **B** | 26. | **C** |
| 3. | **D** | 9. | **B** | 15. | **A** | 21. | **C** | | |
| 4. | **C** | 10. | **C** | 16. | **B** | 22. | **B** | | |
| 5. | **B, F** | 11. | **A** | 17. | **B** | 23. | **C** | | |
| 6. | **A** | 12. | **A** | 18. | **D** | 24. | **A** | | |

## Answers and Explanations

### 1.   A

You may be tempted to take the 60 minutes of the "golden hour," subtract the 10-minute response time and the 30-minute hospital transport time and arrive at 20 minutes, but that does not factor in the amount of time that transpired before you were dispatched. This will be the sum of the minutes spent until someone finds the patient, dials and is connected to the dispatch center, and the lag time while dispatch processes the incoming information and dispatches your unit. This amount of time is a variable and is dependent on a number of factors. In addition, once you arrive at the trauma center, medical personnel will triage the patient and stabilize him in the emergency department before sending him to the operating suite, which will add more minutes. (D) may sound logically correct. However, if you properly treat all of these injuries on the scene, you will definitely exceed the "golden hour."

### 2.   A

The correct answer is (A). The main difference between level 1 and level 2 trauma centers is that level 2 may have 24-hour availability of general surgeons but they may not necessarily be in-house.

### 3.   D

The temptation is always to treat the most noticeable condition first, such as the active bleeding or the obvious fracture. However, you first and foremost must be concerned with the patient's survival; without an airway, she will be dead in minutes. In addition, the patient's cervical spine must be stabilized prior to any other treatments to minimize the danger of damaging the spinal cord. Answer choice (D) takes care of both those things and must be the priority in this scenario.

### 4.   C

The correct answer is (C) in this tricky question. The others are all correct treatments of hypovolemic shock. Trendelenburg position, which is what (C) describes, is contraindicated with head injuries and no longer recommended for treatment in shock as a general rule.

**5.   B, F**

Children are not able to compensate as long as adults (F), so time is of the essence in treating a very sick or injured pediatric patient. Due to their smaller body frame and greater share of adipose (fat tissue), depending on their developmental stage, there may be no obvious evidence of external trauma (B) to signal underlying bleeding or damage. While some children may have a lower pulse rate (C), higher pain tolerance (E), or faster bone-healing time (G), these are not hard and fast rules. For instance, adolescents 12–18 years old typically have pulse rates between 60–100, much like adults. The statement that the ribs better protect the abdominal organs in children (D) is just false. The thoracic and abdominal cavities are two separate spaces, with ribs being located in the thoracic cavity. Although all children get bruises at some point, multiple bruises in various stages of healing (A) suggest the possibility of abuse.

**6.   A**

The correct answer is hemothorax (A) due to the skin condition, mechanism of injury, and lack of breath sounds over the patient's right lower lung, which indicates potential internal bleeding. Spontaneous pneumothorax (B) is incorrect, as the patient's condition was not spontaneous; it was the result of direct, blunt trauma. Although the patient does have a deep contusion (C), this condition does not account for the absent breath sounds; this is not the best answer out of those given. Likewise, the scenario says nothing specific about rib fractures, so flail chest injury (D) is not the best answer.

**7.   C**

An avulsion is partial or complete tearing of a piece of skin. (A) is an amputation, (B) is a laceration, and (D) is a contusion.

**8.   C**

You need to visualize what you're dealing with to be able to intervene properly. Applying a tourniquet to minimize extremity blood flow is not an acceptable procedure for this injury. You may well want to administer supplemental oxygen after you've done a proper assessment, but the assessment is the important thing at this stage.

**9.   B**

The correct next procedure is to apply a sterile occlusive dressing. Answer choices (A) and (C) will do nothing to seal the opening in the pleural space that air is escaping from, which is what is causing the frothy blood. The danger here is that this patient will develop a tension pneumothorax or hemothorax. You may request an ALS intercept to assist with advanced life support measures; however, you would do this after you have taken care of the life-threatening conditions, such as the gross hemorrhage.

**10.   C**

The EMT holding stabilization of the head is always responsible for directing the movement of the patient.

**11.   A**

The amputated extremity should be wrapped in a sterile wet dressing, placed into a cool container, and transported with the patient to the appropriate facility. Attempting to secure it to the patient's hand with gauze and tape will only delay transport and not have any long-term benefit. Placing it directly onto an ice pack could cause it to freeze and the tissue to die. There is no reason to transport it separately either.

**12.   A**

The correct answer is (A), because a pencil through the cheek will interfere with respiration. The other answers will not impede the airway and should be left for the emergency department to treat.

**13.   C**

The correct answer is airway compromise. The nature of the explosion and the fact that his face is burned gives him a high probability that he inhaled the flame and smoke from the explosion. The danger of infection is less problematic than the risk of his airway swelling shut. A secondary explosion has hopefully been minimized by the fire department's securing of the scene.

**14. B**

Calculate this answer using the rule of nines. The anterior and posterior parts of the arm each make up 4.5% of body surface area. "Circumferential" means all the way around, so you should add together both parts for a total of 9% BSA. If you got this question wrong, please go back and reference the chart in the chapter again.

**15. A**

For a sucking chest wound, the priority is to prevent continuous entry of excess air into the thoracic cavity by applying an occlusive dressing (A). We do not suction this type of wound (B), as it would involve suctioning out the air already within the cavity along with any blood that may be there. Although you should absolutely be concerned with the ABCs, ventilation assistance with a BVM (C) is not the first action in this case, as there is no mention of the patient being unresponsive and no respiratory rate is given in the scenario.

**16. B**

The correct answer is scene safety. All of the other answer choices become concerns once you have determined that the patient is not being energized by the wire he is lying across.

**17. B**

While any of the devices listed may be used, the traction splint is the preferred device for this injury.

**18. D**

It is important to read the question and get a picture of what is being described. You could stop with the upper arm and deduce that the correct answer is a broken humerus, but the anterior displacement of the shoulder is the key that this is a dislocation or fracture of the shoulder joint.

**19. D**

The correct answer is (D). To test for motor movement, ask the patient to wiggle their toes/finger and grip your fingers. Sensory function is tested by asking which finger or toe the EMT is touching or whether the patient feels pain when performing any commands.

**20. B**

The correct answer is (B). The case describes 3 or more adjacent broken ribs on the same side; by definition, a flail chest is 3 or more adjacent ribs that are broken in 2 or more places. Chest rise with exhalation and fall with inhalation is the opposite of what happens in normal breathing. This opposite chest movement is called paradoxical motion. The clavicle (A) is up at shoulder level, not in the thoracic cavity. Bell chest (C) is a growth abnormality seen in some newborns; it would not be seen in an adult MVA patient. Multiple rib fracture (D) indicates that more than one rib is broken, but it doesn't necessarily indicate that each rib is broken in at least 2 places; it is not the most correct answer. Dyspnea (C and D) is disordered or dysfunctional breathing; it can be caused by paradoxical motion, but it is not the most correct answer.

**21. C**

This is a combination of an open wound and a fracture, and both must be treated. At this point of the scenario, you have already done DCAP-BTLS. Although you will want to check for a pedal pulse, the key here is that the wound is still actively bleeding. Irrigation of the wound may or may not be advisable due to a number of conditions, which is why (C) is the best answer.

**22. B**

In applying the splint, you may have occluded an artery supplying blood to the foot. The other answers are all possibilities, but you have to correct the problem that was caused by applying the splint too tightly or incorrectly.

**23. C**

The patient is talking to you, so you know that there is an airway and that the patient is breathing. Before extricating her from the vehicle, your next priority is to secure the head and neck. Whether a long or short backboard is used, either way, the neck must be secured in a properly sized C-collar. There is no indication for a jaw thrust to be used in this scenario.

**24. A**

The key to this question is that the patient is found originally lying prone and is breathing with an inadequate rate and depth. Because we are not given information as to how the patient ended up in this scenario, (A) is the safest way to manage this patient. (D) would be used only if cervical spine injury can be ruled out, and in this scenario, it would be unsafe to do so. (B) and (C) deal with airway management. However, one EMT needs to hold on to the cervical spine, making (C) incorrect. (B) removes only part of the helmet and an NRB is not appropriate for this type of aggressive airway management.

**25. C**

Pain to the neck as you are applying pressure to the soles of the feet indicates some type of pressure to the spinal cord. All of the other injuries are possible given the MOI; however, there is nothing in the question to indicate that any of these are the correct answer.

**26. C**

Although (A) is definitely a good idea, (C) is the correct answer here as this is an emergent situation where the intestines must remain moist and secured. This patient needs urgent surgical attention. If the proper facility is closer than ALS interception would be, do not delay transport. Never attempt (D).

# PEDIATRICS

Pediatrics is a generalized term that ranges from infant to young adults aged 18 and below. It is important to realize that people in this age bracket are not just little adults. There are very real differences in pediatric anatomy and physiology, as well as psychological and sociological factors, that make the study of pediatrics in the prehospital setting a true specialty. In addition, the EMT must be prepared to deal with the caregivers of this group, who present another dimension to the issue of providing quality care to the younger patient.

## Assessment

The EMT's initial impression of the patient's condition (always relevant) is even more important in the management of a pediatric patient. Take your initial impression seriously. A child who is actually sick looks sick.

Children often lack an understanding of the structure and function of the human body or have an incorrect understanding of the role that organs play. Be sure to explain in very simple terms what is going on with an injury.

Keep in mind that the following guidelines are typically for children under the age of 12. Starting at around 12 years of age, pediatric patients can often verbalize and even assist in the assessment questions and physical exam on their own. Use your judgment to apply these guidelines for pediatric assessment as appropriate:

- When you approach the child, be gentle and kind. Sick children have a very real fear of being sick or even dying. Your presence must be reassuring and not threatening.

- Try to connect with the child's emotions. It helps to get down to the child's eye level or sit alongside on the ground.

- To assess the child's mental status:

  - Announce your presence as you would with an adult patient, and gauge the child's response to voice, touch, or painful stimuli.

  - Depending on the age, you may calculate a GCS score.

  - You must ascertain whether the child's reaction to EMS presence is normal for a child of that age; for example, a toddler who cries as you approach is giving a normal reaction because children this age often cry at the approach of a uniformed stranger.

- To do the physical exam with a very young patient (infant, toddler), start at the feet and work up toward the head.

---

A big difference between adult and pediatric assessment is that the **pediatric physical exam begins at the feet and works toward the head**. This is because touching a child's head can increase anxiety, especially in a preschool-age child, and it is better to have completed the rest of the body before this occurs.

---

When performing interventions and collecting vital signs, it is important that the devices used are properly sized for the patient:

- **Broselow tape**—a color-coded tape measure, standardized and used worldwide for pediatric emergencies:

  - Provides a rapid estimate of the child's weight based on body length

  - Allows EMS to determine proper dosing, sizing for airway equipment, and level of shock voltage when using a defibrillator

  - Tape is marked with colors and a weight (in kilograms, because certain medications are weightbased in the ALS level of care)

- **Handtevy method**—tool that uses both age and length to assess amount of medication needed in pediatric emergencies:
  - Uses both a tape with prewritten dosages and the provider's hands to "count"
  - Associates five age categories (ages 1, 3, 5, 7, and 9) with their corresponding weight (in kilograms) via a finger-counting method on the hand
- **Blood pressure cuffs**, **pulse oximeter probes**, **OPA/NPAs**, and even the **bell of a stethoscope** all come in pediatric sizes; using an adult size in any of these devices will not give an accurate reading for children

Remember that "normal" vital signs are different for children than for adults. Infants, for example, will have normal respiratory rates in the 40s. In an adult patient, this respiration rate would call for positive pressure ventilation support.

To convert pounds to kilograms, use the following formula:

$$\text{Number of kilograms (kg)} = \frac{\text{Number of pounds (lb)}}{2.2046}$$

---

The NREMT exam is unlikely to include calculation questions about dosage. Once you are on the job, however, you may be asked if you know how much a child weighs. Therefore, it is a good idea to know how to convert pounds to kilograms.

---

## Psychological and Social Factors

In performing assessment on a pediatric patient, the EMT must take into consideration psychological and sociological factors characteristic of this population:

- **Toddlers and preschoolers** generally fear separation from their parents or caregivers and may be very suspicious of strangers:
  - They may rebel at being touched or examined by strangers and will be fearful of masks and needles.
  - If one is available, a parent will best provide patient history as the child may be unable to communicate important medical history and medication use.
  - It is helpful to have a stuffed animal or use parents as examples to show the patient what you want to do; this often increases a pediatric patient's willingness to allow assessment.
- **School-age children and adolescents** are generally more social and open to EMT intervention since they have usually begun social interactions in the school setting.
- **Older adolescents** may have to be assessed privately since they might want to keep issues of sexual activity and substance abuse hidden from their parents.

Subsets of the pediatric population:

- **Neonates**—ages birth-4 weeks
- **Infants**—ages 4 weeks-1 year
- **Toddlers**—ages 1-3 years
- **Preschoolers**—ages 3-6 years
- **School-age children**—ages 6-10 years
- **Adolescents**—ages 11-21 years

The age of 21 may be surprising, but this is the official ending point of adolescence as defined by the American Academy of Pediatrics in 2017. Although age 21 is the cutoff for pediatric patient care, note that some chronic pediatric illnesses may continue past that age.

## Physical Factors

The first thing to note with neonates and infants is that they cannot support their necks and heads on their own, so they must always be held in such a way that supports their neck/head. In addition, the differences in pediatric airway anatomy present real concerns to the EMT:

- Neonates and infants have a larger tongue and smaller trachea compared with adults.
- The epiglottis of neonates and infants is comparatively much higher in the airway.
- The heads of younger children are proportionally larger than those of older children and adults, which can present special problems in the case of trauma.

Children do not typically live alone and at a young age are not able to make their own decisions. Therefore, any EMS call involving a pediatric patient will require attention to both the child and the parent/caregiver:

- Children are very perceptive and will quickly pick up on the EMT's confidence or uncertainty. Project a knowledgeable, confident, take-charge approach.
- Parents may have received specialized training for their child's medical care and can thus be an important resource.
- Children who are seriously injured or ill are almost always comforted by the presence of a parent or caregiver. (Exceptions include a parent/caregiver who is abusing the child.)
- The general rule is that a **calm parent will yield a calm child** (similarly, an anxious parent will yield an anxious child); so help to make that happen. If the parent is calm and can convey that calmness to the child, that will go a long way in gaining the child's compliance. Options include:
  - Have the parent hold the child during the assessment procedure.
  - Have the parent ride up front with you.

## Physiological Factors

Compared with those of adults, pediatric vital signs tend to skew higher the younger child is. As the child grows older, the main vital signs of respiratory rate, pulse, and blood pressure begin to move toward what they will be for most of adulthood.

In general, children have a faster heartbeat, faster respiratory rate, and lower blood pressure than adults.

**Table 8.1** Pediatric Vital Signs

| AGE | RESPIRATORY RATE | PULSE | SYSTOLIC BLOOD PRESSURE |
|---|---|---|---|
| Newborn/neonate (age birth–1 month) | 30–50 breaths per min | 120–160 beats per min | 50–70 mm Hg |
| Infant (age 1–12 months) | 20–30 breaths per min | 80–140 beats per min | 70–100 mm Hg |
| Toddler (age 1–3 years) | 20–30 breaths per min | 80–130 beats per min | 80–110 mm Hg |
| Preschool (age 3–5 years) | 20–30 breaths per min | 80–120 beats per min | 80–110 mm Hg |
| School-age (age 6–10 years) | 20–30 breaths per min | 70–110 beats per min | 80–120 mm Hg |
| Adolescent (age 11+ years) | 12–20 breaths per min | 55–105 beats per min | 110–120 mm Hg |

Knowing the normal ranges for each age group can help the EMT recognize whether a child is in distress. If an adult is breathing 30 times per minute, that would be considered tachypneic; however, in a child age 2, that would be considered normal.

## Airway, Breathing, and Circulation

As with an adult, the ABCs of a child must be assessed and corrected first, before proceeding with treatment. Note two things:

- Equipment is available that is specifically sized for the pediatric population. Do not use adult equipment on children.

- Children are not able to compensate as long as adults, so time is of the essence in treating a very sick child.

## Airway

Neonates and infants are nose breathers, so suctioning the nose with a bulb syringe often relieves a child who is having trouble breathing. When you secure the airway, be careful not to hypo-extend or hyperextend the neck and kink the very small airway. A small towel/blanket placed underneath the child's shoulders can help keep the head tilted at a more neutral position than would the full head-tilt, chin-lift technique used with adults.

Correct

Neck slightly extended

Incorrect

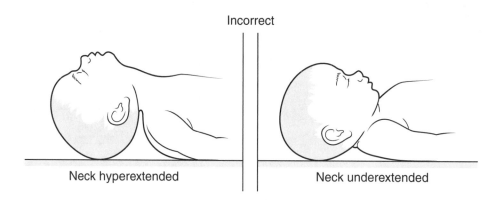

Neck hyperextended　　　　　　　　　Neck underextended

**Figure 8.1** Pediatric Airway Positioning

When inserting an oropharyngeal airway (OPA) or a nasopharyngeal airway (NPA) or when preparing to suction, the proper method of measuring the device is critical. Inserting an oral airway into a pediatric patient is done only in the anatomical position, using a tongue depressor or laryngoscope blade to push the tongue out of the way. If inserting a nasal airway, use lubrication to ease insertion.

The method for measuring is similar to that for an adult, with minor differences and a smaller device. With an OPA, measure from the corner of mouth to the tip of the ear-lobe. With an NPA, measure from the naris to the angle of mandible.

## Breathing

Measure breathing for both rate and quality, and check circulation. It is important to begin oxygen therapy immediately for all children in respiratory distress. If there is severe respiratory distress, provide assistance with ventilation.

Signs of severe respiratory distress are as follows:

- Rates outside of the normal range
- Presence of cyanosis
- Respiratory distress with poor muscle tone
- Seesaw breathing
- Use of accessory muscles in breathing, especially noticeable in the lateral rib view

Special airway concerns in the pediatric population include epiglottitis and croup. The assessment and intervention protocols for these special conditions are state specific. Some states (but not all) allow an EMT to administer epinephrine via nebulizer if croup or epiglottitis is suspected, with permission from medical control.

## Oxygen Therapy

Some services carry masks in pediatric-friendly designs, such as dragons and pandas. Your service may not have these, but at a minimum, it is required to have pediatric-sized nasal cannulas (NC) and non-rebreather masks (NRB). There are also appropriately sized BVMs to deliver more accurate tidal volumes. It is up to the EMT to measure and utilize each piece of equipment properly:

- Neonates and infants will rarely accept an NC or NRB, so administer oxygen therapy with oxygen tubing (called **blow-by oxygenation**):
  - Hold oxygen tubing 2 inches away from the nose and mouth, and simply flow the oxygen over that area.
  - Alternatively, hold a paper cup (also 2 inches away) and blow the oxygen into the cup, creating an oxygen reservoir.
- Older children are much more likely to accept an NC or NRB. Place it as you would for an adult.

In a team-based effort CPR event, the ratio of compressions to breaths should be 15:2 for children, which allows the rescuer to deliver breaths using a BVM at a rate of 20–30 breaths per minute. The volume delivered is also less than when ventilating an adult, so be sure to not overinflate the lungs and to stop squeezing the BVM when you see chest rise.

## Circulation

Checking circulation involves verification of a pulse, skin color and condition, and capillary refill as well as assessing for the presence of any major bleeds.

The absence of pulses is the indication to begin CPR, and the rate and method must be correct for the age of the child:

- Single-rescuer CPR is a ratio of compressions to breath of 30:2.
- Two or more rescuer CPR changes the ratio to 15:2.

In infants, pulse is checked on the brachial artery in the upper arm. In children and teenagers, pulse is checked on the carotid or radial artery.

# Special Conditions

## Seizures

High core body temperatures resulting from infection may cause pediatric seizures. These seizures are referred to as **febrile seizures**. A febrile seizure can be confirmed by checking the patient's forehead for a higher-than-normal temperature. If skin temperature is normal or below normal, the cause of the seizure may be hypoxia, poisoning, trauma, hypoglycemia, or some other cause.

The patient's seizure history and medications should be determined. The patient's airway must be secured, the patient must be transported on their side, and oxygen therapy must be initiated. If the patient feels warm to the touch, a cool, damp towel applied to the head may be effective in lowering the body temperature enough to cancel the seizure. Remember that following a seizure, the patient will be postictal for a period of time.

## Altered Mental Status

This condition may be caused by a variety of conditions, including seizures, hypoglycemia, poisoning, trauma, hypoxia, and shock.

The treatment regimen is the same as with the adult population: secure the airway, administer oxygen, administer medication per local protocol, and transport to an appropriate hospital, ideally a pediatric-specific emergency department.

## Poisoning and Overdose

Since children are curious, poisoning is a major cause of visits to the emergency department. If you suspect poisoning or overdose, you must make an effort while still on scene to locate the container that holds the substance ingested by the child, as this will give important information as to antidotes and treatment.

If the patient is still responsive, contact medical control to check if activated charcoal may be administered in accordance with local protocols. Activated charcoal is an adsorbent that will help prevent the toxin from being further absorbed into the bloodstream.

If the patient is unconscious, nothing may be given by mouth, as this may cause choking and an occluded airway. Maintain the airway, administer oxygen, and transport priority. Provide CPR if necessary but remember your pediatric ratios.

## Shock (Hypoperfusion)

In the pediatric population, unlike the adult population, shock is rarely a cardiac event. Instead, it is usually brought on by dehydration secondary to a variety of illnesses. Dehydration will usually coincide with hypoperfusion, which is more problematic since young children have a much lower blood supply than adults.

Low blood pressure in a pediatric patient is a late sign of shock and requires a more aggressive approach to treatment than in an adult. In infants and toddlers, decreased urine output and dry crying (crying without tears) are good indicators of dehydration.

Shock in children calls for rapid transport with anti-shock measures as per the local protocols, including the use of an ALS intercept if indicated. These measures routinely include keeping the patient warm, administering oxygen, and rapidly transporting to an appropriate facility.

## Near Drowning

It is important to remember, especially in pediatrics, that no one is dead until they are warm and dead. Just because someone is cold to the touch and unresponsive does not always mean they are deceased, especially if only a short time has passed. A cold, lifeless appearance in a near-drowning victim requires aggressive resuscitation efforts by EMS personnel and rapid transport to a pediatric trauma center.

Good ventilation technique has resulted in the resuscitation of many children thought to be dead from near drowning in cold water. Suction excess fluid as necessary, and maintain proper body temperature using blankets or strategically placed hot packs, or by turning on the heat in your ambulance or transporting unit.

Respiratory distress is also a possibility in children who have suffered a near-drowning experience but were breathing fine after the event. Any victim of a near drowning should be transported to a pediatric emergency department for evaluation if available.

## Child Abuse and Neglect

**Abuse** is when improper or excessive action has caused harm or injury to someone. Abuse may be physical, psychological, or emotional in nature. **Neglect** is insufficient attention or respect to someone with a claim to that attention.

Although these concepts can be subjective, the EMT must always err on the side of the patient: **if there is any suspicion of abuse or neglect, it must be reported to the proper authorities**. Failure to report, in many jurisdictions, is a crime in itself and can subject the EMT to criminal and civil penalties.

Some examples of possible neglect or abuse include:

- Infant left in a locked auto (*obvious neglect*)

- EMS intervention to a house where there is no adult present and small children are left alone (*very suspicious but not clear-cut neglect*; explore why this has occurred)

- Multiple EMS interventions to the same address or same patient (*very suspicious*)

- Unexplained bruises, injuries inconsistent with the explanation, conflicting stories of how the injury occurred, fresh burns, fear in the face of the child, and dismissiveness by the parents (*very suspicious*)

- Child who appears malnourished, unsafe, or living in unhealthy living conditions, or with untreated chronic illnesses (*very suspicious and could be considered both neglect and abuse*)

- Infant who presents with CNS deficiencies (*suspicious for shaken baby syndrome*, in which violent shaking has damaged the spinal cord):

  - Often results in death of the infant

  - Your run report must be clear and concise about the facts of the call to assist authorities in the proper disposition of the situation

If you suspect abuse or neglect, it is not your job to accuse the parents or caregivers. Your main focus is to care for the patient:

- You will certainly need to report your suspicions (and supporting evidence) to the authorities, usually the local police, but that is done later.

- Make sure you report this directly by online form, telephone report, or orally to appropriate personnel, i.e., do not rely on anyone else to communicate the information. In many states, EMS staff are considered "mandatory reporters," and they must fill out appropriate paperwork besides their PCR. This is necessary since this agency's interaction with the parent and patient is critical for getting the child appropriate help.

- You should also share this information with the receiving facility to ensure that the patient receives proper treatment.

- Finally, some states require that their children's health and safety agencies be notified of suspected abuse or neglect. Each state has a different reporting system, and you must follow the appropriate procedure.

---

### KEY TAKEAWAY

EMS falls under what is typically called a "mandated reporter," i.e., emergency personnel are responsible for notifying the proper authorities if there is suspected abuse of vulnerable populations, particularly children.

---

## Sudden Infant Death Syndrome

Few calls are more traumatic in EMS than "child not breathing." These cause a heightened state of distress in everyone, from the EMS provider to the 911 caller to the caregiver.

According to the CDC, each year there are about 3,400 sudden, unexpected infant deaths in the United States. These deaths occur in infants <1 year old and may have no immediate known cause.

Sudden infant death syndrome (SIDS) is a condition in which a previously healthy infant is found in the crib not breathing and the postmortem can find no cause for the death. It is important to remember that the patients in these calls include the parents of the child. Proper care means that someone must intervene with them, even if it requires calling for more personnel to the scene or a second rescue.

Many states require resuscitation efforts to be undertaken, even in the presence of biological death indicators such as rigor mortis and postmortem lividity, if for no other reason than to assure the parents that everything possible has been done for their child. Although nothing will compensate for the loss of a child, a professional, assuring demeanor toward the parents may provide a small measure of comfort in this traumatic situation.

## Special Needs Infants and Children

Many infants and children with chronic conditions are cared for at home by their parents and visiting health care workers. Emergencies in this population are common, and 911 is often called. EMS is usually the service to respond and intervene.

---

While EMT courses rarely go into detail on the emergency treatment of children with special needs, the well-versed EMT tries to keep abreast of these procedures so that interventions are correct.

---

Common conditions among this population include:

- **A tracheostomy tube surgically implanted in the trachea:**
  - A tracheostomy tube may become plugged with mucus, which may cause the child to present with difficulty breathing. Suction the tube in the same manner as you would suction fluid from the oropharynx.
  - Suction for no more than 5 seconds at a time, and administer oxygen to the tube between suctioning attempts.
  - In the event of respiratory failure, use the tube to administer positive-pressure ventilation directly to the trachea while blocking the nose and mouth. A Yankauer rigid tip does not fit typically, so use a soft French catheter.
  - If a tube becomes dislodged or is removed by the patient, the stoma or opening can be used to ventilate and may have to be suctioned, especially if bleeding is present because of the removal of the tube.

- Do not attempt to replace a tracheostomy tube that has been removed or dislodged. Instead, transport the child to the nearest pediatric care facility.
- Look for signs of infection, such as swelling and redness around the site.

**Figure 8.2** Tracheostomy Tube with Suction

- **Chronic respiratory failure, possibly connected to a home ventilator:**
  - Parents are usually well instructed in the use of a home ventilator and often have a backup in place. If you are called and none of the devices operate properly, be prepared to ventilate the patient manually with an oxygen-supplied bag-valve mask and transport priority to the nearest facility.
- **Gastrostomy tubes** are implanted directly into the stomach for children who cannot be fed by mouth:
  - If you see that the tubes have become dislodged or plugged and the parents have not been trained in their reinsertion, transport the patient to a pediatric hospital for proper management
  - En route, support the child's breathing.
- **Shunts** are tubes that are placed inside the skull to divert excess fluid to either the stomach or to a reservoir on the side of the neck. If this device fails, the patient will present with signs of brain injury, such as:
  - Change in mental status.
  - Seizures.

- Nausea/vomiting.

- Loss of motor control.

If you find that the shunt has failed, transport the patient to the nearest facility right away. While en route, support the airway and assist in respiration. *This is a severe condition.*

- **Central IV lines** have been placed into the larger veins of the torso in order to supply medication that is needed on a regular basis. If you encounter complications from these lines, transport the patient to a pediatric hospital for proper management. While en route, support the airway, assist in respiration, and control any bleeding.

- **Autism and sensory disorders:**

  - Children on the autism spectrum range from low to high functioning. Some children may be nonverbal and sensitive to any changes in their immediate environment, and the presence of EMS would fit into that category. Other children on the spectrum may be the complete opposite. Every child is unique in not only their level of disability but also in how they react to the EMT.

  - The caregiver is often the "gateway" into gaining trust to allow the provider to do an assessment.

  - Aim to make the child as comfortable as possible by explaining everything you are doing. Include the caregiver as well.

  - Use lights and sirens cautiously, as they may make certain children more reactive or exacerbate symptoms.

  - Remember that not all autistic children are low functioning. If they are older, speak with them in age-appropriate language, and give them respect and time to answer your or your partner's questions.

## Trauma

Trauma, especially motor vehicle trauma, is the number one cause of death in the pediatric population. Head injuries and internal organ injuries are common, while bone injuries are less common:

- **Head injuries** are common because a child's head is proportionally larger than the rest of the body.

- **Organ injuries** are common because the pliability of the child's bones means that the internal organs are not well protected (unlike adults, whose stronger bones provide more protection to the internal organs).

- **Bone injuries** are less common because the pliability of the child's bones means they are less likely to be fractured from blunt-force trauma.

Assessment of pediatric trauma is the same as for adults except that you should begin the physical exam at the feet and work toward the head (in the case of a conscious patient).

Treatment of pediatric trauma is the same as for adults, although pediatric-specific equipment must be used to protect the child as much as possible. Examples of equipment that is available in pediatric sizes include:

- Traction splints
- Immobilization board
- C-collars
- Padded board splints

When transporting a child, use a pediatric-specific harness. (Several types are available, so know which one your municipality uses.) A transporting harness mimics a car seat and is a much safer transport option for children.

Use a car seat attached to the stretcher only as a last resort.

## KEY TAKEAWAY

When transporting a child, it is imperative that the child **not ride on the caregiver's lap** while secured to the stretcher. This arrangement has resulted in many injuries to both caregiver and child. Prevent this avoidable harm by using the appropriate equipment, which should be provided by your service.

# Practice Set

1. A pediatric patient who is 4 years old is categorized as a/an

   A. neonate.

   B. infant.

   C. toddler.

   D. preschooler.

2. An adolescent is defined as being in which age range?

   A. 6–12 years old

   B. 11–21 years old

   C. 13–18 years old

   D. 10–15 years old

3. The airway of an infant is proportionally _____ the airway of an adolescent.

   A. smaller than

   B. larger than

   C. the same size as

   D. inverse to

4. A 6-month-old infant presents with difficulty breathing. Which characteristic of the child may account for this?

   A. Proportionally larger head

   B. Proportionally larger trachea

   C. Obligatory nose breather

   D. Higher respiratory rate

5. For a pediatric patient under the age of 1 in respiratory distress, which of the following pieces of equipment is preferred to help clear secretions in the nasopharynx?

   A. Non-rebreather mask

   B. Vacuum suction unit

   C. Bulb syringe

   D. Magill forceps

6. Which set of vital signs is considered normal for a neonate?

   A. Pulse 140, respirations 40

   B. Pulse 140, respirations 80

   C. Pulse 80, respirations 40

   D. Pulse 80, respirations 60

7. While performing the physical assessment on a 3-year-old who fell off a wall and whose parents are not yet on scene, you begin to palpate his neck, and he begins to cry and tries to pull himself away from you. This action indicates which of the following?

   A. Possible child abuse

   B. Possible carotid artery bruise

   C. Possible pneumothorax

   D. Possible cerebrovascular accident

8. Which of the following techniques should be used to open the airway of a 1-year-old in respiratory arrest?

   A. Head-tilt, chin-lift

   B. Modified jaw thrust

   C. Heimlich maneuver

   D. Valsalva maneuver

9. Which of the following should NOT be used to administer oxygen to a pediatric patient?

   A. Pediatric face mask

   B. Paper cup and oxygen tubing

   C. Blow-by technique

   D. Oxygen-powered manual respirator

10. You should begin the physical examination of a pediatric patient at the

    A. head.

    B. shoulders.

    C. buttocks.

    D. feet.

11. The pulse that should be checked on an infant is located at the

    A. radial artery.

    B. brachial artery.

    C. carotid artery.

    D. femoral artery.

12. The most common cause of seizures in the pediatric population is

    A. poisoning.

    B. hypoxia.

    C. fever.

    D. epilepsy.

13. SIDS stands for

    A. sudden idiopathic dyspnea syndrome.

    B. shaken infant death syndrome.

    C. sudden infant development syndrome.

    D. sudden infant death syndrome.

THIS PAGE INTENTIONALLY LEFT BLANK

## Answer Key

| | | | | |
|---|---|---|---|---|
| 1. **D** | 4. **C** | 7. **B** | 10. **D** | 13. **D** |
| 2. **B** | 5. **C** | 8. **B** | 11. **B** | |
| 3. **A** | 6. **A** | 9. **D** | 12. **C** | |

## Answers and Explanations

**1. D**

A 4-year-old is a preschooler. Neonates are 1 day to 4 weeks old, infants are 4 weeks to 1 year old, and toddlers are 1 to 3 years old.

**2. B**

You have to read this question and all of the answers carefully. The American Pediatric Association classifies adolescence as 11–21 years of age. Each answer contains partially correct ranges, but (B) is the most correct.

**3. A**

The infant's airway is proportionally smaller than that of the adolescent. Please note the presence of the key word *proportionally*.

**4. C**

Since neonates and infants are obligatory nose breathers, the accumulation of mucus in the nasopharynx would cause dyspnea. The size of the head has nothing to do with breathing, making (A) incorrect. Pediatric patients have a relatively smaller trachea, making (B) incorrect. Answer choice (D), while having to do with respirations, would not be directly related to causing dyspnea.

**5. C**

A bulb syringe is used to apply gentle suction and clear the nasal passages of mucus, which will facilitate breathing. A non-rebreather mask (A) is used for high-flow oxygen administration, a vacuum suction unit (B) is too powerful to be used on a children this age, and Magill forceps (D) are used to remove foreign bodies from the oropharynx and trachea.

**6. A**

Normal pulses for a newborn are in a range from 100–180. Respiratory rates are in a range of 30–60. If you were sure of the pulse range, you could eliminate the last two answers and focus on answer choice (A) and (B).

**7. B**

A carotid artery bruise would be painful to the touch and would increase the child's anxiety level. Child abuse (A) is a tempting answer, except that the patient's response is fairly normal given the patient's age; a 3-year-old child should be suspicious of strangers. There is nothing in the question that would indicate a pneumothorax (C) or CVA (D).

**8. B**

The head-tilt, chin-lift (A) may cause the airway of an infant to kink and obstruct; therefore the modified jaw thrust is the preferred method. The Heimlich maneuver (C) is used to dislodge the airway obstruction of an adult, and the Valsalva maneuver (D) is taught to patients with supraventricular tachycardia.

**9. D**

An oxygen-powered manual respirator should not be used in the pediatric population due to the risk of lung rupture from overpressure. Pediatric face mask (A), paper cup and oxygen tubing (B), and blow-by technique (C) are all methods of pediatric oxygen delivery.

**10. D**

Starting at the feet is the reverse of the physical examination technique for an adult. The reason for starting at the feet is that when you begin to examine the head, the anxiety level of the child will increase. If you have already examined the rest of the body, you will be in a good position to finish quickly and with a minimum of anxiety for the patient.

**11. B**

The brachial artery is the most accessible at this age.

**12. C**

Although the other answer choices are all causes of seizures, most pediatric seizures are caused by high core temperatures.

**13. D**

Be sure to read the question and all of the answers before selecting one. Many people will answer (C) and not even read (D) simply because the first two words are part of the correct answer. However, choice (D) is the correct answer.

# AMBULANCE OPERATIONS

All professional-grade EMTs know that failure to plan is planning to fail. Every successful call depends on being physically and emotionally prepared to face the stresses of sudden illness, injury, hysteria, chaos, and even death. In addition, each on-duty EMT must be dressed in the uniform prescribed by the service. A professional appearance is vital if the EMT is to be taken seriously as a medical provider.

## Preparing for a Call

In preparation for a call, there are two things that need to be completed: an equipment check and a truck check.

Depending on your service, you may have only one partner or a multiple-person crew. The checks should be divided equally among all members. (If on an ALS unit, the paramedic will likely check their own equipment/drug box, while the EMT will check everything else.)

Whichever way the work is divided, the following things must be completed *prior to* your first call.

## Equipment Check

Apart from being physically ready for an emergency call, it is important to check your equipment to make sure all items are ready to go. You might get a standardized checklist from your service, but it will soon become second nature to know what equipment should and should not be on your truck. Many EMS providers can do the checklist from memory, but you may also be required to submit a physical checklist to your supervisor for each shift.

The following is a list of basic items that all EMS professionals should be checking at the beginning of each shift, but be aware that this list is not comprehensive:

- Check that medications are full and not expired.
- Check that oxygen tanks as well as regulators are full and in working condition.
- Restock any supplies that may not have been restocked by previous crew.
- Make sure there are various sizes and adequate amounts of PPE available for the crew.
- Verify there are enough cleaning supplies on the unit for cleaning after each call.
- Verify that street maps or GPS machines are working correctly.
- Check that protocols are up-to-date and you are informed of any changes.
- If your service still uses paper forms, check that you have the proper paperwork in adequate amounts.
- If your service uses ePCRs, make sure the computer is charged and has a charging cable.
- Confirm that all radio equipment and company phones are charged and working.

### KEY TAKEAWAY

While not common, it has happened that EMTs have arrived on scene with empty oxygen bottles and dead batteries in their AEDs. Make sure that checking your equipment becomes an automatic part of your routine.

A basic life-support EMS unit must have at least two licensed/certified EMTs on board, one to drive and one to perform patient care. It is common procedure throughout a shift that the two EMTs rotate duties. In the event of a serious call, it is preferable for two licensed/certified EMTs to be in the patient care compartment while a certified driver takes over operation of the unit.

If the EMT is part of an ALS unit, there will be a minimum of one EMT and one paramedic onboard. In systems that have multiple personnel on a unit, patient care typically falls to the paramedic first, who then will complete an assessment and determine what level of care the patient requires.

Regardless of how many people are on the unit, the EMT is a vital part of the team. That includes sharing responsibilities that are not always patient care related: stocking, restocking, navigation, and radio or computer operations.

## Truck Check

At the beginning of your shift, you will be briefed by the personnel going off duty as to the truck and the condition of supplies. At that point, you should begin your truck check, as follows.

**Table 9.1** Truck Check Components

| AREA TO CHECK | COMPONENTS |
|---|---|
| Physical truck components | • Fluid levels are adequate (i.e., oil, windshield fluid, brake fluid)<br>• Emergency lights are operational<br>• Tires are inflated adequately<br>• Sirens are in working order<br>• Doors lock and unlock properly<br>• Seat belts are in working order<br>• Truck exterior is washed and cleaned |
| Medical supplies | • Medications are not expired<br>• Administration units are intact, i.e., lancets for glucose monitoring, nasal atomizers (if available), syringes for drawing up medications<br>• Bandaging supplies are stocked in proper amounts<br>• PPE supplies are available for every crew member |
| Medical equipment | • Stretcher is in working order and cleaned<br>• Batteries are charged and in operating order for equipment, such as:<br>  — AED or cardiac monitor<br>  — Pulse oximeter<br>  — Blood glucometer<br>  — Portable suction unit<br>  — Automatic stretcher battery (if used) |
| Communication devices (each crew member may have a portable radio and/or a direct-connect cell phone) | • All battery-run radios and phones are in working order; all rechargeable radios and phones are fully charged<br>• Radio channels are in working order, and radio communications are able to be heard in both directions<br>• If using ePCR equipment, log-on works and software can be accessed with a wireless or hardwired connection<br>• If using paper charts, stock is available |

*(Continued)*

**Table 9.1** Truck Check Components (*Continued*)

| AREA TO CHECK | COMPONENTS |
|---|---|
| Crew roles and responsibilities | • Within your crew, be clear about duties and responsibilities so that the execution of your next call will be flawless<br>• Share issues that you feel need addressing; trust is essential in a successful EMT team so that in the field you can focus on the challenge at hand:<br>  — Partners don't always get along, and that can impede ideal patient care; try to iron out any problems, and advise management if necessary<br>  — If you are unsure about how to do a certain procedure, be honest about it, especially if working with an ALS partner; do not just try to "wing it," as that isn't safe; ask your partner for direction or explain that you cannot complete the task; wait until after the call has completed to learn the task; most senior or experienced providers will not mind teaching<br>  — You will be spending long hours with your partner; everyone has personal preferences about what time to eat, how to prepare the chart, and even critical thinking on patient care; smooth out these issues beforehand so they are nonissues on your calls<br>  — Your partners are your team; emotions will run high at times, but what matters most is patient care; collaborate with your partners to give the best possible care |

Once your truck and equipment checks are done, be sure to notify the dispatch center with the names of the personnel onboard for the shift. This will alert dispatch that you are ready and available to start taking calls.

## From Dispatch to Arrival on Scene

After a call is received by the dispatcher, the responding unit is notified. (*How* the unit is notified depends on the individual service: loudspeaker, radio, direct-connect cell phone, or in person if the dispatch center and the unit are at the same location.) The dispatcher will relay the following information to the responding EMS unit:

- Location of the call
- Nature of the illness or injury
- Special information that may be useful to the responders

The name of the caller and a callback number are not normally broadcast to the responding unit, although the dispatcher does take that information.

## En Route to the Scene

When a call is received by EMS from the dispatcher, the following steps take place:

- The crew chief acknowledges the call, repeating back the location and nature of the emergency; clarification is provided if needed.
- The crew then responds quickly and enters vehicle; all personnel secure themselves with seat belts as the driver starts the engine.
- Before beginning to move, the driver checks that all doors are closed and all personnel are ready to go.

Professional emergency vehicle drivers are physically and mentally fit at all times and are alert to their surroundings and circumstances.

---

Not all EMTs are vehicle drivers. **Emergency vehicle operation** is a separate course from your EMT-Basic education, with special certification. However, certification is often a condition of employment. Additionally, some services will not employ EMTs until they are age 21 due to driving liability rules.

---

In addition to understanding how to operate an emergency vehicle properly, the driver must:

- Be intimately familiar with the vehicle being driven, especially with its particular quirks.
- Anticipate the unexpected.
- Avoid danger on the road at all costs, i.e., do not let the rush of adrenaline or excited radio traffic overcome your common sense and duty to drive safely.
- Tolerate other drivers on the road who may not yield the right-of-way in spite of the EMS lights and sirens.

All states give certain privileges to emergency vehicles, such as being allowed to drive over the speed limit; however, there are some obvious limitations (with risk of penalty). The general idea is that emergency vehicles must drive with **due regard** for the safety of others. They must:

- Provide adequate warning to others by using the warning devices.
- Control the speed of the vehicle to allow other motorists time to react to warnings.
- Use emergency lights and sirens judiciously and only as stated in state protocols.
- Use extreme caution for cross traffic when approaching any intersection, regardless of the traffic control. (Some drivers actually push through a red stoplight into the path of an oncoming ambulance, thinking the ambulance is behind them.)

- Be aware that other emergency vehicles may be operating in priority mode at the same time you are and attempting to assert their right-of-way.
- Park the ambulance in a normal manner and not on the sidewalk (unless necessary) or in the fire lane.
- Always stop for a school bus with its red lights activated. Emergency vehicles never have the right-of-way in those situations.
- Use a police escort only if your EMS team is unfamiliar with the location of the receiving facility. Vehicles often inadvertently block the path of the ambulance traveling behind a police escort.

In the event of an accident, the driver—not the senior EMT—is responsible for the operation of the vehicle and is personally liable in the event of an accident.

## Arrival on Scene

Once the unit is on scene, notify the dispatcher of this fact and give an update if the information you received was incorrect or incomplete. If the number of patients exceeds the capacity of the unit to handle, additional units must be requested at this time and mass casualty incident (MCI) procedures must be initiated.

The driver must position the vehicle safely and far enough away if the scene is hazardous or could become so. The following should then occur:

- The crew chief should scan the scene for safety issues before committing the crew to a course of action, e.g., weapons, lack of police, electrical hazards, hazardous materials, and collapse dangers.
- Once the scene is determined to be safe, approach and assess the patient. If there is a potential hazard, such as a vehicle on fire, move the patient first to safety before doing the assessment. Attempt an appropriate level of cervical spine stabilization, but do not hinder the patient's prompt removal from the unsafe scene.
- Once the patient is safely away from the hazard, begin assessment based on whether it is a trauma or medical scenario, and initiate proper treatment.
- Once the patient is properly triaged and treated, the next step is transport to an appropriate facility (unless it was earlier determined to be a load-and-go injury and you are already en route).

## Moving and Lifting Patients

Identifying and treating patients is always seen as the main goal of prehospital emergency medicine. However, extricating patients from the circumstance that you find them in and transporting them to an appropriate medical facility is often where the real art of this type of medical practice is demonstrated.

When lifting a patient, always do so safely. This requires exact communication with all of those involved. Before attempting to lift a patient, be sure you and your partners have a plan as to how this will be accomplished. For example, if you are moving a patient from a hospital bed to a stretcher, it is often easier to accomplish this by sliding the patient and the sheets of the bed right onto your stretcher. If there are multiple sheets beneath the patient, be sure that you all know whether you are taking all of them or just the top one. It is critical when lifting a patient secured to a backboard or even in raising the stretcher from its lowered position to the transport position that the lifting be done in a coordinated manner. Failure to do so may tip the patient right off the stretcher and complicate their injuries.

When lifting a patient from a low to a high position, either on a board or on a stretcher, always use your legs to lift, not your back. This necessitates squatting to a kneeling position and keeping the weight close to your body. Your feet should be far enough apart to give you good balance in both squatting and standing positions. You should grip the stretcher, backboard, or sheets with both hands, using your entire hands and not just your fingers.

The EMT must know their own limitations. If the patient weighs more than can safely be handled by the crew on the scene, additional help must be summoned. Remember, all patient transfers must be done with the safety of the crew and patient as a primary consideration.

## Transferring Patients

There are three types of patient transfer, and each of these can be subdivided into trauma and nontrauma:

- Emergency transfer
- Urgent transfer
- Nonurgent transfer

An **emergency transfer** occurs when speed is the primary consideration because the patient and rescuer are in immediate danger:

- The most common example of this is when a motor vehicle has been involved in an accident, the driver is behind the wheel and unconscious, and the vehicle is on fire. The usual precautions for cervical spine stabilization are secondary to removing the patient from the immediate danger.
- This type of extrication is accomplished by whatever method removes the patient from the danger as quickly as possible. If the patient is not trapped, grabbing the patient beneath the arms and pulling headfirst, while trying to cradle the head and neck against your torso as you do so, is the best method.

An **urgent transfer** occurs when the situation is unstable but not critical:

- In the same scenario as just described but with only smoke issuing from the engine compartment and no fire visible, you may have time to take some precautions to minimize spinal injury.
- One EMT should attempt to stabilize the patient by holding their head from the rear, if possible, while the second EMT applies a cervical collar. Then, with coordinated motion, the EMTs should pivot the patient so that they may be pulled from the vehicle by the long axis of the body onto a spine board, which can be placed right on the seat of the vehicle (if possible) to minimize patient motion.
- Once the patient is on the spine board, the patient can be moved away from the vehicle to a safe place as quickly as possible and receive the appropriate treatments.

In the **nonurgent transfer**, when there is no discernible danger, the patient should be stabilized in a Kendrick Extrication Device (KED) or a similar type of stabilization device prior to being extricated.

There are two basic types of equipment available for patient transfer.

The main piece of equipment used to effect transfers and lifting is the **main ambulance stretcher**, which has an adjustable height. This stretcher comes in three configurations:

- The 1-person-loading stretcher allows one person to place the stretcher from its uppermost position into the ambulance as the wheeled undercarriage folds in by itself.

- The 1 1/2-person-loading stretcher has a wheel assembly at the head of the stretcher so that once the stretcher is engaged inside the truck, it enables one person to lift the stretcher and patient. The second person has to lift only the undercarriage to its resting position beneath the stretcher.

- The 2-person-loading stretcher requires 2 EMTs to stand on either side and lower it down into position. These 2 EMTs then lift the stretcher into the truck and together roll it into place.

When a full-size ambulance stretcher cannot be brought to the patient, a **folding stretcher (stair chair)** is used. The patient is secured in a sitting position and then carried to a place where transfer can be made to a main stretcher.

If the patient cannot be placed in a sitting position (e.g. a back or neck injury), they must be secured to a backboard and then transported to the main stretcher.

Once the patient has been loaded into the ambulance, the crew should notify dispatch that they are en route to the receiving facility.

### Air Transfer

Local protocols often dictate when air transport is indicated and how it is to be used. The decision may be made by the incident commander or by the applicable medical control. The driving factors will be the trauma score of the patient and the projected transport time via land vehicle.

Unfortunately, in the real world, many other factors affect the handling of the emergency. Helicopters will not fly in a snowstorm (when EMS calls are frequent and often serious), and helicopters are not always available when they were expected to be. The crew chief must make a decision based upon all of these considerations.

If air transfer does happen, the crew chief must establish a safe landing zone for the helicopter, using the following criteria:

- Must be at least $100 \times 100$ feet, fairly level, and paved/grass-covered if possible
- Must be able to accommodate a nearby fire truck (required for landing)
- Must be free from overhead obstructions, particularly electrical wires
- Must have emergency lighting if at night and unlit

There are many hazards surrounding the use of a helicopter. If possible, the best practice is to have a designated helicopter landing zone along with live trainings to prepare for the real-world events.

When working with helicopters, always follow certain safety rules:

- Never approach a helicopter until instructed to do so by the pilot or a helicopter crew member.
- Always approach a helicopter from the front or side in view of the pilot while keeping your head down. Do not approach from the rear unless instructed to do so by a crew member.
- If the helicopter is on a slight slope, be aware that the clearance of the main rotors will be dangerously low on the uphill side and may be unapproachable there.
- Follow the instructions of the pilot/crew members carefully. Since helicopter engines are often left running to save time, the blades are often rotating as the patient is loaded/unloaded. It is imperative that you do exactly as the crew requests.

The last step is reporting: you (EMT) and your crew should notify the incoming flight team of the patient's status and specific needs. Doing this will allow them time to determine which equipment they wish to offload from the aircraft and bring to the patient versus what to leave on board.

Once the patient has been loaded, following the flight crew instructions, the ambulance crew is now free to end their portion of the call and begin the charting and decontamination process. This is one of the instances in which the ambulance crew often does not do a final handover to hospital personnel, as they have now transferred the patient care to a higher level of care and provider. At this point, once the ambulance has been restocked and cleaned, the crew may notify dispatch that they are available for another emergency call.

## En Route to the Receiving Facility

Once en route to the receiving facility, the driver notifies dispatch of that fact, and the EMT responsible for treating the patient collects the information necessary to notify the receiving facility. It is important to paint as clear a picture as possible so that the receiving facility knows the condition of the patient en route and can prepare accordingly. Additionally, while en route, do the following:

- Comfort the patient and provide assurance that optimal care is being given. A patient will quickly sense if you are unsure of yourself, so be confident in your communication.
- Continue to monitor vital signs throughout the trip.

## Communication Basics

Providing emergency medical services is a joint effort involving many people. The success of an endeavor is predicated upon clear and precise communications between the elements of the EMS system:

- EMS calls usually begin with a phone call to an emergency dispatcher. This call may be to a dedicated emergency line, a 911 call center, or even a routine phone line.
- The dispatcher is responsible for accurately taking down the location and nature of the call and, if qualified, giving prearrival instructions.
- This information may be relayed to a second dispatcher who actually dispatches the nearest appropriate EMS unit, usually by two-way radio, and who is responsible for transmitting the information received by the call taker.
- The EMS unit will give updates and changes in status back to the dispatcher, such as "en route," "arrive on scene," etc.

## Communications Technology

The EMT is also responsible for notifying the receiving hospital of patient information and, in many cases, for seeking guidance from a physician as to performing procedures described in the applicable protocols.

Historically this task was done by two-way radio but is now often done by cell phone.

It goes without saying that clear communication between all personnel involved in the EMS system is paramount. This is accomplished through the following:

- Communications equipment should be checked at the beginning of each shift to ensure its proper functioning.
- Backup systems (and redundant systems) are needed so that all elements of public safety can communicate with each other as needed, even in the event of a large-scale disaster.
- When communicating via radio, know exactly what it is you want to communicate before starting to speak:
    - Speak slowly and clearly, using proper terminology.
    - When listening to / receiving information, remember to release the push-to-talk (PTT) switch.
    - If your system is using radio repeaters to allow for long-range communication, you may have to wait a few seconds before transmitting, which also delays the reception of incoming radio traffic.

EMS uses different types of radio systems to transmit information to each other or to receiving hospitals:

- **Simplex** transmits and receives messages on the same frequency.
- **Duplex** transmits and receives messages on different frequencies, which are referred to as a channel.

- **Multiplex** has the capability to transmit 2 signals at the same time. An example would be when a paramedic can both talk to the physician and transmit an EKG at the same time.

- **Repeater** receives a signal and retransmits it. Repeaters are used to extend transmissions so that the signal can cover longer distances or be received on the other side of an obstruction such as a mountain or valley. This is how units may stay in contact with their base station from many miles away and still be heard clearly.

With two-way radio, various EMS units may share a common frequency. In those cases, be mindful of radio courtesy. If someone transmits while another unit is already transmitting, both conversations may become unintelligible.

---

Research has shown that a **lack of communication among public safety units** is highly problematic and significant during major disasters. EMS systems must take these issues into account when designing and utilizing communications systems.

---

## Confidentiality and Speaking with a Receiving Facility

When communicating over public safety radio, be sure to maintain patient confidentiality. Radio frequencies are open to (and often monitored by) the general public and news media, so be sure not to reveal a patient's name or other identifying information. Keep all information neutral.

A good idea of information to include in a radio report without compromising confidentiality is the following:

- Age and gender of patient
- Chief complaint
- Last or most relevant set of vital signs recorded
- Treatment given or in progress with the patient's response to it
- Any orders, such as asking to administer certain medications, from medical control
- Medical history or medications pertinent to the situation
- Estimated time of arrival (ETA) to facility if transporting

As you become more experienced and confident in your radio reporting style, you will come up with a basic setup of a radio report that will address all the bullet points shown and last approximately 2–3 minutes or less. A sample radio report could sound like:

"This is EMS unit 27 en route to your hospital with a 5-minutes ETA. I am transporting a 67-year-old male BLS, alert and oriented $\times 4$, who is complaining of a hand laceration due to a fall from a stepladder with no loss of consciousness. He is not currently on any blood thinners. His last set of vitals are BP of 132/76 mm Hg, respiratory rate of 18, pulse rate of 86, and $SpO_2$ of 100% on room air. Bleeding is controlled by pressure and bandages. Do you require anything further? See you in 5 minutes."

When you arrive at the receiving facility, the triage nurse may or may not have received your report. So you will tell the nurse in person what you already told the person on the radio and will then follow the nurse's directions to discharge your patient to the emergency department's care.

## Radio Codes

Radio codes are specific words or numbers assigned to each medical issue or injury a patient could be experiencing. It is a way to protect confidentiality over the radio frequencies in case other people are listening. Confidential information should be passed by more secure transmissions, such as cell phones.

Radio codes vary from location to location and even from service to service. Dispatch systems that use confidential codes for sensitive calls, such as attempted suicide or sexual assault, should make sure that all trainees are well versed in the codes and how they are used. For example, a service may dispatch your unit as follows:

- You are dispatched to a code 19, which could mean respiratory distress.
- You would then respond code 7, which means "en route with lights and sirens."
- When you get on scene, you would radio dispatch and say you are code 10, meaning "you have arrived."
- When you transport the patient, you would say that you are code 20, meaning "en route to the hospital."

As you can see, this can be very confusing and time-consuming, especially if the EMT is not completely familiar and comfortable with the meaning of each code.

If you are working for a company that still uses radio codes, it is up to you as the EMT to be familiar with and know how to use them properly.

---

### KEY TAKEAWAY

One service may use a completely different set of radio codes than another service <10 miles away. Therefore, the National Incident Management System (NIMS) prohibits the use of radio codes during a multiple-agency operation. During an event that involves more than one agency, personnel are required to use "plain English," which allows all communication to be easily understood. Since this policy (law) has been implemented, many EMS services are starting to adopt this policy as their standard.

---

# Patient Drop-Off and Postrun

During transport, while patient care is being performed, the EMT must also be thinking about what to communicate in the prehospital radio report (before arrival at the receiving facility) and in the hospital bedside handover report (upon arrival).

The **prehospital radio report** (done orally via radio or cell phone; not written) does the following:

- Provides a brief rundown of how long the hospital has before the ambulance will arrive
- Age and gender of the patient
- Description of the medical or trauma problem the patient is experiencing
- Treatment the patient was given (by EMTs) upon arrival at the scene and response to it
- Additional resources that may be required at the hospital, e.g., security for a combative behavioral patient or additional personnel to help with CPR if the patient is in cardiac arrest

## Patient Drop-Off

Once at the receiving facility, the driver notifies dispatch of their arrival and goes to the rear of the vehicle to assist in removing the patient. The patient is brought to the triage area and transferred to hospital care by the direction of the receiving nurse or physician. A **complete oral report** (or **bedside handover report** [or just bedside report]) is given to the initial hospital caregiver along with a copy of the PCR (in written or electronic format) containing the pertinent information from the assessments, vital signs, and EMT interventions.

Patient care is then transferred to the hospital staff. Once the EMT has confirmed that the hospital staff have all the information they need, only then is prehospital care terminated. The EMT may then move to the cleaning and resupplying of the ambulance.

Remember that unless the EMT has given a report and gained confirmation that hospital personnel (of an equal or higher level of certification) will continue care of the patient, the EMS provider may not leave their patient. This is considered abandonment and poor provider judgment. EMS providers must assure that another medical provider steps in and continues care for their patients, not just leave their patients on a hospital bed and hope someone comes along or checks on them. Legally speaking, there could also be prosecution for this act if charges are pressed by the patient or hospital.

## Postrun

Once you are back at the station, do the following:

- Restock the truck if that wasn't already done at the hospital.
- Complete the run report after obtaining the times from the dispatcher.
- File the run report according to local protocols regarding confidentiality of patient care information.
- Restock the disposable supplies.
- Clean linens that are used for the stretcher.

Once everything has been cleaned, disinfected, and restocked, the unit is available for another run. The last step is to notify dispatch that the unit is back in service.

# Special Situations

## Air Medical Transport

As mentioned earlier in the chapter, situations sometimes arise where the time required to travel by ground in the ambulance would unacceptably delay treatment of a patient or where access to a patient can't be obtained by emergency units in general.

In these cases, it is up to the provider to determine if air medical transport is warranted based on knowledge of the area and personal judgment. Mobilizing air medical transport is not a simple and quick option, so it should be reserved for high-priority and rapid-transport patients. You must weigh the severity of the situation against the distance needed to obtain definitive care.

The following are some examples of medical or trauma incidents where enlisting the help of air medical transport may be appropriate:

- Remote or rural location far from hospital and time is of the essence
- Head injury with altered mental status or GCS <10
- Penetrating injuries to the body cavity
- Extensive burns:
  - Second- and third-degree
  - Involving airway or breathing
  - Covering >30% of body surface area

If the decision is made to mobilize air medical transport, the following steps are required before the air unit can land and assume patient care:

- A landing zone must be established in an open area 100 feet × 100 feet that is free of major debris, overhead wires, heavy foliage, and bright lights.
- An updated patient condition report must be communicated by radio to the incoming air medical crew.

Once the helicopter is ready to land, land personnel must follow specific safety protocols when approaching. Helicopter blades are often still spinning, and it can take an extended amount of time to power them up or down. Precautions for the crew working in the landing zone include:

- Wear a hard helmet and/or eye protection in case of flying debris
- Approach the helicopter only when directed by air crew to do so
- Keep your head down when approaching

Alternatively, the air medical crew may direct you not to approach at all. Instead, they may come meet you away from the blades, bring their own equipment, and transfer the patient to their stretcher. It is at their discretion to decide what is appropriate at the time.

Keep in mind that in times of weather issues such as heavy rain or snow, air medical may not fly at all. In that case, you will have to transport via ground ambulance.

## Weapons of Mass Destruction

It is a sad truth in the post-9/11 world that EMS providers will be on the front line of a terrorist attack involving weapons of mass destruction (WMDs). These weapons fall into five categories and are remembered by the acronym **CBRNE** (pronounced "SeeBurn-E"):

- **C**hemical
- **B**iological
- **R**adiological
- **N**uclear
- **E**xplosives

The primary concern of the responding EMS personnel should be for their own safety. Dangers from these types of attacks are not always apparent, however, so EMS personnel must always be on high guard.

These types of attacks require the intervention of personnel with specific training that falls beyond the scope of this exam. However, all public safety personnel must be aware of weapons of mass destruction and be prepared to provide backup support as needed in the event of a terrorist event.

**Table 9.2** CBRNE Categories

| CATEGORY | COMPONENTS |
|---|---|
| Chemical | • Blistering agents (mustard gas, lewisite)<br>• Nerve agents (sarin, tabun)<br>• Blood agents (cyanogen chloride, hydrogen cyanide)<br>• Choking agents (phosgene, chlorine) |
| Biological | • Anthrax<br>• Tularemia<br>• Smallpox<br>• Ricin<br>• And other bacterial and viral agents |
| Radioactive | • Explosive device that releases radioactive isotopes to pollute an area with radiation<br>• Dispersed by so-called dirty bomb |
| Nuclear | • Major explosive device with resultant radiological contamination; profoundly devastating<br>• Explosion is created by changing atoms (either split or fused to create new atoms), which causes extremely significant destruction within seconds or minutes |
| Explosive | • Bombs—regular, pipe, pressure cooker<br>• Improvised explosive devices (IED)<br>• Anything that can burst apart and cause widespread damage with intent to harm |

## Mass Casualty Incidents

Any incident that involves more patients than a single unit can handle is considered to be a mass casualty incident (MCI). This can be as few as 2–3 people or as many as 100+.

After determining that the scene is safe, whoever was on scene first must analyze the number and severity of patients.

### Doing Triage

Triage identifies the most severely injured patients with the greatest chance of surviving. It helps to sort a large number of people in an unemotional way into categories, in what is likely to be a very emotional and chaotic event.

Triage can be difficult because minimal treatment is provided throughout the process, which can be very counterintuitive for EMS providers who, by their very nature, want to help as many people as possible. In an MCI, the greatest good needs to be offered to the greatest amount of people.

This ideology works efficiently to separate patients into various categories quickly. However, it can be quite emotionally traumatic for those doing triage, especially if dealing with children. Acknowledging this part of the job is half of the mental battle but is important to know. It is one thing to learn about the system. However, it is quite a different thing to do it in real life, where you may have the very real job of declaring a patient deceased even if they are taking shallow breaths.

The crew on scene is often referred to as "command." They will be in charge of getting the triage process started and also directing incoming units where to stage or how to approach the scene. Once more assistance is on scene, dedicated treatment and sorting areas should be identified and set up so that patients can start flowing through them.

There are a few methods of triage, and each service uses a different one. However, the most common methods include:

- **START**—Simple Triage and Rapid Treatment
- **JumpSTART**—pediatric-specific level of START triage
- **SALT**—Sort, Assess, Lifesaving Interventions, Treatment/Transport

Regardless of the system used, patients are identified by a color system. This can be achieved by commercially made triage tags, colored tape, or other means. The most commonly used colors are the following:

- **Red**—requires immediate transport
- **Yellow**—urgent, but transport can be delayed
- **Green**—non-life-threatening injuries; "walking wounded"
- **Black/gray**—deceased or injuries are too extensive
- **White**—no injuries

### Awaiting Transport

Once patients have been triaged, the patients need a place to await transport. During this time, some initial treatment may be started if resources are available:

- On smaller scenes, the arriving ambulance crews might be directed to a specific area to find their patients.
- With larger events, a treatment area and loading area should be identified and constructed. This can be accomplished with tents, colored tarps, or chalked-off areas.

Finally, consider where the patients should be transported. An MCI can overwhelm local hospitals, especially smaller ones. Notify nearby hospitals immediately, i.e., as soon as an event has been identified. Doing so will give them time to prepare for multiple patients at once. Keep in mind the following questions:

- How many patients require transport?
- How many hospitals are available to receive these patients, and what is each hospital's capability? In other words, is it a trauma center? A community hospital? A pediatric-specific facility?
- How many EMS units are available to assist with the transports?

# Practice Set

1. Ambulances should be supplied with

    A. only those supplies that the service can afford.

    B. all the supplies necessary for the operations for which the ambulance is licensed.

    C. an emergency childbirth kit.

    D. safety equipment mandated by the licensing authority.

2. Due regard is best described as

    A. forcing people to pull over for you when using lights and sirens.

    B. following local traffic rules, even during an emergency.

    C. making sure your ambulance is in working order.

    D. slowing down at stop signs and then proceeding through the intersection.

3. As you begin your shift, you receive an emergency dispatch for a patient in respiratory distress at a local nursing home. You have not yet performed the mandatory truck check. What should you do?

    A. Disregard the check and let the next shift do it.

    B. Do not respond to any calls until the check is completed.

    C. Respond to the call and perform the check when you return in service.

    D. Have the driver perform the check while you assess the patient.

4. Which of the following does NOT rely on an electrical battery?

    A. Pulse oximeter

    B. Portable oxygen tank

    C. Glucometer

    D. Portable suction unit

5. Your EMS radio announces, "Rescue 1, respond to 123 Main Street for a man fallen off a ladder with head laceration, possibly unconscious, time out 15:30 hours." Your response to dispatch should be

    A. "10-4."

    B. "Roger."

    C. "Rescue 1 responding emergently to 123 Main Street for a male, possibly unconscious, with a head laceration."

    D. "Rescue 1 responding with 2 EMTs, basic life support only, lights and sirens, to 123 Main Street in Anytown for a male who has fallen off of a ladder and has a possible skull fracture. We are responding at 15:31 hours. Do you copy, dispatch?"

6. The yellow triage tag color most commonly means

    A. patient is soon to be deceased without treatment.

    B. patient has a serious injury but can wait to be transported by another responding unit.

    C. patient needs to have additional airway maneuvers done.

    D. patient needs to be transported immediately.

7. You respond emergently to a motor vehicle accident. Once arriving on scene, you notice that a car has struck a fuel tank truck broadside, and liquid is running downhill toward you. The best place to park your ambulance is

   A. at the spot you first noticed the liquid.

   B. past the vehicle, uphill from the liquid spill.

   C. beside the vehicle to expedite patient care and transfer.

   D. 250 feet from the crash.

8. When should you notify the receiving facility of a critically ill patient?

   A. At the time of dispatch

   B. At the conclusion of the rapid assessment

   C. En route to the hospital

   D. Never

# Answer Key

| | | | | | | | |
|---|---|---|---|---|---|---|---|
| 1. | **B** | 3. | **C** | 5. | **C** | 7. | **B** |
| 2. | **B** | 4. | **B** | 6. | **B** | 8. | **C** |

# Answers and Explanations

## 1.  B

The minimum list of supplies is usually mandated by the licensing authority. However, the service should be carrying everything necessary for the operations for which the ambulance is licensed, whether basic life support, advanced life support, pediatric transport, neonate transport, etc. Answer choices (C) and (D) are partially correct since any BLS ambulance should have those items, but choice (B) is the best answer.

## 2.  B

Regardless of whether lights or sirens are being used, an emergency vehicle operator must always follow local traffic rules and posted speed limits, which makes (B) the answer. Certain allowances may be afforded to EMS by local police, such as driving over the speed limit within reason. However, these allowances are not always guaranteed, and it is up to the driver to exercise caution in all operations of the vehicle. (C) is part of the shift truck check. (A) and (D) are dangerous maneuvers that should not be used.

## 3.  C

The check should be performed by each shift and not be relegated to the next shift (A). Patient care is always a priority, so it would be inappropriate to neglect the response to a priority call (B). A call for respiratory distress is going to require both crew members, so (D) is incorrect as well.

## 4.  B

The portable oxygen tank does not rely on an electric battery. (A) and (C) are definitely battery operated. (D) is questionable since portable suction units can be either electrically or manually operated. Again, all answers must be read and the best answer chosen.

## 5.  C

If the information was not heard properly, the unit could respond to the wrong location, so repeating the dispatch information is always prudent. (A) and (B) are merely acknowledgments. (D) is too long, relays back information that is not pertinent, and attempts a diagnosis without even seeing the patient. This ties up the radio frequency unnecessarily.

## 6.  B

The correct answer is (B). The patient may have serious injuries but is stable enough to be transported later by an additional unit.

## 7.  B

The uphill parking place will put your vehicle out of the path of this potentially dangerous spill. (A) is incorrect because the liquid is continuing to spill and will soon be underneath your vehicle, putting the ambulance directly in a hazardous situation. (C) is incorrect since parking that close to a leaking fuel truck is dangerous to the vehicle, crew, and patient. (D) is incomplete and should be discarded.

## 8.  C

En route to the receiving facility is the correct answer. (A) is incorrect since at the time of dispatch, you do not have enough information. (B) is incorrect since after the rapid assessment, you still do not have all of the required information.

# FULL-LENGTH PRACTICE TEST AND EXPLANATIONS

# Answer Sheet

Remove (or photocopy) this answer sheet and use it to complete the practice test. See the answer key following the test when finished. For an analysis of your score, see Your Practice Test Score following the Answers and Explanations section.

1. Ⓐ Ⓑ Ⓒ Ⓓ   31. Ⓐ Ⓑ Ⓒ Ⓓ   61. Ⓐ Ⓑ Ⓒ Ⓓ   91. Ⓐ Ⓑ Ⓒ Ⓓ   121. Ⓐ Ⓑ Ⓒ Ⓓ
2. Ⓐ Ⓑ Ⓒ Ⓓ   32. Ⓐ Ⓑ Ⓒ Ⓓ   62. Ⓐ Ⓑ Ⓒ Ⓓ   92. Ⓐ Ⓑ Ⓒ Ⓓ   122. Ⓐ Ⓑ Ⓒ Ⓓ
3. Ⓐ Ⓑ Ⓒ Ⓓ   33. Ⓐ Ⓑ Ⓒ Ⓓ   63. Ⓐ Ⓑ Ⓒ Ⓓ   93. Ⓐ Ⓑ Ⓒ Ⓓ   123. Ⓐ Ⓑ Ⓒ Ⓓ
4. Ⓐ Ⓑ Ⓒ Ⓓ   34. Ⓐ Ⓑ Ⓒ Ⓓ   64. Ⓐ Ⓑ Ⓒ Ⓓ   94. Ⓐ Ⓑ Ⓒ Ⓓ   124. Ⓐ Ⓑ Ⓒ Ⓓ
5. Ⓐ Ⓑ Ⓒ Ⓓ   35. Ⓐ Ⓑ Ⓒ Ⓓ   65. Ⓐ Ⓑ Ⓒ Ⓓ   95. Ⓐ Ⓑ Ⓒ Ⓓ   125. Ⓐ Ⓑ Ⓒ Ⓓ
6. Ⓐ Ⓑ Ⓒ Ⓓ   36. Ⓐ Ⓑ Ⓒ Ⓓ   66. Ⓐ Ⓑ Ⓒ Ⓓ   96. Ⓐ Ⓑ Ⓒ Ⓓ   126. Ⓐ Ⓑ Ⓒ Ⓓ
7. Ⓐ Ⓑ Ⓒ Ⓓ   37. Ⓐ Ⓑ Ⓒ Ⓓ   67. Ⓐ Ⓑ Ⓒ Ⓓ   97. Ⓐ Ⓑ Ⓒ Ⓓ   127. Ⓐ Ⓑ Ⓒ Ⓓ
8. Ⓐ Ⓑ Ⓒ Ⓓ   38. Ⓐ Ⓑ Ⓒ Ⓓ   68. Ⓐ Ⓑ Ⓒ Ⓓ   98. Ⓐ Ⓑ Ⓒ Ⓓ   128. Ⓐ Ⓑ Ⓒ Ⓓ
9. Ⓐ Ⓑ Ⓒ Ⓓ   39. Ⓐ Ⓑ Ⓒ Ⓓ   69. Ⓐ Ⓑ Ⓒ Ⓓ   99. Ⓐ Ⓑ Ⓒ Ⓓ   129. Ⓐ Ⓑ Ⓒ Ⓓ
10. Ⓐ Ⓑ Ⓒ Ⓓ   40. Ⓐ Ⓑ Ⓒ Ⓓ   70. Ⓐ Ⓑ Ⓒ Ⓓ   100. Ⓐ Ⓑ Ⓒ Ⓓ   130. Ⓐ Ⓑ Ⓒ Ⓓ
11. Ⓐ Ⓑ Ⓒ Ⓓ   41. Ⓐ Ⓑ Ⓒ Ⓓ   71. Ⓐ Ⓑ Ⓒ Ⓓ   101. Ⓐ Ⓑ Ⓒ Ⓓ   131. Ⓐ Ⓑ Ⓒ Ⓓ
12. Ⓐ Ⓑ Ⓒ Ⓓ   42. Ⓐ Ⓑ Ⓒ Ⓓ   72. Ⓐ Ⓑ Ⓒ Ⓓ   102. Ⓐ Ⓑ Ⓒ Ⓓ   132. Ⓐ Ⓑ Ⓒ Ⓓ
13. Ⓐ Ⓑ Ⓒ Ⓓ   43. Ⓐ Ⓑ Ⓒ Ⓓ   73. Ⓐ Ⓑ Ⓒ Ⓓ   103. Ⓐ Ⓑ Ⓒ Ⓓ   133. Ⓐ Ⓑ Ⓒ Ⓓ
14. Ⓐ Ⓑ Ⓒ Ⓓ   44. Ⓐ Ⓑ Ⓒ Ⓓ   74. Ⓐ Ⓑ Ⓒ Ⓓ   104. Ⓐ Ⓑ Ⓒ Ⓓ   134. Ⓐ Ⓑ Ⓒ Ⓓ
15. Ⓐ Ⓑ Ⓒ Ⓓ   45. Ⓐ Ⓑ Ⓒ Ⓓ   75. Ⓐ Ⓑ Ⓒ Ⓓ   105. Ⓐ Ⓑ Ⓒ Ⓓ   135. Ⓐ Ⓑ Ⓒ Ⓓ
16. Ⓐ Ⓑ Ⓒ Ⓓ   46. Ⓐ Ⓑ Ⓒ Ⓓ   76. Ⓐ Ⓑ Ⓒ Ⓓ   106. Ⓐ Ⓑ Ⓒ Ⓓ   136. Ⓐ Ⓑ Ⓒ Ⓓ
17. Ⓐ Ⓑ Ⓒ Ⓓ   47. Ⓐ Ⓑ Ⓒ Ⓓ   77. Ⓐ Ⓑ Ⓒ Ⓓ   107. Ⓐ Ⓑ Ⓒ Ⓓ   137. Ⓐ Ⓑ Ⓒ Ⓓ
18. Ⓐ Ⓑ Ⓒ Ⓓ   48. Ⓐ Ⓑ Ⓒ Ⓓ   78. Ⓐ Ⓑ Ⓒ Ⓓ   108. Ⓐ Ⓑ Ⓒ Ⓓ   138. Ⓐ Ⓑ Ⓒ Ⓓ
19. Ⓐ Ⓑ Ⓒ Ⓓ   49. Ⓐ Ⓑ Ⓒ Ⓓ   79. Ⓐ Ⓑ Ⓒ Ⓓ   109. Ⓐ Ⓑ Ⓒ Ⓓ   139. Ⓐ Ⓑ Ⓒ Ⓓ
20. Ⓐ Ⓑ Ⓒ Ⓓ   50. Ⓐ Ⓑ Ⓒ Ⓓ   80. Ⓐ Ⓑ Ⓒ Ⓓ   110. Ⓐ Ⓑ Ⓒ Ⓓ   140. Ⓐ Ⓑ Ⓒ Ⓓ
21. Ⓐ Ⓑ Ⓒ Ⓓ   51. Ⓐ Ⓑ Ⓒ Ⓓ   81. Ⓐ Ⓑ Ⓒ Ⓓ   111. Ⓐ Ⓑ Ⓒ Ⓓ   141. Ⓐ Ⓑ Ⓒ Ⓓ
22. Ⓐ Ⓑ Ⓒ Ⓓ   52. Ⓐ Ⓑ Ⓒ Ⓓ   82. Ⓐ Ⓑ Ⓒ Ⓓ   112. Ⓐ Ⓑ Ⓒ Ⓓ   142. Ⓐ Ⓑ Ⓒ Ⓓ
23. Ⓐ Ⓑ Ⓒ Ⓓ   53. Ⓐ Ⓑ Ⓒ Ⓓ   83. Ⓐ Ⓑ Ⓒ Ⓓ   113. Ⓐ Ⓑ Ⓒ Ⓓ   143. Ⓐ Ⓑ Ⓒ Ⓓ
24. Ⓐ Ⓑ Ⓒ Ⓓ   54. Ⓐ Ⓑ Ⓒ Ⓓ   84. Ⓐ Ⓑ Ⓒ Ⓓ   114. Ⓐ Ⓑ Ⓒ Ⓓ   144. Ⓐ Ⓑ Ⓒ Ⓓ
25. Ⓐ Ⓑ Ⓒ Ⓓ   55. Ⓐ Ⓑ Ⓒ Ⓓ   85. Ⓐ Ⓑ Ⓒ Ⓓ   115. Ⓐ Ⓑ Ⓒ Ⓓ   145. Ⓐ Ⓑ Ⓒ Ⓓ
26. Ⓐ Ⓑ Ⓒ Ⓓ   56. Ⓐ Ⓑ Ⓒ Ⓓ   86. Ⓐ Ⓑ Ⓒ Ⓓ   116. Ⓐ Ⓑ Ⓒ Ⓓ   146. Ⓐ Ⓑ Ⓒ Ⓓ
27. Ⓐ Ⓑ Ⓒ Ⓓ   57. Ⓐ Ⓑ Ⓒ Ⓓ   87. Ⓐ Ⓑ Ⓒ Ⓓ   117. Ⓐ Ⓑ Ⓒ Ⓓ   147. Ⓐ Ⓑ Ⓒ Ⓓ
28. Ⓐ Ⓑ Ⓒ Ⓓ   58. Ⓐ Ⓑ Ⓒ Ⓓ   88. Ⓐ Ⓑ Ⓒ Ⓓ   118. Ⓐ Ⓑ Ⓒ Ⓓ   148. Ⓐ Ⓑ Ⓒ Ⓓ
29. Ⓐ Ⓑ Ⓒ Ⓓ   59. Ⓐ Ⓑ Ⓒ Ⓓ   89. Ⓐ Ⓑ Ⓒ Ⓓ   119. Ⓐ Ⓑ Ⓒ Ⓓ   149. Ⓐ Ⓑ Ⓒ Ⓓ
30. Ⓐ Ⓑ Ⓒ Ⓓ   60. Ⓐ Ⓑ Ⓒ Ⓓ   90. Ⓐ Ⓑ Ⓒ Ⓓ   120. Ⓐ Ⓑ Ⓒ Ⓓ   150. Ⓐ Ⓑ Ⓒ Ⓓ

# Practice Test

1. Which of the following is an example of an unsafe scene for an EMT to enter?

   A. 54-year-old male with difficulty breathing

   B. 23-year-old female with abdominal pain

   C. 18-year-old male with a gunshot wound to the chest

   D. 4-year-old male with leg pain

2. The arterioles connect the _____ and the capillaries.

   A. veins

   B. venules

   C. arteries

   D. vena cavae

3. Which of the following patients is at greatest risk for hypothermia?

   A. 30-year-old firefighter

   B. 70-year-old librarian

   C. 45-year-old EMT

   D. 11-year-old skier

4. Which of the following is NOT one of the 5 stages of grief?

   A. Denial

   B. Anger

   C. Crying

   D. Acceptance

5. The zygomatic bones are located in the

   A. chest.

   B. lower leg.

   C. back.

   D. face.

6. A 62-year-old female who was the unrestrained driver in a car crash complains of difficulty breathing. This patient's medical history includes COPD, and she has an implanted pacemaker. You auscultate diminished lung sounds and bowel sounds in the left base. The patient's vital signs are found to be $SpO_2$ of 96% on room air, pulse of 68, respiratory rate of 22, and blood pressure of 142/70 mm Hg. Which of the following should you do FIRST?

   A. Administer supplemental oxygen.

   B. Assist with the administration of the patient's prescribed inhaler.

   C. Wrap the patient's chest circumferentially with an ACE bandage to help with pain reduction.

   D. Assist ventilations with a BVM connected to oxygen.

7. When using air transport, the EMT should approach a helicopter

   A. from the uphill side.

   B. from the rear.

   C. only when instructed to do so by a helicopter crew member.

   D. under no circumstances but instead allow the crew to come to them.

8. Which of the following should be noted as insignificant in conducting the patient assessment?

   A. Medication bottles

   B. Comments of bystanders and family members

   C. Physical condition of the patient

   D. Patient's medical insurance

9. Which of the following is NOT a component of the Glasgow Coma Scale?

   A. Eye opening

   B. Verbal response

   C. Motor response

   D. Grimace response

10. You have an EMT student riding with you today. She is studying for an upcoming test and cannot remember a legal term. She recalls that you must have 4 elements in order to prove this type of claim. She knows that the 4 elements are duty, breach of duty, proximate cause, and harm caused. What term is she studying?

    A. Abandonment

    B. Gross negligence

    C. Simple negligence

    D. Malpractice

11. The head is _____ to the chest.

    A. inferior

    B. anterior

    C. superior

    D. posterior

12. Which of the following are responsibilities of the emergency medical dispatcher (EMD)? Select the 4 answer options that are correct.

    A. Assign incident command at mass casualty operations.

    B. Triage and prioritize calls that come in.

    C. Coordinate with other public safety agencies as needed.

    D. Provide medical direction to providers on scene.

    E. Provide medical instructions to callers.

    F. Handwrite name and number to pass along to crews.

    G. Inform providers which hospitals are on "divert" status.

13. There are _____ vertebrae in the lumbar section.

    A. 5

    B. 7

    C. 12

    D. 14

14. Signs and symptoms of post-traumatic stress disorder (PTSD) include the following EXCEPT

    A. loss of sexual desire.

    B. loss of appetite.

    C. loss of interest in work.

    D. loss of spontaneity.

15. What does the letter "G" in the Apgar score represent?

    A. Grating

    B. Grimace

    C. Guarding

    D. Gurgling

16. You are dispatched to a motor vehicle accident on a local city street. You respond emergently and arrive on scene with suitable precautions. The police are also on scene. There is one victim, a female seated in the car. Her car backed into another car as she was pulling out of her driveway at low speed. As you approach, she advises you that she is 36 weeks pregnant with her first child. She says she has no injuries, is not hemorrhaging, and is not in any pain; however, she wishes to be checked out at the hospital. In what position should she be transported?

    A. Trendelenburg

    B. Fowler

    C. Left lateral recumbent

    D. Right lateral recumbent

17. You respond to an 18-year-old male who is threatening suicide. The fire department states that before you arrived, the patient told them that he wanted to kill himself. Now the patient says he does not want to hurt himself but he just wants to be left alone. Which of the following is the most appropriate treatment?

    A. Explain the risks of staying at home with suicidal thoughts, and then have the patient sign a refusal form if he appears mentally competent.

    B. Inform the patient that because he told the fire department that he wants to hurt himself, he will have to go to the hospital. Have the police department assist you with ensuring that the patient is transported to the hospital.

    C. Find out if the patient can make an appointment with his personal doctor, and then confirm that he does have an appointment before you clear the scene and return to the station.

    D. Since the patient did not tell you personally that he wants to kill himself, you must allow him to make his own decisions. Explain to him that he needs to get mental health assistance.

18. Your patient is an 87-year-old male who is complaining of chest pain and difficulty breathing. Vital signs are blood pressure of 134/82 mm Hg, pulse rate of 96, respiratory rate of 22, and $SpO_2$ of 93% on room air. He describes pain that is 8/10, constant, and radiating to his left arm. This patient has no allergies but does have a significant cardiac history. Which of the following treatments would be indicated for this patient? Select the 3 answer options that are correct.

    A. Administer 325 mg of aspirin, chewed.

    B. Deliver 4 LPM of oxygen on nasal cannula.

    C. Place an oral airway adjunct.

    D. Assess his blood glucose level.

    E. Apply the AED pads.

    F. Administer 0.4 mg of nitroglycerin sublingually.

19. A neonate will normally have _____ pulse rates and respiratory rates than an infant.

    A. higher

    B. lower

    C. more irregular

    D. less irregular

20. Most EMTs are injured at which of the following types of calls?

    A. Domestic violence calls

    B. Motor vehicle accidents

    C. Industrial accidents

    D. In-station accidents

21. All veins other than the pulmonary vein are blood vessels that carry deoxygenated blood _____ the heart.

    A. into

    B. away from

    C. toward

    D. from the lungs to

22. Which of the following is NOT a type of muscle?

    A. Voluntary

    B. Involuntary

    C. Cardiac

    D. Regulatory

23. Which of the following is NOT a component of the SAMPLE history?

    A. Signs and symptoms

    B. Allergies

    C. Medications

    D. Pulse rate

24. When should EMS communication equipment be checked?

    A. Daily

    B. Monthly

    C. Weekly

    D. At the start of every shift

25. The first thing to consider when arriving on scene of an emergency call is

    A. scene safety.

    B. universal precautions.

    C. airway.

    D. breathing.

26. A bull's-eye or star pattern in a windshield that was caused during a motor vehicle crash indicates that the patient may suffer from what kind of serious injury?

    A. Laceration to the scalp

    B. Broken nose from the impact

    C. Concussion

    D. Cervical and spinal damage

27. Once you have determined that the scene is safe and you are wearing the proper universal precautions, the next thing to be checked is

    A. airway.

    B. breathing.

    C. circulation.

    D. level of consciousness.

28. Which of the following is NOT a level of consciousness?

    A. Alert

    B. Conscious

    C. Active

    D. Oriented

29. Perfusion in patient assessment refers to the amount of

    A. fluid in the lungs.

    B. oxygen in the hemoglobin.

    C. urine in the bladder.

    D. blood in the heart.

30. Your patient has a core body temperature of 91° Fahrenheit. This temperature indicates what stage of hypothermia?

    A. Severe

    B. Moderate

    C. Mild

    D. Irreversible

31. You are dispatched to a residence for a man down. You respond emergently and arrive on scene wearing suitable precautions. The scene is safe, and the patient's wife advises you that he is undergoing chemotherapy for lung cancer. The patient presents on the primary assessment as unresponsive reflex. His airway is open, he is breathing spontaneously at a rate of 12, and he has a weak, thready pulse rate of 100. A non-rebreather mask is placed onto the patient at a flow rate of 15 LPM. Your transport time to the nearest hospital emergency department is 30 minutes, but there is an ALS unit 15 minutes out. Your next step should be which of the following?

    A. Call for an ALS intercept.

    B. Begin priority transport.

    C. Administer 0.3 mg epinephrine subcutaneously.

    D. Request an air transport.

32. The letter "Q" in the acronym OPQRST stands for

    A. quantity.

    B. quality.

    C. quasi.

    D. quick.

33. After the focused trauma assessment is completed on a serious trauma patient, the assessment should be rechecked every

    A. 2 minutes.

    B. 3 minutes.

    C. 5 minutes.

    D. 15 minutes.

34. Which of the following best describes an indirect-force injury?

    A. When an object strikes a person and transfers all of its energy to the point of impact

    B. When a force is applied to one region of the body but causes an injury in another region of the body

    C. When a patient has a medical condition that causes weakened bones to fracture

    D. When a penetrating injury leads to a fracture or other musculoskeletal injury

35. In the mnemonic DCAP-BTLS, the letter "B" stands for

    A. bruising.

    B. brittleness.

    C. burns.

    D. broken.

36. A patient viewed from the side is bisected by the

    A. midaxillary line.

    B. midclavicular line.

    C. midsternal line.

    D. horizontal plane.

37. You are dispatched to a man who has fallen from a garage roof. You respond emergently and arrive on scene wearing suitable precautions. The scene is safe. The patient is a 32-year-old male who is conscious but confused as to what events happened to cause the injury. You are holding stabilization while your partner completes the focused trauma assessment. Which device should be applied following the focused assessment of the head and neck?

    A. Head blocks

    B. Hare traction device

    C. NRB mask

    D. Cervical collar

38. The Good Samaritan Act is a

    A. religious doctrine.

    B. statute that minimizes liability for undertaking certain actions.

    C. good deed done by an EMT.

    D. law that protects EMTs 100% of the time from getting sued.

39. While en route to the hospital with a critically ill patient, how often should you repeat vital signs as part of the ongoing assessment?

    A. Every 1 minute

    B. Every 3 minutes

    C. Every 5 minutes

    D. Every 10 minutes

40. The "U" in the mnemonic AVPU means

    A. uniform.

    B. unequivocal.

    C. unknown.

    D. unresponsive.

41. Which of the following should never be given over the two-way radio system?

    A. The location of a call

    B. The nature of a call

    C. The patient's name

    D. The EMT's name

42. Which of the following is NOT a required part of a prehospital care report?

    A. Patient's name

    B. Patient's date of birth

    C. Patient's gender

    D. Patient's medical insurance

43. You are dispatched to the local high school for an eye injury. You respond emergently and arrive on scene. The scene is safe, and you are wearing suitable precautions. You are directed to the nurse's office, where you find a 16-year-old male with a pencil stuck in his left eye. All vital signs are normal, and there is no other injury. You should dress and bandage

    A. his left eye.

    B. both eyes.

    C. his entire upper head.

    D. nothing; a dressing is not indicated.

44. Which of the following situations do you NOT have to report if you become aware of it?

    A. Child abuse

    B. Sexual abuse

    C. Elder abuse

    D. Alcohol abuse

45. When is the umbilical cord cut?

    A. Immediately after the baby is delivered

    B. When it ceases pulsing

    C. When the placenta is delivered

    D. At the hospital

46. Which of the following is NOT a sign or symptom of hypovolemic shock?

    A. Hypotension

    B. Excessive thirst

    C. Tachypnea

    D. Hypertension

47. A competent patient may refuse which of the following procedures?

    A. Cervical stabilization with a cervical collar

    B. Spinal immobilization with a spine board

    C. Medication administration

    D. All of the above

48. Which of the following oxygen delivery devices normally provides 24–40% oxygen when attached to supplemental oxygen?

    A. Nasal cannula

    B. Simple face mask

    C. Non-rebreather mask

    D. Bag-valve mask

49. SIDS normally occurs between the ages of

    A. 0 and 1.

    B. 1 and 2.

    C. 2 and 3.

    D. 3 and 4.

50. An impaled object should never be removed unless

    A. ordered to do so by police on scene.

    B. requested by the patient.

    C. it interferes with airway management.

    D. it is longer than 12 inches.

51. An EMT must check which of the following when administering pharmaceuticals?

    A. Temperature of drug

    B. Contraindications

    C. Side effects

    D. Expiration date

52. Your patient is experiencing severe respiratory difficulty due to pulmonary edema. In which of the following positions would you expect to see this patient?

    A. Semi-Fowler position

    B. Trendelenburg position

    C. Tripod position

    D. Reverse Fowler position

53. The contraction of the ventricles produces the _____ pressure in the arteries.

    A. diastolic

    B. systolic

    C. arterial

    D. static

54. On a cold, winter day, you respond to a local pond for an ice fisherman who fell through the ice. You arrive on scene, and you observe a male lying supine in cold and wet clothes; the patient has no pulse or respirations. A scuba diver advises that your patient has been underwater for the 30 minutes it took the diver to suit up and effect the rescue. You should next

    A. pronounce the patient dead.

    B. immediately begin CPR.

    C. place the patient into the truck, remove his wet clothes, and begin to warm him.

    D. request an ALS intercept.

55. You are dispatched to a local health club for a male with difficulty breathing. You respond emergently and arrive on scene. The scene is safe, and you are wearing suitable precautions. You observe a 30-year-old male patient with obvious dyspnea who is pale and mildly diaphoretic. He has a history of asthma, blood pressure of 150/80 mm Hg, pulse of 110, and respiratory rate of 24. His pulse oximetry saturation is 88% on room air. Which of the following oxygen delivery devices should you apply?

    A. Nasal cannula

    B. Simple face mask

    C. Bag-valve mask

    D. Non-rebreather mask

56. In the scenario in question 55, to what flow rate will you set your oxygen regulator?

    A. 4 liters per minute

    B. 10 liters per minute

    C. 15 liters per minute

    D. 20 liters per minute

57. Which of the following is NOT a landmark for a lung field you would auscultate in question 55?

    A. Anterior midclavicular

    B. Posterior base

    C. Inferior vena cava

    D. Right midaxillary

58. Which of the following foods is/are highly suspect in anaphylaxis?

    A. Nuts

    B. Seafood

    C. Eggs

    D. All of the above

59. Which of the following is NOT a classic symptom of a heart attack?

    A. Chest pain

    B. Dyspnea

    C. Denial

    D. Headache

60. The beginning of obstetrical labor is the

    A. discharge of the placenta.

    B. fertilization of the ovum.

    C. discharge of the cervical mucus plug.

    D. rupture of the amniotic sac.

61. Which of the following is useful in absorbing toxins in the stomach?

    A. Activated charcoal

    B. Ipecac syrup

    C. Oxygen

    D. Aspirin

62. Labor concludes with

    A. the delivery of the baby.

    B. the delivery of the placenta.

    C. the delivery of the umbilical cord.

    D. the delivery of the amniotic sac.

63. You are dispatched to a call for chest pains. You respond emergently, the scene is safe, and you are wearing protective equipment. Your patient is a female in her sixties, seated at the kitchen table. She is guarding her chest with one hand and tells you she has crushing chest pain of sudden onset. She has a history of cardiac problems and is currently on nitroglycerine paste and diltiazem (Cardizem). Her pulse is weak and thready. Which of the following drugs should you NOT administer?

    A. Aspirin

    B. NTG

    C. Epinephrine

    D. Oxygen

64. The preferred method of ventilating a patient in respiratory arrest in the prehospital setting is a

    A. manual ventilator.

    B. face mask.

    C. BVM.

    D. BVM with oxygen reservoir.

65. You are dispatched to a local restaurant for a man down. You arrive on scene and observe a male in full cardiac and respiratory arrest. You and your partner perform CPR for 2 minutes and then convert his heart rhythm with the AED; his pulse is 65 and blood pressure is 90/60 mm Hg. After 2 minutes, he begins to have spontaneous respirations and his gag reflex returns, so you remove the oropharyngeal airway. You finish your assessment and begin transport to the nearest emergency department 15 minutes away. At 10 minutes from the hospital, he suddenly lapses into unconsciousness and again has no pulse or spontaneous respirations. Your next step should be which of the following?

    A. Begin chest compressions.

    B. Begin rescue breathing.

    C. Shock with the AED.

    D. Request an ALS intercept.

66. You are dispatched to a residence for an unconscious male. You respond emergently with suitable precautions, and the scene is safe. You find an adult male lying on the kitchen floor with spontaneous respirations and with carotid and radial pulses. He is conscious and responsive to verbal stimuli with a patent airway and no difficulty swallowing. You measure his blood sugar with a glucometer and get a reading of 45. He is probably suffering from

    A. postictal seizure.

    B. hypoglycemia.

    C. hyperglycemia.

    D. hypovolemia.

67. A confused 22-year-old male has an 8-inch, full-thickness laceration diagonally across his right thigh, sustained in a fight with someone who had a knife. His skin is pale and diaphoretic, and you observe a steady flow of dark-red blood oozing from the wound onto the carpeted floor. The carpet under his leg is saturated. You should suspect which of these?

    A. Minor hemorrhage

    B. Arterial hemorrhage

    C. Massive hemorrhage

    D. Capillary hemorrhage

68. Presentation of the cord from the vagina before delivery of the baby is called

    A. presenting cord.

    B. prolapsed cord.

    C. breech cord.

    D. premature cord.

69. You are dispatched to a local clinic for a child convulsing. You respond emergently while wearing suitable precautions and arrive on scene. The nurse on scene advises that the mother brought her 2-year-old male child in for not feeling well, and as the nurse began to examine him, he began to seize. His vital signs are BP of 100/60 mm Hg, pulse rate of 80, respirations of 18 prior to the seizure, and a rectal temperature of 105 degrees Fahrenheit. You suspect the patient is having a/an _____ seizure.

    A. tonic-clonic

    B. postictal

    C. febrile

    D. anaphylactic

70. Which of the following indicates the normal blood glucose range in adults?

    A. 0–40 mg/dL

    B. 40–80 mg/dL

    C. 80–120 mg/dL

    D. 120–160 mg/dL

71. Another term for heart attack is

    A. myocardial infarction.

    B. congestive heart failure.

    C. mitral valve defect.

    D. left bundle branch block.

72. You are dispatched to a call for a possible allergic reaction. You are directed to a restaurant table where a male in his twenties is clutching his throat in severe respiratory distress. His partner tells you that he is allergic to nuts and nut products, but he has not had anything other than grilled steak with sautéed vegetables. Which drug do you want to administer following your initial assessment?

    A. Benadryl 50 mg tablet

    B. Epinephrine 0.3 mg intramuscular

    C. Nitroglycerin spray sublingual

    D. Oxygen 2–6 LPM via non-rebreather

73. You and your partner arrive on scene of a female having a seizure. When you enter the room, you witness the patient's muscles tensing up and remaining rigid. What is this period of the seizure called?

    A. Tonic

    B. Clonic

    C. Generalized

    D. Postictal

74. A motor vehicle accident in which one vehicle strikes another broadside is also referred to as a _____ crash.

    A. front-end

    B. rear-end

    C. T-bone

    D. rollover

75. You are dispatched to a local residence for a female acting strangely. You respond while emergently wearing suitable precautions and arrive on scene simultaneously with the police. The house is extremely cold inside, and the patient is a female in her sixties wearing heavy clothing. She responds to your questions in a faint, intelligible voice, and as you feel her neck for a carotid pulse, she is cold to the touch. Your treatment of this patient should include all of the following EXCEPT

    A. placing the patient into a warm environment.

    B. applying heat packs to the groin, axillary, and cervical regions.

    C. advising the patient to drink hot coffee.

    D. removing any wet clothing.

76. The blood component that carries the antibodies the body uses to fight infection is/are

    A. hemoglobin.

    B. leukocytes.

    C. plasma.

    D. platelets.

77. You are dispatched to a residence for an unconscious patient. You respond emergently and arrive on scene wearing universal precautions. You establish that the scene is safe. The firefighters on scene advise that they have removed the victim from his garage where his car was running. The patient has labored breathing and his face is cyanotic, but his lips and tongue are bright red. Which poison should you suspect?

    A. Carbon dioxide

    B. Carbon monoxide

    C. Gasoline

    D. Narcotic overdose

78. To which of the following treatment facilities would you transport the patient in question 77?

    A. Nearest level 1 trauma center

    B. Nearest level 3 trauma center

    C. Nearest emergency department

    D. Nearest facility with a hyperbaric chamber

79. On a hot summer day, you are dispatched to a road race site for a runner down. You respond emergently and arrive on scene to find a 25-year-old male lying unconscious on his back in his running clothes. He skin is red, dry, and very hot to the touch. His pulse is 120, respirations are 20, and blood pressure is 100/60 mm Hg. Which condition should you suspect?

    A. Heat cramps

    B. Heat exhaustion

    C. Heatstroke

    D. Heat overdose

80. Which should you immediately do for the patient in question 79?

    A. Request transport priority.

    B. Request an ALS intercept.

    C. Administer oxygen 6 LPM via nasal cannula and monitor his $SpO_2$.

    D. Transfer him to a cooler location and apply wet cloths to his head.

81. A phobia is

    A. a feeling of sadness or worthlessness.

    B. an alternating feeling of euphoria and depression.

    C. an irrational fear.

    D. a mistrust of everyone and everything.

82. Tuberculosis is an example of a/an _____ pathogen.

    A. airborne

    B. bloodborne

    C. contact-borne

    D. fluid-borne

83. Which of the following poisons could be vomited without danger?

    A. Bleach

    B. Kerosene

    C. Alcohol

    D. Ammonia

84. You are dispatched to a person in the water at a local reservoir. You respond emergently and arrive on scene before the police and fire units. You observe a male yelling for help 100 yards from shore. You should immediately

    A. jump into the water and swim to the victim.

    B. check for a boat nearby so you can row to the victim.

    C. throw a life preserver to the victim.

    D. advise dispatch that you will need a rescue boat.

85. The EMT should ask the patient to do which of the following prior to administration of a bronchodilator?

    A. Hold their breath for 5 seconds

    B. Exhale deeply

    C. Inhale rapidly 3 times

    D. Pant

86. You are dispatched to the scene of a 12-year-old female who has been struck by a car in her neighborhood. Police on scene are unable to reach her parents. What legal doctrine enables you to treat the girl?

    A. Explicit consent

    B. In loco parentis

    C. Informed consent

    D. Refusal of consent

87. You respond for a female who is having a behavioral emergency. The patient is not able to leave her house until she checks each door 5 times to make sure it is locked properly. This demonstrates which of the following types of behavior?

    A. Schizophrenia

    B. Psychosis

    C. Obsessive-compulsive disorder

    D. Impulse-control disorder

88. Which of the following is the most common mental illness experience in the United States?

    A. Depression

    B. Manic-depressive illness

    C. Obsessive-compulsive disorder

    D. Bipolar mood disorder

89. At which stage of hypothermia does loss of consciousness normally occur?

    A. Mild

    B. Moderate

    C. Severe

    D. Irreversible

90. Most behavioral emergency calls are

    A. violent.

    B. nonviolent.

    C. exaggerated.

    D. transferred.

91. Which of the following obstetrical conditions usually presents with painless, bright-red bleeding?

    A. Abruptio placenta

    B. Multipara

    C. Placenta previa

    D. Supine hypotensive syndrome

92. Apgar scores are taken at 1 minute and _____ minutes postpartum.

    A. 2

    B. 5

    C. 10

    D. 20

93. The normal respiratory rate for an adult is

    A. 6–12 times per minute.

    B. 12–20 times per minute.

    C. 15–25 times per minute.

    D. 20–40 times per minute.

94. The heart contains _____ chambers.

    A. 1

    B. 2

    C. 3

    D. 4

95. Which of the following is the primary effect of chronic bronchitis on the airway?

    A. Failure of the hemoglobin to be able to carry oxygen

    B. Increased mucus production in the bronchial tree

    C. Increased bronchial dilation

    D. Decreased carbon dioxide production

96. What is the minimum number of people required to safely restrain a violent patient in 4-point soft restraints?

    A. 2

    B. 3

    C. 4

    D. 5

97. In which of the following situations should a police escort be used with EMT transport?

    A. Transport of a critical patient

    B. Transport of a mother and child postpartum

    C. Unfamiliarity with the location of the hospital

    D. Transport of a police officer injured in the line of duty

98. The normal gestation period for a human fetus is

    A. 12 weeks.

    B. 24 weeks.

    C. 40 weeks.

    D. 52 weeks.

99. The liquid component of the blood is called

    A. hemoglobin.

    B. leukocytes.

    C. plasma.

    D. platelets.

100. Obstetrical crowning is when

    A. the mother's amniotic sac ruptures.

    B. the baby's head becomes visible in the birth canal.

    C. labor pains are <5 minutes apart and last >1 minute.

    D. the baby cries for the first time.

101. How many vertebrae make up the spinal column?

    A. 23

    B. 29

    C. 33

    D. 45

102. A patient who presents with hyperthermia, erratic behavior, super strength, and a history of illegal drug usage is most likely suffering from

    A. bipolar disorder.

    B. excited delirium.

    C. schizophrenia.

    D. panic disorder.

103. You are dispatched to a call for a "possible heart attack" to a residence along with an ALS rescue that is 10 minutes out. You respond emergently and arrive on scene 4 minutes after being dispatched. The scene is safe, and you are wearing appropriate universal precautions. You observe a male in his seventies lying supine on the living room floor, cyanotic, and with his eyes open. You open his airway and note that he is not breathing. You administer 2 breaths, which inflate his lungs. You check for a carotid pulse, and there is none. You advise your partner to begin chest compressions. What is your next step?

    A. Continue rescue breathing and compressions pending arrival of ALS.

    B. Place 15 LPM NRB.

    C. Apply the AED and follow the directions.

    D. After 1 minute of CPR, place the patient onto a backboard and transport priority.

104. Which of the following vehicles has the right-of-way over an ambulance?

    A. Police car with flashing lights operating

    B. Fire truck with flashing lights operating

    C. School bus with flashing red lights operating

    D. Utility truck with flashing yellow lights operating

105. The ulna is located in the

    A. lower arm.

    B. lower leg.

    C. chest.

    D. face.

106. You are dispatched to a female in labor. You observe a female in her twenties lying in bed with her knees drawn up and her upper body supported by pillows in a semi-Fowler position. She advises you that this is her third pregnancy, that her water has broken, and that the pains are less than a minute apart. You examine her vaginal area, and as she experiences another contraction, you see the top of the baby's head in the birth canal. You should next

    A. prepare for immediate delivery.

    B. place the mother onto the stretcher left lateral recumbent and transport priority to the nearest obstetrical unit.

    C. bind the mother's legs together to slow delivery while you do a full assessment.

    D. boil water.

107. In the scenario in question 106, the next contraction delivers the baby's head. You notice the cord wrapped around the baby's neck. You should next

    A. clamp the cord.

    B. place 2 fingers between the cord and the baby's neck.

    C. cut the cord.

    D. request an ALS intercept.

108. Your patient is a 34-year-old female with a history of illness for the last 2 weeks. She tells you, "I'm not getting better, and it's getting harder to breathe. I also don't have a lot of energy. My doctor gave me some antibiotics, but I don't think they're working." According to the SIRS criteria, which of the following would NOT contribute to this patient's likelihood of developing sepsis from a prolonged infection?

    A. Systolic blood pressure of 76 mm Hg

    B. Heart rate of 86

    C. Respiratory rate of 32

    D. Temperature of 95.2°F

109. If an EMT makes an error while writing a paper prehospital care report (PCR) narrative, which of the following should be done?

    A. Disregard the error, and continue with the narrative.

    B. Destroy the document.

    C. Cross out the error, write a correction, and date and initial the correction.

    D. Write a new narrative, and staple it to the old narrative.

110. Why are the bottom two ribs called floating ribs?

    A. They are not connected to the sternum.

    B. They are not connected to any other bony structure.

    C. They are suspended in fluid.

    D. They are not really ribs.

111. All calls for behavioral emergencies should also have a/an

    A. ALS intercept.

    B. police response.

    C. second rescue.

    D. fire department response.

112. What is the maximum Apgar score?

    A. 5

    B. 8

    C. 10

    D. 12

113. A patient has a blood glucose level of 45 mg/dL. This is considered what type of emergency?

    A. Hyperglycemia

    B. Hypoglycemia

    C. Diabetic ketoacidosis with hyperventilation

    D. Hyperglycemic hyperosmolar nonketotic coma

114. Victims of sexual assault should initially be assessed and treated by

    A. EMTs of the same gender if possible.

    B. police officers trained in sexual assault.

    C. registered nurses.

    D. rape crisis counselors.

115. Which route describes placing medication into the cheek mucosal area?

    A. Oral

    B. Sublingual

    C. Buccal

    D. Tympanic

116. Which of the following incident types is the most common EMS trauma call?

    A. Falls

    B. Shootings

    C. Stabbings

    D. Motor vehicle accidents

117. In treatment of severe trauma, what is the recognized time standard from injury to the operating room?

    A. 30 minutes

    B. 60 minutes

    C. 180 minutes

    D. 240 minutes

118. How many liters of blood are in the average adult human's circulatory system?

    A. 2 to 3

    B. 3 to 4

    C. 4 to 5

    D. 5 to 6

119. The most common cause of seizures in the infant population is

    A. epilepsy.

    B. high fever.

    C. poisoning.

    D. mother's use of illegal drugs while pregnant.

120. You are dispatched to a residence for a man with a lacerated arm. You respond emergently and arrive on scene wearing suitable precautions; the police are on scene. Your patient is lying on the ground behind the house with a series of lacerations around his lower arm. He is bleeding profusely with a steady flow but does not appear to be spurting. He is intoxicated and belligerent. You attempt to control the bleeding with pressure bandages, but he continues to hemorrhage. Which procedure is the best next option?

    A. Hemostatic agent

    B. Tourniquet

    C. Pressure bandage

    D. Oxygen at 15 LPM NRB

121. The most common cause of dyspnea in the infant is

    A. foreign bodies.

    B. mucus.

    C. congenital birth defects.

    D. SIDS.

122. What is the most desirable characteristic the EMT wants in a dressing?

    A. Size

    B. Shape

    C. Sterility

    D. Elasticity

123. Which of the following statements pertaining to refusal to treat or transport is NOT true?

    A. The treatment and transport options must be explained.

    B. The consequences of refusal must be explained.

    C. The patient may not change their mind after they have signed a refusal form.

    D. The signature of the patient must be witnessed by a disinterested third party.

124. You are dispatched to a motor vehicle accident on the highway. You respond emergently and arrive on scene wearing suitable BSI gear. The police and fire department are on scene. Your patient is a male lying next to his wrecked car. He has been collared and placed onto a spine board by the fire department. He is responsive to painful stimuli with BP of 100/60 mm Hg, pulse of 120, and respirations of 18. He is pale and clammy. Your treatment of this patient should include all of the following EXCEPT

    A. focused trauma assessment en route.

    B. prevention of heat loss.

    C. administration of high-flow oxygen.

    D. Fowler position.

125. Which of the following is NOT a type of open wound?

    A. Abrasion

    B. Incision

    C. Bruising

    D. Laceration

126. One of the side effects of nitroglycerin tablets is

    A. hypotension.

    B. hypertension.

    C. diaphoresis.

    D. tachypnea.

127. Wounds to which of the following anatomical areas should be treated with occlusive dressings?

    A. Head

    B. Neck

    C. Abdomen

    D. Genitals

128. You are dispatched along with the fire department to a report of a person on fire behind a residence. You respond emergently and arrive simultaneously with the fire department. A woman tells you her husband was lighting his charcoal grill with gasoline and there was an explosion. The patient is an adult male who is conscious, alert, and oriented times 3. He states he was trying to light the grill when the gasoline exploded. He denies any dyspnea. The physical exam reveals second-degree burns to both arms, with no other burns. What percentage of the patient's body surface area is burned?

    A. 9%

    B. 18%

    C. 27%

    D. 20%

129. In the scenario in question 128, what priority is this patient?

    A. Nonpriority

    B. Critical

    C. Moderate

    D. Fatal

130. Naloxone is a drug given for the following drug overdose (OD) and in what dosage?

    A. Heroin OD, 2 mg total IN

    B. Opioid OD, 6 mg total IN

    C. LSD OD, 2 mg total IN

    D. NSAID OD, 4 mg total IN

131. You are dispatched to the high school football field for a player injured. You respond emergently and arrive on scene wearing suitable precautions. The coach tells you that he suspects a fractured fibula in this player. The patient is conscious, alert, and oriented times 3, and his only complaint is severe pain in his lower leg. Where must the suspected fracture site be splinted?

    A. Below the injury

    B. Above and below the injury

    C. Above the injury

    D. Over the injury

132. Your patient is a 32-year-old female who was stabbed with a long, serrated bread knife in a domestic dispute with her significant other. She is presenting with an abdominal evisceration of the intestines with significant bleeding and respiratory distress. Which of the following are appropriate treatment for this patient's condition? Select the 2 answer options that are correct.

    A. Attempt to replace the intestines into the abdominal cavity.

    B. Maintain the patient's body temperature.

    C. Apply a dry pressure dressing.

    D. Apply a moist, 4-sided occlusive dressing.

    E. Apply a dry, 4-sided occlusive dressing.

    F. Irrigate the whole area with sterile water.

133. The letter "M" in the acronym SAMPLE stands for

    A. menstrual period.

    B. medications.

    C. most active symptom.

    D. movement.

134. The epiglottis in a pediatric patient is _____ in the airway than in an adult patient.

    A. lower

    B. higher

    C. more anterior

    D. more posterior

135. In which of the following injury situations should you apply a cervical collar?

    A. Head trauma secondary to a rear-end motor vehicle collision

    B. Fall from a garage roof

    C. Neck pain as a result of a football injury

    D. All of the above

136. You are ventilating with a BVM an unresponsive 37-year-old female who is in respiratory arrest. The spouse states that the patient was out drinking tonight. After coming home, she passed out on the bed, and he couldn't wake her up. The patient has a history of drug and alcohol abuse. The spouse says she is not currently taking any medications that he knows of. Which of the following should you use to ensure that you are delivering adequate tidal volume with a BVM? Select the 2 answer options that are correct.

    A. Look for chest rise and fall.

    B. Fully deflate the BVM after delivering each breath.

    C. Assess a pulse oximeter.

    D. Auscultate for bronchial breath sounds when delivering breaths.

    E. Look for skin color change.

    F. Hook up the BVM to 15 LPM oxygen.

137. You are dispatched to a 2-car motor vehicle accident and respond emergently. You arrive on scene wearing the appropriate precautions, and the scene is safe. Your patient is in a vehicle that was struck broadside by another vehicle traveling at a high rate of speed. He was not restrained and is complaining of dyspnea. His shirt is ripped and bloody, and you notice that he has an open wound that is gurgling and foaming. This patient is most at risk for

    A. hypovolemic shock.

    B. pneumothorax.

    C. subdural hematoma.

    D. myocardial infarction.

138. Patients with open abdominal injuries are at greater risk for which of the following?

    A. Hypertension

    B. Infection

    C. Sudden cardiac death

    D. Peritonitis

139. A patient aged 8 months is defined as a/an

    A. neonate.

    B. toddler.

    C. infant.

    D. preschooler.

140. If a tourniquet is applied to control bleeding, at what point should it be loosened?

    A. Every 5 minutes

    B. Every 10 minutes

    C. Every 15 minutes

    D. At the hospital

141. You are called to respond, with police, to a local residence for a psychological evaluation. You respond emergently with suitable precautions, and when you arrive, the police have secured the scene. A male in his thirties is pacing around the room anxiously. He is not cooperative or responsive to your questions. The police advise that his psychiatrist has requested his transport to the nearest emergency department for medical evaluation prior to admission to the psychiatric facility. As the patient hears this, he attacks the police officer but is quickly subdued. The police officer advises you that the patient's psychiatrist has approved the use of restraints. What is the most appropriate way to restrain this patient?

    A. Prone with hands behind his back and ankles drawn up to his wrists

    B. Supine with hands behind his back and ankles secured to the stretcher

    C. Supine with both hands and ankles secured to the stretcher

    D. Prone with handcuffs attached to both the wrists and ankles

142. You are dispatched to a local nursing home for a patient who has fallen. You respond emergently with suitable precautions, and the scene is safe. You find an 82-year-old female lying supine on the floor, conscious and alert, complaining of pain to her hip. You note that her right leg is rotated outward. What splinting device should you use?

    A. Traction splint

    B. Pelvic binder

    C. Padded board splint

    D. Backboard

143. Which of the following types of bleeding is the most severe?

    A. Capillary

    B. Venous

    C. Arteriole

    D. Arterial

144. Aspirin is indicated for which of the following conditions in EMS protocols?

    A. Headache

    B. Chest pain

    C. Abdominal pain

    D. Leg and arm pain

145. All of the following persons are routinely allowed to access a prehospital care report EXCEPT

    A. the patient.

    B. the receiving physician.

    C. the police.

    D. the EMT who wrote the report.

146. Which of these is the abbreviation of the book used to identify hazardous materials?

    A. EEG

    B. ERG

    C. ENT

    D. EKG

147. Which of the following pregnancies will normally have a longer labor period?

    A. First

    B. Second

    C. Third

    D. Fourth

148. At the scene of a motor vehicle accident, it is MOST important for the ambulance to be parked

    A. downhill and downwind of the scene.

    B. in a way that protects the scene.

    C. in a way that helps to load the patient into the back doors.

    D. without obstructing the police investigation.

149. The cervix is fully dilated and the baby "drops" into the birth canal in which stage of labor?

    A. First

    B. Second

    C. Third

    D. Fourth

150. Which of the following is an example of implied consent?

    A. Patient who agrees to be transported to the emergency department

    B. Pediatric patient whose parent allows them to be treated and transported

    C. Unconscious patient who was discovered alone by a passerby

    D. Patient who is diagnosed with schizophrenia and refuses transport

# Answer Key

| | | | | | | | | | |
|---|---|---|---|---|---|---|---|---|---|
| 1. | **C** | 31. | **A** | 61. | **A** | 91. | **C** | 121. | **B** |
| 2. | **C** | 32. | **B** | 62. | **B** | 92. | **B** | 122. | **C** |
| 3. | **D** | 33. | **C** | 63. | **C** | 93. | **B** | 123. | **C** |
| 4. | **C** | 34. | **B** | 64. | **D** | 94. | **D** | 124. | **D** |
| 5. | **D** | 35. | **C** | 65. | **A** | 95. | **B** | 125. | **C** |
| 6. | **A** | 36. | **A** | 66. | **B** | 96. | **A** | 126. | **A** |
| 7. | **C** | 37. | **D** | 67. | **C** | 97. | **C** | 127. | **B** |
| 8. | **D** | 38. | **B** | 68. | **B** | 98. | **C** | 128. | **B** |
| 9. | **D** | 39. | **C** | 69. | **C** | 99. | **C** | 129. | **C** |
| 10. | **B** | 40. | **D** | 70. | **C** | 100. | **B** | 130. | **A** |
| 11. | **C** | 41. | **C** | 71. | **A** | 101. | **C** | 131. | **B** |
| 12. | **B, C, E, G** | 42. | **D** | 72. | **B** | 102. | **B** | 132. | **B, D** |
| 13. | **A** | 43. | **B** | 73. | **A** | 103. | **C** | 133. | **B** |
| 14. | **D** | 44. | **D** | 74. | **C** | 104. | **C** | 134. | **B** |
| 15. | **B** | 45. | **B** | 75. | **C** | 105. | **A** | 135. | **D** |
| 16. | **C** | 46. | **D** | 76. | **B** | 106. | **A** | 136. | **A, D** |
| 17. | **B** | 47. | **D** | 77. | **B** | 107. | **B** | 137. | **B** |
| 18. | **A, B, F** | 48. | **A** | 78. | **D** | 108. | **B** | 138. | **B** |
| 19. | **A** | 49. | **A** | 79. | **C** | 109. | **C** | 139. | **C** |
| 20. | **B** | 50. | **C** | 80. | **D** | 110. | **A** | 140. | **D** |
| 21. | **C** | 51. | **D** | 81. | **C** | 111. | **B** | 141. | **C** |
| 22. | **D** | 52. | **C** | 82. | **A** | 112. | **C** | 142. | **D** |
| 23. | **D** | 53. | **B** | 83. | **C** | 113. | **C** | 143. | **D** |
| 24. | **D** | 54. | **B** | 84. | **C** | 114. | **A** | 144. | **B** |
| 25. | **A** | 55. | **D** | 85. | **B** | 115. | **C** | 145. | **C** |
| 26. | **D** | 56. | **C** | 86. | **B** | 116. | **D** | 146. | **B** |
| 27. | **D** | 57. | **C** | 87. | **C** | 117. | **B** | 147. | **A** |
| 28. | **C** | 58. | **D** | 88. | **A** | 118. | **D** | 148. | **B** |
| 29. | **B** | 59. | **D** | 89. | **C** | 119. | **B** | 149. | **B** |
| 30. | **A** | 60. | **C** | 90. | **B** | 120. | **A** | 150. | **C** |

# Answers and Explanations

**1. C**

Any dispatch to a call with violence involved, such as a gunshot wound, must be secured by police prior to EMS involvement. The other calls give no indication of being unsafe scenes.

**2. C**

The path of blood flow goes from the heart to the aorta to the arteries to the arterioles to the capillaries to the venules to the veins to the vena cava to the heart.

**3. D**

The very young and the very old are at greatest risk for hypothermia.

**4. C**

Crying may be a response to the depressive stage of grief, but it is not a stage of grief. Denial, anger, and acceptance are among the 5 stages. The missing stages from this list are depression and bargaining.

**5. D**

The zygomatic bones are the cheekbones. Zygomatic fractures are very common among males in their twenties and thirties, often as a result of blunt trauma.

**6. A**

While past medical history is important, it is a distracter in this question. Regardless of the history, if your patient is complaining of difficulty breathing from a traumatic injury, your *first* step should always be to administer supplemental oxygen (A). You may then move on to the next treatment step, such as assistance with a prescribed inhaler (B) or, if the patient decompensates, perhaps even ventilation assistance with BVM (D). Circumferentially wrapping the patient's chest (C) is not good practice in general as it limits chest expansion, which can reduce tidal volume.

**7. C**

Helicopters are dangerous vehicles, and they have safety rules. Do not approach from the uphill side because of the danger of the rotors (A). Do not approach from the rear because of the tail rotor (B). Do not approach until instructed to do so by a helicopter crew member so that the patient loading can be coordinated safely. Not approaching the helicopter (D) may be impractical due to patient care concerns.

**8. D**

Medication bottles, (A), observer comments (B), and the patient's physical condition (C) are all significant in conducting patient assessment. A patient's medical insurance is not a consideration when treating emergency patients.

**9. D**

Eye opening (A), verbal response (B), and motor response (C) are all components of the Glasgow Coma Scale (GCS). It describes a patient's level of consciousness after a traumatic brain injury using best motor response, best verbal response, and eye opening. Grimace response is not part of the GCS measurement.

**10. B**

In order to prove simple (or "ordinary") negligence, there must be 4 elements: duty, breach of duty, proximate cause, and harm caused.

**11. C**

Superior refers to an upper region. So the head is considered superior to the chest, while the chest is considered inferior to the head. Anterior is the front, and posterior is the back.

## 12. B, C, E, G

The EMD prioritizes and triages calls to make sure each call is appropriately staffed (B) and coordinates with other public safety agencies as needed (C). EMDs are also in a position to report which hospitals may be full or on "divert" status, which is very helpful for providers to know to avoid wasting resources by being turned away from or having to wait for ED beds to be available (G). EMDs can provide limited medical instructions to callers based on designated assessment questions such as how to operate an AED or provide CPR prior to EMS arriving (E). They do not, however, provide medical direction to providers (D); this is done by physicians. Nor do they assign a specific person as incident command at MCIs (A); this is done on scene and by the providers. The EMD conducts official communications by radio, not telephone, and providing name and number to crew members (F) is not an EMD responsibility.

## 13. A

The correct answer is 5. It is a common question on the National Registry to ask how many vertebrae are in each section of the spine. For review, the cervical section of the spine has 7 vertebrae, the thoracic 12, the lumbar 5, the sacral 5, and the coccyx 4.

## 14. D

Loss of spontaneity is not a characteristic symptom of PTSD. The other answer choices are all symptoms of PTSD, and if they last longer than a few days, the EMT should be referred for professional help.

## 15. B

A baby's ability to make a facial expression ("to grimace") is indicative of its ability to function in the outside world. A grimace response or reflex irritability describes a response to stimulation, such as a mild pinch. None of the other answer choices are indicators in the Apgar score. Grating refers to rubbing of two organs together, guarding is when one protects a portion of the body with one's hands, and gurgling is the sound one makes when there is fluid in the oropharynx.

## 16. C

Unless contraindicated by some other condition, females in their third trimester of pregnancy should be transported on their left side. This will prevent the weight of the child from compressing the inferior vena cava and causing circulatory problems, which could lead to impairment of consciousness and other complications. Trendelenburg is when the legs are elevated to help combat hypotension, and Fowler position is seated upright.

## 17. B

Because the patient has already expressed the desire to harm himself to a public safety official, the patient must be evaluated by a physician. If the patient refuses to go, the police may have to place the patient into protective custody to have him transported to the hospital.

## 18. A, B, F

Your patient is most likely experiencing a myocardial infarction (MI), or heart attack, and his systolic blood pressure is above 100 mm Hg. He is therefore indicated to take aspirin (A) and nitroglycerin (F). Because this patient has respiratory difficulty and $SpO_2$ under 94%, you should administer oxygen (B). Checking the patient's blood glucose level (D) is not the best intervention for a patient with respiratory difficulty and $SpO_2$ under 94%. In a conscious patient, you normally would not place either an OPA (C), which could stimulate a gag reflex, or AED pads (E), which are not needed at this time (though you may need them later if the patient becomes unresponsive).

## 19. A

Neonates have higher pulse rates and respiratory rates than infants. There is no change in regularity between neonates and infants.

## 20. B

Most EMT injuries on the job occur during treatment of injured patients at motor vehicle accidents. Thus, EMTs should be more alert to the dangers posed by being on the streets and highways. The other situations also present dangers that need the EMT's awareness, but the MVA is the leading cause of injury.

**21. C**

Veins carry blood toward the heart. The vessels that carry blood away from the heart are the arteries.

**22. D**

The three types of muscles are voluntary, involuntary, and cardiac. There is no such thing as a regulatory muscle.

**23. D**

SAMPLE stands for Signs and symptoms, Allergies, Medications, Pertinent past history, Last oral intake, and Events leading up to this situation. Pulse rate is a vital sign.

**24. D**

Communication equipment should be checked at the start of every shift. No self-respecting EMT would like to find out 2 hours into the shift that their radio was not working and that calls were missed.

**25. A**

Before anything else is done, you must be certain that the scene is safe place for you to operate. Universal precautions should already be in place prior to arrival on scene.

**26. D**

Although all of these injuries may be possible with this type of scenario, the most serious injury is spinal damage, particularly in the cervical region (D). In order to produce the bull's-eye or star pattern, the patient would have struck their head against the windshield with a significant amount of force. This would have been both a direct and an indirect force directed down his spinal cord, which may have damaged vertebrae along the way.

**27. D**

Once the scene is determined to be safe and the EMT is wearing proper precautions, the EMT must assess the patient's level of consciousness.

**28. C**

Answers (A), (B), and (D) are all descriptions of levels of consciousness.

**29. B**

Perfusion refers to the percentage of oxygen that a red blood cell can carry to the cells and is measured by the use of the pulse oximeter. This is a vital sign for determining how efficiently the lungs are transferring oxygen to the red blood cells and how well the heart is pumping those cells throughout the body. Basic EMS does not have the diagnostic capabilities to determine the other answers.

**30. A**

A core body temperature 91°F (32.8°C) indicates mild hypothermia. A body temperature of 82.4–89.6°F (28–32°C) indicates moderate hypothermia, and a body temperature <82.4°F (28°C) indicates severe hypothermia. Irreversible hypothermia (D) is not considered a stage of hypothermia.

**31. A**

This patient would benefit from an ALS intervention considering his underlying medical problem and weakened lungs. His pulse is weak and thready, and he is unresponsive. He is indeed a priority patient, but priority transport (B) would require much more time than ALS (30 min versus 15 min). Also, ALS can perform more advanced airway and cardiac management. Epinephrine (C) would be used only if the assessment gave some indication that his level of consciousness was caused by an allergic reaction. A helicopter (D) is not appropriate since the amount of time spent taking off and landing would delay arrival at the emergency department.

**32. B**

OPQRST stands for Onset, Provocation, Quality, Radiation, Severity, and Time. This question also reinforces the need to read the question carefully, since the words *quality* and *quantity* are very similar.

**33. C**

Good patient assessment requires that vital signs and assessment observations be checked and tended every 5 minutes since a patient's condition can change very rapidly.

### 34. B

Answer choices (A) and (D) describe a direct-force injury. Answer choice (C) describes a pathological fracture.

### 35. C

The mnemonic DCAP-BTLS is used in the focused assessment of a trauma patient and stands for Deformity, Contusions, Abrasions, Punctures, Burns, Tenderness, Lacerations, and Swelling.

### 36. A

The midaxillary line runs through the underarm of the patient, dividing the anterior plane from the posterior plane.

### 37. D

The proper order for securing a cervical spine is the following: First, perform a focused assessment to find any bleeding, step-offs, bones out of place, tracheal deviation, JVD, pain, or abnormal sensations. Next is placement of a properly sized C-collar (D). After that, the partner who is holding the C-spine must not let go (even with the collar on) until the person is fully secured to a long or short backboard device. If using a long backboard, then head blocks (A) are appropriate, but that is not what this question is asking. There is no mention of a femur fracture, so hare traction (B) is incorrect. Although the patient may require oxygen, nothing here states that, so an NRB mask (C) is not appropriate.

### 38. B

The Good Samaritan Act was passed to encourage people to render aid by minimizing the liability for such acts.

### 39. C

While 5 minutes is the standard, vital signs should be retaken anytime there is any change in the patient's condition. Changes in the patient's condition will be noted only if the patient's ongoing assessment is constant and not just performed at a predetermined interval.

### 40. D

AVPU stands for Alert, Verbal, Pain, Unresponsive and is used to assign a level of consciousness to a patient. A patient who does not awaken when yelled at and doesn't respond to a vigorous rubbing of the sternum is considered unresponsive.

### 41. C

Patient confidentiality laws mandate that the patient's name and specific medical information be kept confidential. Broadcasting a patient's name over the radio, which is monitored, would be a violation of this confidentiality. (A) and (B) are important information when responding to a call.

### 42. D

While some reports do have spaces for medical insurance information for use by billing services, this information is not required for the patient care report.

### 43. B

When bandaging an eye injury, you must cover both eyes to prevent the sympathetic movement of the uninjured eye from causing further injury to the injured eye. In the absence of other injuries, there is no need to bandage the entire upper head.

### 44. D

All states mandate reporting by medical providers to the appropriate state agency if they become aware of child abuse (A). Some states also require reporting of sexual abuse (B), elder abuse, (C) and spousal abuse, but that is not yet universal. Alcohol abuse (D) could require multiple visits by emergency responders. (Alcoholics are prone to self-harming behaviors, altered mental status, falls with subsequent injuries, or driving while under the influence.) However, alcohol abuse is considered a regular type of medical emergency and would not require mandatory reporting.

**45. B**

Once the cord ceases pulsing and the baby is breathing on their own, it is safe to cut the cord. If the cord is cut before the pulsing has ceased, there is a danger of the mother exsanguinating (bleeding). By waiting until the placenta is delivered, there is no increased danger to the mother or neonate. Waiting until the hospital would also not be a problem. However, in order to treat the neonate properly, it would be easier to have the baby separated from the placenta.

**46. D**

Dropping blood pressure (A), excessive thirst (B), and tachypnea (C) are all symptoms of hypovolemic shock, along with tachycardia, or fast heart rate. Hypertension (D) is not seen in shock.

**47. D**

A competent and conscious patient may refuse any medical procedure or transport.

**48. A**

The nasal cannula is a lightweight, easy-to-use device that provides 24–40% oxygen. It is given when patients are stable and when a low flow of oxygen is required. The simple face mask provides 35–55% oxygen. A patient who requires low-flow oxygen would most likely find the nasal cannula more comfortable than the face mask since the nasal cannula requires only an insertion into the nose (as opposed to both the mouth and nose). The non-rebreather mask provides 90–100% oxygen; and the bag-valve mask provides nearly 100% oxygen.

**49. A**

SIDS normally occurs in the neonate and infant populations, although toddlers are also occasionally at risk.

**50. C**

An impaled object should never be removed unless it interferes with managing the airway or performing chest compressions.

**51. D**

The expiration date must always be checked. The other answers should also be checked, but expiration date (D) is one of the "5 Rights" to be checked in drug administration.

**52. C**

A patient with severe respiratory difficulty due to pulmonary edema would most likely present in the tripod position. A patient with respiratory difficulty due to pulmonary edema would not find any relief in the Trendelenburg position or the reverse Fowler position and would generally find only moderate relief in the semi-Fowler position.

**53. B**

The systolic pressure in the arteries occurs when the ventricles contract and force the blood through the circulatory system. Diastolic pressure occurs when the heart is relaxing between contractions. Arterial pressure is the general pressure in the arteries.

**54. B**

The patient may still be resuscitated since his vital signs may have been suppressed by sudden immersion in cold water, a condition referred to as the mammalian diving reflex. EMS personnel cannot normally pronounce people dead, although state protocols do usually allow EMTs to assume death has occurred if certain signs and symptoms, such as rigor mortis and postmortem lividity, are present. You will want to warm the patient by cutting away his clothing and placing him into a warm truck, but your priority should be beginning CPR. You may request an ALS intercept, but it is imperative that basic life support begin immediately.

**55. D**

The patient is hypoxic and needs high-flow oxygen. The device that will provide the most flow is the non-rebreather, which delivers 90–100% oxygen to the patient. The other devices deliver less oxygen: the nasal cannula (A) 24–40% and the simple face mask (B) 40–60%. A BVM (C) would be inappropriate here as the patient is still alert, and although his oxygen levels are low and concerning, his respiratory rate is not excessively high or low. A non-rebreather mask is the best choice.

**56. C**

The maximum flow rate for the full non-rebreather is 15 liters per minute.

**57. C**

The inferior vena cava is a blood vessel that returns deoxygenated blood to the heart and has little to do with auscultation of breath sounds.

**58. D**

Any food product may be implicated in anaphylaxis, or an allergic reaction.

**59. D**

Headache (D) is not a symptom of a myocardial infarction (MI). All of the other answers, including denial (C), are symptoms of an MI.

**60. C**

The first stage of labor begins when the mucus plug is discharged from the cervix. Labor ends following the delivery of the placenta, or afterbirth. Fertilization of the ovum is the beginning of gestation, or pregnancy. The amniotic sac usually, but not always, ruptures during the first stage of labor after the mucus plug is discharged.

**61. A**

Activated charcoal is very effective at absorbing toxins in the stomach before they can be absorbed into the bloodstream. Ipecac syrup (B) causes vomiting. Oxygen (C) is used for respiratory problems. Aspirin (D) is an analgesic and is used only in chest pain protocols in EMS.

**62. B**

Labor concludes with the delivery of the placenta.

**63. C**

Epinephrine is indicated in cardiac arrest but not in the treatment of chest pain, nor is it in most BLS protocols. Aspirin (A) and oxygen (D) are always indicated in the treatment of sudden chest pain. Medical control may order nitroglycerin (B) if state protocols allow.

**64. D**

A bag-valve mask with an oxygen reservoir is the most effective method of ventilating a patient in the prehospital setting. A manual ventilator (A) is unwieldy in the prehospital setting, and a face mask (B) is not as effective in ventilating as a bag-valve mask. The oxygen reservoir also makes the percentage of oxygen much higher than the other prehospital devices do.

**65. A**

If an arrest reoccurs, compressions need to be resumed due to the patient's lack of pulse and breathing. Because he is not breathing on his own, (B) is inappropriate. Rescue breathing is used when a patient is breathing at inadequate rates on his own (ideally with the use of a simple face mask or BVM). An AED is a plausible answer; however, it would need to analyze the heart first before allowing the shock button to be pressed. ALS intercept is also a possibility, but the best answer is (A).

**66. B**

This patient is having a diabetic emergency caused by low blood sugar, or hypoglycemia. Normal blood sugar is 80–120. Postictal seizure (A) meets the symptoms except for the low blood sugar; hyperglycemia (C) is high blood sugar, which is definitely not the case here; and hypovolemia (D) would be caused by loss of blood volume, which is not suggested here.

**67. C**

The only option that makes sense is massive hemorrhage, and you can reach this answer by the process of elimination. Arterial bleeding (B) is characterized by a spurting flow of blood, not oozing. Pale skin, diaphoresis, and the saturated carpet indicate a problem beyond minor bleeding (A). Capillary bleeding (D) is typically easily controlled and is more likely in injuries such as abrasions.

**68. B**

When the cord presents first, there is great danger that the cord will be compressed between the vaginal walls and the baby's head, cutting off circulation and oxygen to the baby. This is also technically a breech delivery, but prolapsed cord is the more correct terminology.

**69. C**

Most infant seizures are caused by a high temperature, or fever. Tonic-clonic (A) refers to the extremely jerky movements of a full-blown seizure. Postictal (B) is the state of unconsciousness that follows the tonic-clonic portion of the seizure. Anaphylactic (D) refers to an allergic reaction.

**70. C**

Normal blood glucose ranges from 80–120 mg/dL in adult patients.

**71. A**

A heart attack occurs when a coronary artery is blocked and, as a result, a portion of the heart muscle becomes ischemic from lack of oxygen, or infarcts. The other answers are all cardiac conditions but not literally a heart attack.

**72. B**

This patient is exhibiting symptoms of an allergic reaction and needs the immediate intervention of epinephrine, an intervention allowed to EMTs by many state protocols. Even if he has not knowingly ingested any known allergen, the food he has eaten may have been prepared with a nut product, and this may be the cause. Oxygen (D) may be indicated but not in low-flow amounts. Epinephrine is the best answer.

**73. A**

The tonic (A) part of a seizure is when the muscle becomes rigid and stays that way for a period of time, and the clonic (B) part is when the uncontrollable jerking happens. The term *generalized* (C) refers to a seizure category, while postictal (D) is the phase after a seizure occurs.

**74. C**

A vehicle struck broadside is referred to as a T-bone crash. All these crashes may be serious or fatal, but the best answer is T-bone.

**75. C**

Unless a medication in liquid form is to be given to the patient by mouth, most EMS systems do not allow for the administration of oral liquids, such as hot coffee, as part of patient care. The reason is that hot liquids could have unintended consequences. All of the other answer choices would be done to treat this patient's hypothermia.

**76. B**

Leukocytes, or white blood cells, are the body's primary mechanism for combating infection and disease. Hemoglobin is the protein that carries oxygen in blood. Plasma is the fluid part of blood. Platelets are what bind together to form clots.

**77. B**

The telltale sign of carbon monoxide poisoning is bright-red lips and tongue. Carbon dioxide (A) is not directly poisonous but can cause anoxia since it displaces oxygen in the air. Gasoline (C) is a petroleum distillate. A narcotic overdose (D) will not cause bright- red lips.

**78. D**

Carbon monoxide poisoning is best treated by a hyperbaric chamber. Such a chamber forces oxygen into the hemoglobin under pressure and displaces the carbon monoxide. State protocols and medical control naturally dictate the proper course of action. A level 1 trauma center (A) has the equipment and staff to deal with all cases of trauma. In contrast, a level 3 trauma center (B) has minimal equipment and staff and will often stabilize a patient in preparation for transfer to a level 1 center.

**79. C**

The patient's condition indicates that his sweating mechanism has been compromised and his temperature is dangerously high. This condition is called heatstroke. Heat cramps (A) are muscle aches caused by hyperthermia. Heat exhaustion (B) is impaired consciousness brought on by hyperthermia but without the disruption of the sweating mechanism. Heat overdose (D) is not a medical term.

## 80. D

This patient needs to be cooled immediately; then transport (A) would take place. An ALS intercept (B) is a possibility, but the priority is to cool the patient to prevent seizures, possible brain insult, and death. While oxygen administration (C) is indicated in a patient with heatstroke, the first step is cooling the patient. Oxygen should be administered (at whatever liters per minute are adequate per the patient's presentation and SpO$_2$ level) to a minimum of 94% saturation for proper oxygenation.

## 81. C

Phobias are irrational fears. A feeling of sadness or worthlessness is often the result of clinical depression. The alternating feelings of euphoria and depression are symptomatic of bipolar disorder. A mistrust of everyone and everything is paranoia.

## 82. A

Tuberculosis is transmitted by an airborne bacteria.

## 83. C

Alcohol (C) can be vomited without danger. The other answer choices can do more harm coming back through the esophagus than they caused going down. Vomiting caustic bleach (A) or ammonia (D) could severely damage the delicate and thin tissues of the esophagus. (Additionally, note that if mixed together, bleach and ammonia would cause a chemical reaction and toxic fumes, which should never be inhaled.) Vomiting kerosene (B) or any other petroleum product could aspirate the product into the lungs.

## 84. C

You must begin with the fastest step that does not risk your own safety: throwing a life preserver. Then check for a nearby boat (B). If there is no boat, you should notify dispatch to send one (D). You should never attempt to swim to a victim (A) as a first step. Even if you are confident in both your swimming ability and your ability to actually rescue a drowning person, this method of water rescue should be used only as a last resort.

## 85. B

Prior to the administration of a bronchodilator, the EMT asks the patient to exhale deeply to remove as much air from the lungs as possible and then to inhale the vapor deeply into the lungs for maximum effect.

## 86. B

In loco parentis (B) is the Latin term for "in place of parents" and is a type of implied consent. Explicit consent (A) is not a type of consent in EMS. Informed consent (C) is not appropriate as the child is a minor and is unable to provide that type of consent for treatment. Refusal of consent (D) is not an option here.

## 87. C

Patients who lack the ability to resist a temptation or who cannot avoid acting on an impulse have an impulse-control disorder. Obsessive-compulsive disorder (OCD) is a form of impulse-control disorder (D). Schizophrenia (A) is a mental illness characterized by periods of psychosis. Psychosis (B) is loss of contact with reality, which might involve seeing or hearing things that other people cannot see or hear (hallucinations).

## 88. A

Depression is the leading cause of mental illness in people ages 15–44, and it is the most common mental illness of the answer choices listed. Anxiety disorders (not listed as an option) are the second most common mental illness in the United States.

## 89. C

Unconsciousness usually occurs in the severe stage of hypothermia. Mild hypothermia is marked by shivering as the body tries to raise its temperature. The moderate stage is when consciousness and judgment begin to become impaired and there is a loss of motor functions. In severe hypothermia, unconsciousness sets in and the extremities begin to freeze.

## 90. B

Most behavioral emergency calls are nonviolent, but the EMT must always be prepared to deal with violent patients.

**91. C**

Placenta previa usually presents with painless, bright-red bleeding. Abruptio placenta (A) presents with severe pain and dark-red bleeding. Multipara (B) simply means the patient has been pregnant multiple times. Supine hypotensive syndrome (D) does not present with bleeding.

**92. B**

Apgar scores are taken at 1 and 5 minutes postpartum to check on the health of the baby and determine whether emergency care is needed, such as suctioning the airways. The 1-minute score assesses the newborn's heart rate, color, and muscle tone at 1 minute of life. The 5-minute score reassesses those things a few minutes later.

**93. B**

Most texts give the normal adult respiratory rate as 12–20 times per minute. None of the other answers would be considered normal.

**94. D**

The 4 chambers are the left and right atria and the left and right ventricles.

**95. B**

The hallmark sign of chronic bronchitis is the excessive mucus production that occurs in the bronchial tree. Chronic bronchitis patients do not have a failure of the oxygen-carrying capacity of the hemoglobin, and there is an increase in carbon dioxide production. Because of the increased mucus production, the bronchioles become constricted, not dilated.

**96. A**

Ideally, 5 people are needed: one person for each limb and one to apply the restraints. However, the minimum number needed is 2.

**97. C**

Use of a police escort is not a common practice, and it has been statistically shown to be more hazardous than not using one. The reason is that citizen drivers likely don't realize that *both* a police car and an ambulance are passing. So they pull back into traffic too early and cause congestion or even a collision. Use a police escort only when you are unfamiliar with the hospital and the GPS is not working.

**98. C**

The normal gestation period is 9 months from conception, or 40 weeks.

**99. C**

Plasma is the liquid part of the blood that carries the other components through the circulatory system. The other components are hemoglobin, or red blood cells; leukocytes, or white blood cells; and platelets.

**100. B**

Crowning is when the baby's head becomes visible. The mother's amniotic sac and the baby's crying have nothing to do with this term. Labor pains that are <5 minutes apart but longer than 1 minute are an indication that delivery is imminent.

**101. C**

There are a total of 33 vertebrae in the spinal column, so answer choice (A) is correct. There are 7 cervical, 12 thoracic, and 5 lumbar bones (all individual), along with 5 in the sacrum (fused) and 4 in the coccyx (fused).

**102. B**

Excited delirium is the extreme overstimulation of the body and nervous system, typically caused by illegal drug usage. Bipolar disorder (A) is the same as manic-depressive syndrome. Schizophrenia (C) is a long-term mental disorder involving a breakdown in the relation between thought, emotion, and behavior. In panic disorder (D), the patient becomes overly anxious about a situation that does not warrant that sort of response.

**103. C**

Application of the AED may diagnose a dysrhythmia, which may then be treated by a countershock and restore a normal heartbeat, or it may advise to continue CPR. Administration of epinephrine in this instance is an ALS intervention. Since ALS has already been dispatched, you should maintain your patient with CPR pending their arrival, but your first step is to apply the AED.

**104. C**

A school bus with flashing red lights has the right-of-way over all other vehicles, including ambulances. Police cars and fire trucks have the same rights-of-way as ambulances but no additional privileges.

**105. A**

The ulna is one of the two bones in the lower arm.

**106. A**

Crowning is indicative of imminent delivery. Attempting to transport the mother (B) at this point will result in delivery in the back of the ambulance. The legs should never be bound together (C); this would harm both the mother and the baby. Boiling water (D) is what you send anxious onlookers to get to keep them out of the way.

**107. B**

If the baby presents with the cord wrapped around the neck, you must either unwrap the cord or open the baby's airway by relieving the pressure of the cord around the neck. Clamping (A) or cutting (C) the cord will impair the circulation of the baby and may cause the mother to bleed out.

**108. B**

The correct answer is (B). SIRS criteria state that a heart rate above 90 would be a positive finding; the question asks for which one is NOT a contributing factor. A respiratory rate of 32 (C) and a temperature of 95.2°F (35.1°C) (D) are within the SIRS criteria. Systolic blood pressure of 76 mm Hg (A) is part of the qSOFA score, not the SIRS criteria.

**109. C**

A PCR is a legal document, so changes may be made only by the person who is writing the narrative. The changes must be noticeable and documented. They are best made by crossing out (with a single line through the error) and then adding one's own initials and the current date in that same location. Disregarding the error (A) would compound the error by suggesting that it was the actual assessment or treatment given. Destroying the document (B) would break the serial change of reports required for authenticity. Writing a new narrative and stapling it to the old (D) would cause confusion as to which narrative was correct, especially if the forms became separated.

**110. A**

The bottom two ribs (called floating ribs) are not connected to the sternum. The other ribs are all connected to both the sternum and the spinal column.

**111. B**

While most behavioral calls are nonviolent, the potential for violence exists and warrants police presence. ALS units may have the ability to administer sedatives to violent patients and might be included, but police would still be necessary. A second rescue or the fire department would be necessary only if more personnel was necessary to restrain the patient.

**112. C**

Either 1 or 2 points is given for each of the 5 elements of the Apgar score, for a maximum of 10.

**113. C**

The normal range for blood glucose is 80–120 mg/dL. Low blood sugar, or hypoglycemia (B), is the correct answer. Hyperglycemia (A) is a condition where there is an excessive amount of sugar in the blood. Diabetic ketoacidosis (C) is a condition resulting from too little insulin in the body; as a result, ketones are produced that turn the blood acidic, and the body attempts to compensate with faster breathing. Hyperglycemic hyperosmolar nonketotic coma (D) occurs when a person's blood glucose levels are too high for a long period, leading to severe dehydration and confusion; 45 mg/dL is lower than the normal range, not higher.

#### 114. A

Victims of a sexual assault may be suspicious of EMTs of the same gender as their attacker and might prefer to share sensitive information with an EMT of their own gender. Police officers and rape crisis counselors are important in the follow-up treatment of these victims, as are registered nurses. However, initial prehospital care should be done by an EMT, preferably one of the same gender.

#### 115. C

Buccal (C) means relating to the cheek. Neither oral (A) nor sublingual (B), meaning "under the tongue," is specific to the cheek, even though both refer to the mouth. Tympanic (D) refers to an area in the ear canal.

#### 116. D

The most common EMS trauma call is for motor vehicle accidents.

#### 117. B

Numerous studies have shown that survivability increases dramatically if a patient with severe trauma can have surgical intervention within the "golden hour," or 60 minutes.

#### 118. D

The average adult human has 5 to 6 liters of blood.

#### 119. B

A high temperature is the most frequent cause of pediatric seizures, followed by epilepsy, poisoning, and drug exposure to the fetus while in the mother's uterus.

#### 120. A

Look at the presentation of the bleeding. Although the information does state that the bleeding is profuse, it also states that the bleeding is a steady flow and not spurting. Steady flow indicates a venous bleed, so a hemostatic agent (A) is appropriate to stanch the blood flow. Unlike a tourniquet (B), a hemostatic agent doesn't have the potential of causing tissue damage. (If your service does not carry hemostatic agents, a tourniquet can be used, but it is less preferred for a venous bleed.) A hemostatic agent has more stopping power than just a pressure bandage (C). Blood that was pressurized and spurting would indicate a possible arterial bleed, which would require a tourniquet without delay.

#### 121. B

Since neonates and infants are nose breathers, upper respiratory infections cause mucus buildup, which causes difficulty breathing in that population. Foreign bodies (A) and birth defects (C) can also cause dyspnea, but mucus is the most common cause. Sudden infant death syndrome, or SIDS (D) is a condition in which a previously healthy infant is found dead with no explicable cause.

#### 122. C

As EMTs work in all types of situations outside of a consistently clean environment that is the hospital, sterility is a big consideration. Nonsterile equipment or dressings can introduce bacteria into the patient's bloodstream, which could have serious consequences later. The most important feature of a dressing is that it comes in an unopened package. Size and shape are important, too, but less important than sterility. Elasticity is not a factor unless specifically aiming for a compression type of bandage.

#### 123. C

A patient may always change their mind, even after signing a refusal. When a patient refuses treatment or transport, all options must be explained (A) as well as the possible medical consequences (B). The signature of the patient on the refusal form should be witnessed by a disinterested third party (D) to attest to the facts of the refusal.

#### 124. D

Fowler position (seated upright) is not indicated for hypovolemia. Trendelenburg position (feet raised above the level of the head) would be used for treatment of shock, along with retention of body heat (B) and administration of oxygen (C). A trauma assessment should be performed en route (A).

#### 125. C

Bruising is a type of closed wound; the skin is not open to the outside. Abrasions, incisions, and lacerations are all types of open wounds.

### 126. A

NTG (nitroglycerin) is a potent vasodilator, which accounts for its effectiveness in relieving chest pain caused by reduced blood flow in the carotid arteries. It consequently may lead to lowered blood pressure, or hypotension.

### 127. B

A wound in the neck that may leak air into the body should be dressed with an occlusive dressing to keep air from entering and contributing to a pneumothorax. Wounds to the head, abdomen, and genitals may be treated with ordinary dressings.

### 128. B

By the rule of nines, each arm is 9% of the body surface, so both arms are a total of 18%.

### 129. C

Second-degree, or partial-thickness, burns are critical if they involve an entire body part. A second-degree burn would normally be considered critical only if it involved >30% of the body surface area.

### 130. A

Naloxone is a drug used for overdoses of opioids, including heroin. The total dosage given via the IN route is 2 mg, making (A) the correct answer; 6 mg total IN (B) is too large a dose. LSD is not an opioid (C). NSAID (D) stands for nonsteroidal anti-inflammatory drug. NSAIDs are not opioids; ibuprofen is an example of an NSAID.

### 131. B

No matter the type of splint you use, the splint must always be secured above and below the injury site (B) for full immobilization. By securing above and below the injury, you are securing the entire bone to limit additional movement. (Never secure a splint directly over a joint, as that could put tension on the ligaments/tendons and limit proper anatomical movement.) You would not splint over the injury (D), as that would be painful for the patient.

### 132. B, D

The correct treatment for abdominal eviscerations is to cover the exposed contents with a moist, sterile dressing with a 4-sided occlusive dressing on top (D). Applying a moist dressing may cause the patient to lose body heat, so it is imperative for the provider to maintain warmth of the abdominal contents and the patient (B); this is also an important treatment for shock. You should not attempt to replace the organs (A) or try to hold the contents in place with a pressure dressing (C). The 4-sided occlusive dressing should be moist, not dry (E). However, irrigation with sterile water (F) is not ideal; a better solution would be sterile saline, which is chemically different from plain, sterile water.

### 133. B

SAMPLE stands for Signs and symptoms, Allergies, Medications, Past history, Last oral intake, and Events leading up to the situation.

### 134. B

The epiglottis is higher in the airway of an infant, which is an important anatomical difference.

### 135. D

Cervical spine injury should be considered in all trauma situations unless you can definitely rule it out. Neck pain brought about by sleeping also calls for immobilization until damage to the spinal cord can be ruled out.

### 136. A, D

When assessing the airway and breathing status of a patient, conscious or not, always check for adequate chest rise and fall (A). When the patient is unresponsive, it becomes imperative to provide enough volume to raise the chest for the patient, who is unable to do so on her own. It is also good practice to make sure that you listen (auscultate) for lung sounds (D) to make sure you are directing the air volume into the lungs versus the stomach. Present lung sounds indicate air is reaching the correct area. Although all of the other answers are part of the respiratory assessment or good practice, they are not the 2 best answer options for this question.

**137. B**

The foaming of a wound to the chest indicates that the pleural cavity has been compromised; as the air pressure builds in the pleural space, it prevents the lung from expanding normally. This condition is referred to as a pneumothorax.

**138. B**

Abdominal wounds are at a high risk for infection if the contents of the gastrointestinal tract spill into the abdominal compartment, especially if the wound is open and exposed to the air and/or bacteria. Hypertension (A), sudden cardiac death (C), and peritonitis (D) are always a possibility in serious injuries, but the best answer is infection (B).

**139. C**

Neonates (A) are aged from birth to 4 weeks, infants (C) from 4 weeks to 1 year, toddlers (B) from 1 to 3 years, preschoolers from 3 to 6 years, school-age children (D) from 6 to 10 years, and adolescents from 11 to 21 years of age.

**140. D**

Once applied, a tourniquet should never be released in the field since serious shock may develop. Therefore, it should be released only after the patient is in the hospital and bleeding can be controlled surgically.

**141. C**

The use of 4-point restraints requires that each limb be restrained. The patient should always be supine so you can intervene immediately should that become necessary for another medical condition, such as cardiac arrest. Patients should never be restrained prone (A and D) or facedown, as this position causes pressure on the diaphragm; this may lead to apnea and sudden death, which would not be apparent with the patient facedown. Furthermore, handcuffs are not approved EMS restraints, and they should be used only by authorized and trained police officers. Likewise, the patient should never be made to lie on his restrained limbs (B) due to the risk of impaired circulation in the extremities.

**142. D**

In order to immobilize a fractured hip properly, the patient must be secured to a long backboard. The other splints would not do this.

**143. D**

A lacerated artery bleeds more readily than other blood vessels due to the higher pressure in the arteries as well as the pulsing action that makes clotting more difficult. Arterioles (C) are smaller arteries and clot more readily than a larger vessel, and capillaries (A) and veins (B) flow at lower pressures that facilitate clotting.

**144. B**

Aspirin is given for chest pain due to its anticlotting action and is listed in most state protocols following the American Heart Association guidelines. Aspirin is also indicated for headache and other pain but not usually in the emergency setting.

**145. C**

The police may obtain a copy of the report only if they obtain either permission from the patient or a search warrant from a judge or magistrate. Note the use of the qualifying word *routinely* in the question.

**146. B**

The correct answer is (B), which stands for *Emergency Response Guidebook*. An electroencephalogram or EEG (A) is a diagnostic test to measure brain waves, while an electrocardiogram or EKG (D) measures heart rhythms. ENT (C) stands for ear, nose, and throat.

**147. A**

A first pregnancy will normally have a longer labor and delivery time than subsequent pregnancies.

**148. B**

The ambulance should be used to protect the scene in order to avoid injury to the EMTs and the patients.

**149. B**

The second stage of labor occurs when the baby is forced out of the uterus by the contractions down into the mother's vagina and ends with the birth of the baby. The first stage of labor (A) is from the expulsion of the mucus plug through full dilation of the cervix. The third stage (C) follows the birth of the baby, when the placenta is delivered. There is no fourth stage of labor (D).

**150. C**

Implied consent means that in the case of a patient who cannot give consent, such as an individual who is unconscious, consent for treatment is implied and constitutes what the average person would want under similar circumstances.

# Your Practice Test Score

The Practice Test in this book is designed to give you experience answering multiple-choice questions about EMT content.

- Recall that the NREMT Cognitive Exam is a CAT, a computer-based test that adapts to your ability. At the start of the exam, the computer assumes you have average aptitude and gives you a medium-difficulty question. After each question that you answer correctly, the computer increases its estimate of your ability and gives you a more difficult question. If, on the other hand, you answer a question incorrectly, you are given an easier question.

- Your score on the real exam is determined by an algorithm that calculates your ability level based not just on what you got right or wrong but also on the difficulty level of the questions you answered.

- As a result, the **paper and pencil practice test here can provide only limited feedback on scoring**.

Additionally, **there is no actual point score on the exam**. Instead, the NREMT governing body aims for a 95% confidence rate. In other words, as a result of you answering questions right or wrong, your exam will be "scored" based on whether there is 95% confidence that you have met minimal entry-level competency.

Therefore, to "score" your practice exam, calculate the percentage of questions you answered correctly:

1. Number of questions right divided by 150 = **decimal score**
2. Multiply your decimal score × 100 = **percentage**
   - Example: 120/150 = 0.8 → 0.8 × 100 = 80%
   - Example: 75/150 = 0.5 → 0.5 × 100 = 50%

| YOUR SCORE | NOW WHAT? |
|---|---|
| 80% or better | You have a good understanding of essential EMT content and are able to use the knowledge and thinking skills required to answer exam-style questions. |
| | Consider scheduling your NR cognitive exam, and remember to study a little bit every day until Test Day to keep it fresh in your mind. |
| 60–79% | You have areas of EMT content that need further review, and/or you may need continued work to master the knowledge and thinking skills required to be successful on the cognitive exam. |
| | If you schedule your cognitive exam now, you may or may not pass it. Keep in mind that you are charged an exam fee for every attempt. |
| 59% or less | You need concentrated study of EMT content and continued practice utilizing the knowledge and thinking skills required to be successful on the cognitive exam. |
| | You should hold off on scheduling your cognitive exam at this time. Dedicate more time to studying the basics. Review your textbook, and then go back through the chapters and practice questions that gave you the most difficulty. |

# EMT-BASIC RESOURCES

# GLOSSARY

## A

**Abandonment:** failure to properly treat an ill or injured person who is in need of emergency medical care

**Abdominal quadrants:** the four sections of the abdomen, using the umbilicus (navel) as the focal point—upper left, upper right, lower left, lower right

**Abrasion:** type of wound in which the epidermis is scraped by an object, causing little blood loss but with increased danger of infection due to the amount of dermis exposed

**Activated charcoal:** charcoal in liquid suspension used to absorb ingested poisons

**Active rewarming:** use of heat packs and heated fluids to rewarm a hypothermic patient

**Acute:** immediate

**Adolescent:** pediatric patient age 13–18

**Advance directive:** medical decisions made by a patient or caregiver in advance, usually in the form of do-not-resuscitate orders

**Afterbirth:** placenta and fetal membranes that are expelled from the mother following delivery of a baby

**Allergic reaction:** severe and unusual response of the body to a foreign substance

**Altered mental status:** inappropriate response to normal stimuli, e.g., being responsive only to voice or only to pain, or being unconscious; also used to describe abnormal behavior

**Alveoli:** sacs in the lung in which oxygen is exchanged for carbon dioxide in the red blood cells

**Amniotic sac:** bag of fluid that surrounds and protects the fetus during pregnancy; usually ruptures prior to delivery

**Amputation:** complete separation of a body part from the body

**Anaphylaxis:** consequence of an allergic reaction, where the body responds with swelling of respiratory tissues and shock

**Aorta:** large artery at the top of the heart carrying blood to all major arteries

**Apnea:** lack of breathing, absence of respiratory activity

**Arteries:** vessels that carry oxygenated blood from the aorta to the arterioles

**Arterioles:** vessels that connect the arteries to the capillaries

**Arteriosclerosis (or hardening of the arteries):** disease process in which the arteries lose elasticity as they become rigid

**Aspiration:** inhaling of foreign substances into the trachea, bronchial tree, and lungs

**Asystole:** cardiac standstill, lack of electrical activity in the heart muscle

**Atria:** the two uppermost chambers of the heart

**Aura:** visual, auditory, olfactory, or other sense of an impending seizure

**Auscultation:** listening for sounds within the body, usually with a stethoscope

**Automated external defibrillator (AED):** device that attempts to overcome certain cardiac dysrhythmias with an electrical countershock; operates by interpreting the cardiac rhythm and responding appropriately without the need for operator interpretation

**AVPU:** acronym used for determining level of consciousness—**A**lert, responsive to **V**erbal, responsive to **P**ain, **U**nresponsive

**Avulsion:** forcible tearing away of tissue as a result of blunt-force trauma

## B

**Bag-valve mask:** respiratory device used to manually support respirations in cases of respiratory distress or apnea

**Bandage:** cloth used to secure a sterile dressing to a wound

**Baseline vital signs:** vital signs taken first and used to track a patient's improvement or decline

**Battle sign:** ecchymosis behind the ears that suggests a basilar skull fracture

**Behavioral emergency:** emergency medical call in which the patient's actions are bizarre and inappropriate

**Bilateral:** refers to both the right and left sides of the body

**Bipolar disorder:** psychiatric condition in which a patient alternates between extremes of euphoria and depression; extremes may last from a few minutes to several months

**Blood pressure:** pressure (in millimeters of mercury) of the blood flow through the arteries

**Blood pressure cuff (sphygmoma-nometer):** device used to measure blood pressure by applying pressure to an artery

**Body substance isolation (BSI):** important act of protection of an EMT from airborne and blood-borne pathogens by the use of personal protective equipment (PPE)

**Brachial artery:** large artery in the upper arm that feeds the entire extremity

**Bradycardia:** heart rate slower than 60 beats per minute

**Bradypnea:** respiratory rate slower than 8 respirations per minute

**Breech birth:** presentation of any part of a fetus other than the head during delivery

**Bronchi:** two tubes that connect the trachea to the bronchioles

**Bronchioles:** smaller tubes that connect the bronchi to the alveoli

**Burn sheet:** large, sterile dressing used to cover burn injuries

## C

**Capillaries:** small blood vessels in which oxygen is given off to the cells for metabolism and waste products are collected

**Capillary refill:** diagnostic sign in which the nail bed is blanched by applying pressure and the time for it to return to normal color is measured; normally <2 seconds

**Cardiac arrest:** condition caused by the heart's failure to pump blood

**Carotid arteries:** large arteries that feed the brain

**Central nervous system (CNS):** brain and spinal cord

**Cerebrovascular accident (CVA) (stroke):** ischemia in the brain caused by either a cerebral hemorrhage or thrombus

**Chief complaint:** illness or injury for which the emergency medical system was activated

**Chronic:** long-term, gradual process

**Chronic obstructive pulmonary disease (COPD):** degeneration of the alveoli by disease processes causing progressive dyspnea; examples are emphysema and chronic bronchitis

**Conduction:** method of heat transfer in which heat is transferred by direct contact between bodies

**Congestive heart failure (CHF):** condition of dyspnea in which fluid backs up into the lungs caused by failure of the heart's pumping action

**Contraindications:** situations in which a drug or protocol should not be used

**Contusion:** hemorrhage that occurs beneath the skin; bruising

**Convection:** method of heat transfer from the body caused by air passing over it

**Convulsion:** seizure activity of the body

**Critical incident stress debriefing (CISD):** discussion of a stressful incident, with the goal of allowing an EMT to deal with the emotions encountered and move on

**Crowning:** appearance of the top of the baby's head in the birth canal during delivery

**Cushing reflex:** increased blood pressure, decreased heart rate, and respiratory changes caused by hypoxia in the brain; indicative of severe head injury

**Cyanosis:** bluish-gray color indicative of poor circulatory perfusion

**D**

**Decerebrate posturing:** when a patient extends arms outward and arches the back; indicates a more severe head injury

**Decorticate posturing:** when a patient flexes arms inward and arches the back; indicates a severe head injury

**Defibrillation:** correction of cardiac fibrillation by electrical countershock

**Dementia:** abnormal behavior brought about by disease of the brain

**Dermis:** intermediate layer of skin between the epidermis and fatty tissue or muscle

**Diabetes:** disease of the pancreas that inhibits the body's ability to process sugars

**Diastolic blood pressure:** pressure in the arteries while the heart is at rest

**Dressing:** sterile pad placed directly onto a wound

**Drowning:** death caused by suffocation in water

**Drug:** any chemical introduced into the body to combat disease

**Dyspnea:** difficulty breathing

**E**

**Ecchymosis:** black-and-blue discoloration caused by subcutaneous hemorrhage

**Endocrine system:** system of the body that produces hormones used in the metabolic process

**Epidermis:** top layer of skin

**Epidural:** layer between the skull and the dura mater of the brain and spine

**Epilepsy (seizure disorder):** disease of the brain that causes seizures

**Epinephrine:** natural hormone that helps the body regulate multiple processes; also a medication used for heart irregularities and anaphylaxis

**Epistaxis:** bleeding from the nose

**Esophagus:** body's tubular passage from the pharynx to the stomach

**Evisceration:** traumatic opening of the abdominal cavity in which the intestines protrude to the outside

**Expressed consent:** formal consent from a competent patient for treatment and/or transport

**Extubation:** removal of a breathing tube

**F**

**Femoral artery:** large artery in the upper leg that feeds the entire extremity

**Femur:** large bone of the upper leg

**Fetus:** child in the uterus before birth

**Fibula:** one of two bones in the lower leg

**Flail segment:** ≥2 ribs broken in ≥2 places

**Fontanel:** soft spot in a baby's skull where bones have not yet fused together

**Fowler position:** position in which patient is sitting upright; normally best for conscious patients with dyspnea

**French catheter:** soft-suction catheter

**Full-thickness burn (formerly known as third-degree burn):** burn that extends through the epidermis and dermis to the tissues below

**G**

**Glucose:** form of sugar used by the body for fuel

**Guarding:** position in which a patient places the hands over the part of the body that is painful

**H**

**Hard catheter:** rigid-suction catheter

**Hazardous material:** any material that is dangerous to one's health or safety

**Head-tilt, chin-lift:** procedure in which the airway of a nontrauma patient is secured; one hand is placed onto the patient's forehead, which is tilted back, while the other hand lifts the chin

**Hives:** itchy, red blotches on the skin associated with allergic reactions

**Hot zone:** in a hazardous materials incident, the area that contains the hazardous material; only personnel in proper protective equipment should enter this zone

**Hyper-:** prefix meaning higher, more, faster

**Hyperthermia:** overheated, having a high temperature

**Hypo-:** prefix meaning lower, below, less, slower

**Hypoglycemia:** low blood sugar

**Hypothermia:** cold, having a low temperature

**Hypovolemia:** low blood volume

**Hypoxia:** low oxygen level

## I

**Immune response:** body's response to a foreign invader

**Implied consent:** assumption that consent would be given for treatment/transport if the patient was conscious

**Incident command system:** system of command and control at a mass casualty or disaster scene

**Indications:** situations in which a drug or protocol should be followed

**Infant:** pediatric patient age 1–12 months

**Ingestion:** process in which an object is taken into the mouth and swallowed

**Inhalation (inspiration):** process in which an object is brought into the lungs through the nose and mouth

**Initial assessment:** first impression of a patient's condition after scene size-up

**Injection:** process in which a substance is introduced into the body by a needle

**In-line stabilization:** holding of the head and neck in a straight-line, neutral position to minimize the danger of damaging the spinal cord during treatment and transport

**Inspiration (inhalation):** process by which an object is brought into the lungs through the nose and mouth

**Insulin:** hormone used by the body to metabolize sugars

**Intercostal muscles:** muscles between the ribs used in the breathing process

**Intracranial pressure (ICP):** pressure within the skull

**Intravenous (IV):** into a vein; giving medication via a vein

**Intubation:** placement of a tube into the trachea to facilitate rescue breathing

## J

**Jaundice:** yellowish appearance of the skin, commonly caused by diseases of the liver

**Jaw-thrust maneuver:** maneuver to open the airway of a trauma patient; head and neck are maintained in a neutral position while the jaw is lifted upward to open the airway

**Joint:** location where two bones meet

## K

**Kinetics:** study of physical laws of motion; used for trauma assessment

## L

**Labor:** process through which a baby is born; begins when the mucus plug blocking the cervix is expelled and concludes with the delivery of the placenta

**Laceration:** wound in which the skin is opened by a cut or tear

**Ligament:** fibrous tissue that connects bones to other bones and facilitates movement at the joints

**Lungs:** organs comprised of small air sacs in which oxygenated air is inhaled and passes into the blood while carbon dioxide waste is removed

## M

**Main stem bronchi:** large tubes connecting the trachea to the lungs

**Malaise:** general feeling of illness

**Mammalian diving reflex:** body's response to sudden immersion into cold water, when vital systems reflexively shut down to preserve oxygen

**Mantoux test:** test for tuberculosis bacteria

**Mass casualty incident (MCI):** a scene with more patients than the initial arriving unit can safely treat and transport

**Mechanism of injury (MOI):** manner in which an injury occurs

**Meconium:** waste product expelled by a distressed fetus during delivery

**Medical control:** the EMT's supervising medical professional(s)

**Medical direction:** protocols and practices given to EMTs by a physician

**Medication:** any substance introduced into a body to affect healing or alleviation of abnormal symptoms

**Meninges:** layers of tissue surrounding the brain and spinal cord

**Metered-dose inhaler:** device prescribed to patients to deliver a prescribed dosage of medication to be inhaled; often prescribed for asthma and other respiratory illnesses

**Minor consent:** permission obtained from a responsible adult for a minor child or incapacitated adult

**Miscarriage:** expulsion of a fetus and products of conception before the fetus is viable

## N

**Nasal cannula:** oxygen delivery device that delivers 2–6 liters per minute into the nasopharynx

**Nasogastric tube:** tube inserted into the nose and down into the stomach to suction possible toxins and/or administer medication directly into the stomach

**Nasopharyngeal airway:** airway device inserted into the nose and nasopharynx

**Nature of illness (NOI):** signs and symptoms of patient's illness

**Negligence:** legally defined as failure to act as a reasonable and prudent person would under similar circumstances

**Neonate:** pediatric patient from age birth to 1 month

**Nervous system:** system of sensory and motor nerves that control the human body functions, both voluntary and involuntary

**Neurogenic shock:** type of shock brought about by damage to the central nervous system that causes vasodilation; results in hypovolemia

**Neurological deficit:** any lessening or absence of the body's nervous system response

**Nitroglycerin (NTG):** medication used for chest pain that causes vasodilation, which increases oxygen flow to the heart

**Non-rebreather mask:** oxygen delivery device that delivers 10–15 liters per minute; the reservoir bag provides 100% oxygen to the patient

## O

**Obstetric:** having to do with delivery or childbirth

**Occlusive dressing:** sterile covering that seals off the wound from air; dressings of impermeable material or impregnated with sterile petroleum jelly

**Offline medical direction:** written standard protocols from an EMS medical director

**Ongoing assessment:** continuous monitoring of a patient while en route to a receiving facility

**Online medical direction:** direct contact with a physician to obtain orders or consultation

**Open fracture:** a broken bone associated with an open wound

**Oral airway:** device that assists in holding the tongue clear of the airway and maintaining a clear passage through the oropharynx

**Oral glucose:** high concentration of sugar given orally to a conscious patient with hypoglycemia

**Orbits:** the openings in the skull for the eyeballs

**Oropharyngeal airway:** specific type of oral airway, shaped like the letter "J" and inserted into the mouth to hold the tongue down

**Overdose:** misuse of any substance by ingesting, inhaling, or absorbing more than needed

**Oxygen:** element used by the body for metabolism, constituting 21% of normal air; supplemental oxygen is often given to assist breathing and metabolism in times of illness/injury

**Oxygen humidifier:** bottle of sterile water placed in-line with oxygen flow to provide moisture and prevent drying out of the pharynx

**P**

**Pallor:** pale or abnormally light skin color

**Palpation:** feeling with the hands and fingers

**Paradoxical motion:** opposite motion from the norm; describes the effect when a flail segment moves in an opposite-to-normal direction during breathing

**Paranoia:** mental illness categorized by deep feelings of persecution

**Paresthesia:** loss of sensation or paralysis in an extremity

**Partial-thickness burn (formerly known as second-degree burn):** burn causing blisters that extends through the epidermis and dermis but not below

**Passive rewarming:** reheating of a hypothermic patient by raising the ambient temperature, removing cold and wet clothing, and applying blankets to utilize the patient's own body heat

**Patent airway:** open, secure airway

**Pathogens:** substances that cause disease

**Patient assessment:** medical examination to determine mechanisms of injury and manner of illnesses

**Perfusion:** physiology of delivery of oxygen to the cells for the metabolic process

**Peritonitis:** infection of the abdominal cavity

**Personal protective equipment (PPE):** any device used by an EMT to protect against airborne and blood-borne pathogens

**Pharynx:** area between the mouth and the epiglottis in which the trachea and esophagus separate

**Phobia:** mental illness manifesting itself in irrational fears

**Physiology:** study of the body's systems and functions

**Placenta:** organ that feeds the fetus during pregnancy; attaches to the wall of the uterus and is discharged after delivery of the fetus

**Plasma:** liquid component of blood

**Platelets:** component of blood that produces the clotting effect

**Pleural space:** space between the outer walls of the lungs

**Pneumothorax:** collapse of the lung caused by air buildup in the chest

**Pocket mask:** device for providing artificial ventilation by allowing an EMT to utilize their own exhalation to inflate a victim's lungs

**Poison:** any substance that inhibits the body's normal processes

**Positive pressure ventilation:** type of ventilation where lungs are inflated by a device that forces in air; may be a mechanical ventilator, pocket mask, or a bag-valve mask

**Postictal state:** state of unconsciousness following a seizure

**Prehospital care report (PCR):** summary of observations and interactions between the emergency medical service and a patient; this document is left with the receiving facility to become a permanent part of the patient's record

**Premature infant:** infant who is delivered before 36 weeks of gestation

**Preschooler:** pediatric patient age 3–6 years

**Pressure point:** place in which an artery crosses a bone and pressure can reduce hemorrhage

**Primary triage:** in an MCI, the first categorization of degree of injury, with the primary goal of identifying the most severely injured patients and prioritizing them for treatment and transport

**Prolapsed cord:** abnormal delivery situation in which the umbilical cord presents from the birth canal before the fetus

**Prone:** position of a body face down

**Protocols:** series of directives approved by a medical director for EMS to follow in given situations

**Pulmonary edema:** fluid in the lungs

**Pulmonary embolism:** blockage in the circulatory system of the lungs caused by a clot or bubble of air

**Pulse:** movement of blood through the arteries caused by contraction of the left ventricle

**Pulse oximetry:** measurement of oxygen perfusion, measured by the infrared signature of red blood cells

**Pulse pressure:** difference between the systolic and diastolic blood pressure

**Pulseless electrical activity (PEA):** random electrical activity of the heart that fails to produce a pulse

**R**

**Raccoon sign:** ecchymosis around the eyes, which may be symptomatic of a basilar skull fracture

**Radiation:** method of heat transfer in which there is no direct contact between bodies

**Rapid extrication:** method of removal of a patient from a hazardous situation without using normal precautions due to imminent danger

**Rapid medical assessment:** method of assessing an unconscious patient from head to toe to ascertain medical problems and to check for injuries

**Rapid trauma assessment:** method of assessing an unconscious patient from head to toe to check for injuries if there is a substantial mechanism of injury

**Reasonable force:** legal definition used to describe the minimum amount of force needed to restrain a patient in order to prevent injury to the patient or others

**Red blood cells:** component of the blood that carries oxygen to the cells

**Repeaters:** radios that amplify a radio signal and enable it to carry longer distances

**Respiration:** inhaling oxygen into the lungs for the metabolic process

**Respiratory arrest:** absence of spontaneous respirations

**Respiratory failure:** inability of the body to bring in adequate oxygen for the metabolic processes

**Retractions:** depressions in the neck and chest cavity indicating use of the accessory muscles for respirations; indicative of respiratory distress

**Right main stem intubation:** placement of an endotracheal tube too far into the trachea and into the right main stem bronchus, resulting in the inflation of only the right lung

**Rigid catheter (tonsil-tip suction):** hard-plastic suction device

**Route:** manner of drug delivery: oral, intravenous (IV), sublingual, buccal, intramuscular, intraosseous, or endotracheal

**Rule of nines:** method for rapidly determining the extent of a burn injury; divides body surface area of an adult body into 11 zones of 9% each

**S**

**SAMPLE:** diagnostic mnemonic that stands for Signs and symptoms, Allergies, Medications, Pertinent history, Last oral intake, and Events leading to current illness or injury

**Scene safety:** primary concern of an arriving EMT that the situation into which they are arriving is as hazard-free as possible

**Scene size-up:** quick assessment of a scene upon arrival to determine scene safety, number of victims, and need for additional or special units

**Schizophrenia:** mental illness categorized by delusions, blunted affect, thought disorders, and sometimes catatonia

**School-age:** pediatric patient age 6–12

**Scope of practice:** medical procedures that are legally permitted based on level of licensure and training

**Secondary triage:** in an MCI, triage of a specific patient's condition to determine treatment and transport

**Seizure:** alteration in neurologic function that can include behavioral changes, muscle tremors, and loss of consciousness

**Semi-Fowler position:** position in which patient is sitting at a 45° angle; normally the best position for conscious patients with mild dyspnea and cardiac symptoms

**Shock:** situation in which cells are not properly oxygenated due to loss of blood; also known as hypoperfusion syndrome

**Side effects:** effects of any drug or procedure other than the intended effect

**Signs:** objective measurements of a body's response to illness and/or injury

**Snoring:** sound made by a partial obstruction of the upper airway

**Soft catheter (French catheter):** suction device of soft plastic

**Sphygmomanometer (blood pressure cuff):** device used to measure blood pressure by applying pressure to an artery

**Spinal column:** bony structure of the back that protects the spinal cord

**Spinal cord:** series of nerves leading from the base of the brain that carry impulses to the muscles and sensory information back to the brain

**Spinal shock:** shock caused by injury to the spinal cord that affects its ability to transmit the necessary nerve impulses for normal perfusion

**Splint:** any device that immobilizes a bone or joint

**Spontaneous abortion (miscarriage):** any termination of pregnancy that occurs before a fetus is able to remain viable

**Staging sector:** section where units are deployed to remain ready to respond to specific assignments at a mass casualty incident

**Standard of care:** level of medical treatment that is normal and expected for a given situation

**Standing orders:** procedures that medical control deems suitable for the EMT to perform under given situations without the need to contact medical control (see Offline medical direction)

**Status epilepticus:** seizures lasting longer than a few minutes or multiple seizures that occur without an intervening period of lucidity

**Sterile:** objects free from pathogens

**Stoma:** opening in the neck bypassing the pharynx to enable breathing

**Stridor:** high-pitched wheezing sound indicating upper airway swelling or obstruction

**Stroke (cerebrovascular accident [CVA]):** brain damage caused by a clot or hemorrhage in the cerebrum or cerebellum

**Stylet:** semirigid rod used to shape an endotracheal tube for insertion

**Subarachnoid hemorrhage:** bleeding between the brain and the arachnoid membrane

**Subcutaneous layer:** layer of tissue directly below the skin

**Subdural hematoma:** bleeding beneath the dura, or outer covering of the brain

**Sucking chest wound:** open wound that extends into the lung cavity, causing deflation of the lung (pneumothorax)

**Sudden infant death syndrome (SIDS):** medical condition affecting infants who die suddenly and without any explanation

**Suicide:** the taking of one's own life

**Superficial burn (formerly known as first-degree burn):** burn that involves only the epidermis; common example is a sunburn

**Supine hypotensive syndrome:** condition seen in late pregnancy where the weight of the fetus impairs the return circulation of blood and causes low blood pressure and inadequate perfusion

**Supply sector:** MCI location where supplies are brought for units to restock

**Syncope:** brief period of loss of consciousness

**Systolic blood pressure:** pressure in the arteries while the ventricles contract

# T

**Tachycardia:** sustained fast heart rate in excess of 100 beats per minute

**Tachypnea:** sustained fast respiratory rate in excess of 20 breaths per minute

**Tendon:** fibrous tissue that connects bones to muscle and facilitates movement at the joints

**Tension pneumothorax:** collapse of a lung where the organs in the chest begin to shift into the space vacated by the collapsed lung

**Tidal volume:** amount of air inhaled in a normal respiratory effort

**Toddler:** pediatric patient age 1–3 years

**Toxin:** substance that poisons the body

**Trachea:** tube connecting the mouth and nose to the lungs

**Tracheostomy:** surgical opening in the neck that allows a patient with an occluded airway to breathe

**Transient ischemic attack (TIA):** condition that causes temporary stroke-like symptoms (up to 24 hours); caused by spasms of the arteries in the brain

**Transportation sector:** in an MCI, the area in which patients are transported to appropriate medical facilities

**Trauma:** sudden injury caused by the application of external forces to a human body

**Treatment sector:** in an MCI, the area in which patients are given initial treatment before transport

**Trendelenburg position:** supine positioning of the body with legs elevated in order to combat shock

**Triage:** process of determining the severity of injuries in order to best utilize available resources; normally there are 4 groups: red for critical patients, yellow for serious patients, green for slightly injured ambulatory patients, and black for patients who are dead or mortally wounded

**Triage sector:** in an MCI, the area in which triage occurs and is controlled; initial triage occurs where the patient is found

**Triage tag:** tag that allows the EMT to mark the patient's status and initial impressions; also used to account for patients as they pass through the various sectors in an MCI

**Tripod position:** position often assumed by patients in severe respiratory distress, i.e., seated with arms to the side and rotated forward to facilitate breathing

# U

**Umbilical cord:** vessel that connects a fetus to the placenta in utero

**Umbilicus:** the navel, i.e., area where the umbilical cord is connected to fetus's abdomen

**Urgent move:** situation in which a patient is moved quickly due to the seriousness of the condition or immediate danger of further injury

**Uterus:** female organ that harbors a fetus during pregnancy

# V

**Vein:** blood vessel that carries blood toward the heart

**Venae cavae:** main veins leading directly into the heart; singular: vena cava

**Ventilation:** passage of air into and out of the lungs

**Ventricles:** the 2 lower chambers of the heart

**Ventricular fibrillation (V-Fib):** cardiac condition in which the heart muscles vibrate rather than contract, resulting in collapse of circulation

**Ventricular tachycardia (V-Tach):** rapid heartbeat that frequently fails to produce a pulse and thus fails to produce perfusion

**Venules:** small blood vessels leading from the capillaries to the veins

**Vital signs:** assessments of an ill or injured patient that are objectively measured, including blood pressure, heart rate, respiratory rate, pupil response, and oxygen saturation

**Voluntary guarding:** contractions of the abdominal wall as a response to pain or injury

## W

**Warm zone:** in a hazardous material incident, the area adjacent to the hot zone where injured patients are moved so that they can receive decontamination, triage, and treatment

**Water chill:** increase in loss of body heat due to presence of water

**White blood cells:** component of the blood that combats infection in the body

**Wind chill:** increase in loss of body heat due to wind speed

**Withdrawal:** body's response to the cessation of use of alcohol or narcotic substances

## X

**Xiphoid process:** bony inferior tip of the sternum

# STATE EMS CERTIFICATION LINKS

**Alabama**

Office of Emergency Medical Services and Trauma
*adph.org/ems*

**Alaska**

Emergency Medical Services
*chems.alaska.gov/EMS/default.htm*

**Arizona**

Bureau of Emergency Medical Services and Trauma System
*azdhs.gov/bems*

**Arkansas**

Emergency Medical Services and Trauma Systems
*healthy.arkansas.gov/programs-services/topics/ems-resources*

**California**

Emergency Medical Services Authority
*emsa.ca.gov*

**Colorado**

Emergency Medical and Trauma Services
*cdphe.state.co.us/em/index.html*

**Connecticut**

Emergency Medical Services
*ct.gov/dph/cwp/view.asp?a=3127&q=387362*

**District of Columbia**

Fire and Emergency Medical Services
*https://fems.dc.gov*

**Delaware**

Emergency Medical Services
*dhss.delaware.gov/dph/ems/paramediceducation.html*

**Florida**

Bureau of Emergency Medical Services
*floridahealth.gov/licensing-and-regulation/emt-paramedics/index.html*

**Georgia**

Emergency Medical Services
*http://ems.ga.gov/*

**Hawaii**

Emergency Medical Services and Injury Prevention System Branch
*https://health.hawaii.gov/ems/home/certification-and-licensure-for-ems-providers-and-personnel/*

**Idaho**

Emergency Medical Services
*idahoemslicense.net/lms/public/portal#/login*

**Illinois**

Emergency Medical Systems and Highway Safety
*idph.state.il.us/ems/index.htm*

**Indiana**

Emergency Medical Services
*in.gov/dhs/4142.htm*

**Iowa**

Bureau of Emergency Medical Services
*https://idph.iowa.gov/BETS/EMS*

**Kansas**

Board of Emergency Medical Services
*ksbems.org*

**Kentucky**

Board of Emergency Medical Services
*http://kbems.kctcs.edu/index.html*

## Louisiana

Emergency Medical Services
*http://ldh.la.gov/index.cfm/page/759*

## Maine

Maine Emergency Medical Services
*state.me.us/dps/ems*

## Maryland

Institute for Emergency Medical Services Systems
*miemsslicense.com/lms/public/portal#/login*

## Massachusetts

Office of Emergency Medical Services
*mass.gov/dph/oems*

## Michigan

Emergency Medical Services
*michigan.gov/ems*

## Minnesota

Emergency Medical Services Regulatory Board
*emsrb.state.mn.us*

## Mississippi

Emergency Medical Services
*ems.doh.ms.gov/ems/index.html*

## Missouri

Emergency Medical Services
*https://health.mo.gov/safety/ems/licensing.php*

## Montana

EMS, Trauma, and Injury Prevention Systems
*https://dphhs.mt.gov/publichealth/emsts*

## Nebraska

Emergency Medical Services
*http://dhhs.ne.gov/Pages/EHS-EMS-Licensing.aspx*

## Nevada

Emergency Medical Services
*http://dpbh.nv.gov/Reg/EMS/dta/Licensing/Emergency_Medical_System_(EMS)_-_Licensing/*

## New Hampshire

Bureau of Emergency Medical Services
*nh.gov/safety/divisions/fstems/ems/index.html*

## New Jersey

Office of Emergency Medical Services
*state.nj.us/health/ems/index.shtml*

## New Mexico

Emergency Medical Services Bureau
*nmems.org*

## New York

Bureau of Emergency Medical Services
*health.state.ny.us/nysdoh/ems/main.htm*

## North Carolina

Office of Emergency Medical Services
*http://facility-services.state.nc.us/EMS/ems.htm*

## North Dakota

Division of Emergency Medical Services and Trauma
*ndhealth.gov/EMS/*

## Ohio

Division of Emergency Medical Services
*ems.ohio.gov*

## Oklahoma

Emergency Medical Services Division
*ok.gov/health/Protective_Health/Emergency_Medical_Services/*

## Oregon

Emergency Medical Services and Trauma Systems
*oregon.gov/oha/ph/providerpartnerresources/emstraumasystems/emstrainingcertification/Pages/index.aspx*

## Pennsylvania

Emergency Medical Services
*health.pa.gov/topics/EMS/Pages/FAQ.aspx*

## Rhode Island

Division of Emergency Medical Services
*https://health.ri.gov/licenses/detail.php?id=284*

### South Carolina

Emergency Medical Services
*scdhec.gov/health-professionals/ems-training-protocols-requirements*

### South Dakota

Office of Emergency Medical Services
*http://dps.sd.gov/emergency_services/emergency_medical_services/default.aspx*

### Tennessee

Emergency Medical Services
*tn.gov/health/health-program-areas/health-professional-boards/ems-board/ems-board/licensure.html*

### Texas

Emergency Medical Services
*dshs.state.tx.us/emstraumasystems/emsdirectory.shtm*

### Utah

Bureau of Emergency Medical Services
*http://health.utah.gov/ems*

### Vermont

Emergency Medical Services
*http://healthvermont.gov/hc/ems/ems_index.aspx*

### Virginia

Office of Emergency Medical Services
*vdh.virginia.gov/emergency-medical-services/education-certification/*

### Washington

Office of Emergency Medical Services and Trauma System
*doh.wa.gov/ForPublicHealthandHealthcare-Providers/EmergencyMedicalServicesEMSSystems/EMSProviderCertification*

### West Virginia

Office of Emergency Medical Services
*wvoems.org*

### Wisconsin

Emergency Medical Services
*dhs.wisconsin.gov/ems/licensing/index.htm*

### Wyoming

Emergency Medical Services
*https://health.wyo.gov/publichealth/ems/ems-program-2/ems-licensure/*

# ANSWER KEY FOR TEST YOURSELF QUESTIONS

## Test Yourself 2.1

While the parents are not on scene to give consent, an EMS professional acting under in loco parentis would be able to render care. This is a Latin phrase meaning "in place of a parent" when dealing with minor children. However, an attempt must be made to reach the parents/guardians (must be documented on the patient care report).

## Test Yourself 3.1

## Test Yourself 4.1

**O**nset: I was lifting weights and all of a sudden, I felt a sharp pain.

**P**rovocation: If I raise my left arm, it gets a lot worse. I've never had anything like this before.

**Q**uality: I felt a sharp pain right here [points to left chest superior to left nipple]. It feels like a tearing sensation.

**R**adiation: The pain doesn't move.

**S**everity: I would rate it about 6 on a scale of 1 to 10.

**T**ime: The pain started right after I finished exercising an hour ago. It's the first time this has happened.

The patient's answers point toward an injury to the pectoral muscle during his exercising rather than to another condition, such as a heart attack.

## Test Yourself 4.2

The RTS score is 11. Guarding loses 1 point on GCS but does not affect the RTS. The only point lost on the RTS is from the low blood pressure.

## Test Yourself 4.3

This is a challenging question. It relies both on hard data (e.g., blood sugar level, GCS) and on the patient's presentation in general. As he is able to answer your questions despite the slurred words and is cooperative with your commands and requests, he is not necessarily "altered." Your best bet is to consult medical command and request permission to administer more glucose (or have the patient speak to a doctor) or to request that ALS come for further evaluation.

This is one of those situations that comes down to ethical and legal critical decision making. Do you think the patient is a danger to himself or others? Could having him sign a refusal at this point be a legal minefield? If he is given more medication, will the issue resolve itself?

## Test Yourself 5.1

You would use a head-tilt, chin-lift maneuver since you can rule out cervical trauma as her fainting episode happened right in front of you. If she struck her head on the ground, you could potentially use the jaw-thrust maneuver. As she has facial and specifically nasal trauma, you would use an OPA. Finally, you would use a hard-tipped suction catheter (Yankauer) tip as her mouth is easily opened.

## Test Yourself 5.2

This is a gray area question. The patient is normally on oxygen at 2 liters per minute (LPM) on a daily basis, but for whatever reason, his oxygen is not on currently. He is not in any obvious respiratory distress, and his $SpO_2$ levels are near the low end of "normal" at 93%. The most correct answer is that if he is normally on oxygen, the EMT should continue this therapy, as perhaps without the oxygen the patient could desaturate.

However, if the patient is not presenting with respiratory difficulty, the EMT may elect not to put on oxygen at first and see how the patient maintains his oxygen levels and adjust accordingly. This is a type of question that requires the EMT to think critically.

## Test Yourself 7.1

All the burns are anterior, so you are working with half of each arm. Remember that the forearm is the lower half of the arm, below the elbow. If the anterior of each arm is 4.5% of body surface area (BSA), then half of the arm for the forearm and hand is 2.25%.

Since the anterior portion of both forearms and hands are involved, this equals 4.5%.

The chest in total is worth 9%. Since only half of the chest is burned, as described in the scenario as the "upper chest," this is 4.5%.

So add these percentages to find the total: 4.5 + 4.5 = 9% total BSA burned.